Imaging Diagnostics in Cancer: A Clinical Guide

Imaging Diagnostics in Cancer: A Clinical Guide

Editor: Nadia Lilley

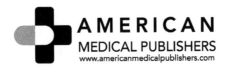

AMERICAN
MEDICAL PUBLISHERS
www.americanmedicalpublishers.com

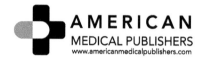

AMERICAN
MEDICAL PUBLISHERS
www.americanmedicalpublishers.com

Cataloging-in-Publication Data

Imaging diagnostics in cancer : a clinical guide / edited by Nadia Lilley.
    p. cm.
Includes bibliographical references and index.
ISBN 978-1-63927-696-7
1. Cancer--Imaging. 2. Cancer--Ultrasonic imaging. 3. Cancer--Diagnosis.
4. Diagnostic imaging. I. Lilley, Nadia.
RC270.3.D53 I43 2023
616.994 075 4--dc23

American Medical Publishers,
41 Flatbush Avenue,
1st Floor, New York,
NY 11217, USA

ISBN 978-1-63927-696-7 (Hardback)

Contents

Preface

Medical imaging is a process of imaging the internal view of the human body for medical intervention and clinical analysis. It depicts the internal structure of the body, which is covered by the skin. It helps in the identification of abnormalities for appropriate diagnosis and treatment of a disease. Medical imaging includes technologies such as magnetic resonance imaging, radiology, ultrasound, radiography, medical photography, elastography, thermography, computed tomography and mammography. Imaging diagnostics are used for detecting cancer and its management in all the phases. Medical imaging is a significant part of clinical protocols related with cancer and it helps in furnishing functional, structural, metabolic, and morphological information. In combination with other diagnostic tools like in vitro fluids and tissue analysis, medical imaging helps in undertaking clinical decisions. Cancer can be detected in the early stages through imaging based on screening, which has substantially decreased the mortality in certain cancers. This book unravels the recent studies on diagnostic imaging and its applications in cancer. Those in search of information to further their knowledge will be greatly assisted by it.

All of the data presented henceforth, was collaborated in the wake of recent advancements in the field. The aim of this book is to present the diversified developments from across the globe in a comprehensible manner. The opinions expressed in each chapter belong solely to the contributing authors. Their interpretations of the topics are the integral part of this book, which I have carefully compiled for a better understanding of the readers.

At the end, I would like to thank all those who dedicated their time and efforts for the successful completion of this book. I also wish to convey my gratitude towards my friends and family who supported me at every step.

Editor

Applications of Computational Methods in Biomedical Breast Cancer Imaging Diagnostics

Kehinde Aruleba [1], George Obaido [1], Blessing Ogbuokiri [1], Adewale Oluwaseun Fadaka [2,*], Ashwil Klein [2], Tayo Alex Adekiya [3] and Raphael Taiwo Aruleba [4,*]

[1] School of Computer Science and Applied Mathematics, University of the Witwatersrand, Johannesburg 2001, South Africa; arulebak@gmail.com (K.A.); rabeshi.george@gmail.com (G.O.); ogbuokiriblessing@gmail.com (B.O.)
[2] Department of Biotechnology, Faculty of Natural Sciences, University of the Western Cape, Private Bag X17, Bellville, Cape Town 7535, South Africa; aklein@uwc.ac.za
[3] Department of Pharmacy and Pharmacology, School of Therapeutic Science, Faculty of Health Sciences, University of the Witwatersrand, Johannesburg, 7 York Road, Parktown 2193, South Africa; adekiyatalex@gmail.com
[4] Department of Molecular and Cell Biology, Faculty of Science, University of Cape Town, Cape Town 7701, South Africa
* Correspondence: afadaka@uwc.ac.za (A.O.F.); arulebataiwo@yahoo.com (R.T.A.)

Abstract: With the exponential increase in new cases coupled with an increased mortality rate, cancer has ranked as the second most prevalent cause of death in the world. Early detection is paramount for suitable diagnosis and effective treatment of different kinds of cancers, but this is limited to the accuracy and sensitivity of available diagnostic imaging methods. Breast cancer is the most widely diagnosed cancer among women across the globe with a high percentage of total cancer deaths requiring an intensive, accurate, and sensitive imaging approach. Indeed, it is treatable when detected at an early stage. Hence, the use of state of the art computational approaches has been proposed as a potential alternative approach for the design and development of novel diagnostic imaging methods for breast cancer. Thus, this review provides a concise overview of past and present conventional diagnostics approaches in breast cancer detection. Further, we gave an account of several computational models (machine learning, deep learning, and robotics), which have been developed and can serve as alternative techniques for breast cancer diagnostics imaging. This review will be helpful to academia, medical practitioners, and others for further study in this area to improve the biomedical breast cancer imaging diagnosis.

Keywords: cancer; breast cancer; diagnostics; imaging; computation; artificial intelligence

1. Introduction

Cancer is a non-communicable disease characterized by abnormal cell proliferation or cell division, with the ability to spread to other parts of the body [1]. Cancer continues to be a major public health problem and has been labeled as a global threat exacerbated by poor lifestyle choices and environmental factors [2,3]. Generally, cancer is classified according to the affected body part or tissue of origin. The most common cancer diseases include but are not limited to lung cancer, ovarian cancer, prostate cancer, head and neck cancer, breast cancer, etc. [4]. Indeed, breast cancer has been considered as one of the most common cancers diagnosed among women around the world. Breast cancer comprises 18%

of the total cases of female cancer and approximately a million new cases are reported in the world every year [5]. Due to the ability of this type of cancer to metastasize to distant organs or lymph nodes, it has been considered to be the leading cause of mortality in females [5,6].

Due to the increase in the numbers of breast cancer over the years, there has been a rise in the number of computational models and algorithms for diagnosis and treatment to assist medical practitioners. A commonly, and frequently, used computational method is artificial intelligence (AI). Many AI related models have been developed for detecting and diagnosing diseases not only for breast cancer or mammography image analysis and classification [7] but for other diseases such as hycobacterium tuberculosis classification (MTC) [8], human immunodeficiency virus (HIV) therapy, screening, identification, and prediction [9], coronavirus disease 2019 (COVID-19) detection and diagnosis [10], etc. These AI models include machine learning, deep learning, and robotics. Rapid improvement in classification and learning algorithms is one of the main reasons these models have been widely used for these purposes with good and efficient results. Therefore, the contribution of this review is to provide a concise overview of past and present conventional diagnostics approaches in breast cancer detection and diagnosis. Further, we gave an account of several AI related computational models that have been developed and can serve as alternative models for breast cancer diagnosis. The remaining part of this paper is organized as follows: The types of biomedical imaging is presented in Section 2. The computational techniques used in breast cancer imaging diagnostics are outlined in Section 3. This section discusses the AI models used in breast cancer diagnosis. Finally, the paper is concluded in Section 4, where some points of future work are recommended.

2. Types of Biomedical Imaging

2.1. Mammography

Mammography is an excellent method used in primary breast imaging. It is used for early detection of abnormalities in the breast, especially those suspicious for breast cancer before it becomes apparent clinically, by using low-dose X-ray imaging to generate the images of the breast [11,12]. According to the United States of America preventive services task force (USPSTF), this type of breast imaging has been helpful in the earlier and better treatment for women over 40 years of age and has decreased breast cancer mortality by at least 30% [13]. Although this imaging approach remains the key for early breast cancer detection and screening, the overall accuracy of the test remains low and second-line accurate imaging techniques are required in some instances to lessen the number of unnecessary excisional biopsies [14,15].

Screening mammography is credited with the examination of an asymptomatic woman and decreases the risk of breast cancer-related death [16,17]. Conventional mammography has limitations in specificity and sensitivity, especially in dense breasts. The sensitivity of this type of imaging in breast cancer diagnostics is about 50 to 85%, depending on the density of the breast. Meanwhile, the sensitivity is below 50% in the dense breast due to tissue superposition; this is a major reason for the false-positive result, which leads to additional imagining and cost and false-negative results due to masking of true lesions [18–20].

In the breast, the normal internal mammary lymph node chain is usually below 5 mm in diameter. Metastases to this chain cannot be easily detected by mammography or ultrasonography clinical examination because they are normally covered by cartilaginous and bony structures of the chest wall [21,22]. The use of mammography in the detection of recurrent breast cancer is a challenging task due to changes in the architecture of the breast, mainly in fibrosis and scarring secondary to radiotherapy and surgery, resulting in difficulties to interpret mammograms. Breast compression is another major challenge faced by this modality due to accompanied pain which could lead to delayed diagnosis. Hence, considering all of the aforementioned mammography limitations, there is a call for alternative and more accurate methods that can resolve the imaging of dense breasts [19,20].

2.2. Tomosynthesis

Due to the limitations of mammography, breast tomosynthesis was introduced to the clinic because of its ability to produce three-dimensional information at a lower dose and its relative cost-effectiveness. Consequently, there has been an upsurge in interest in tomosynthesis. The Food and Drug Administration (FDA) has approved some products that are now in use and on the market [23]. This technique involves using X-ray projection images acquired over an arc to generate image slices for a partially 3D image [24]. Tomosynthesis allows for the generation of an arbitrary number of in-focus planes retrospectively from a series of radiograph projections obtained in a single motion of the X-ray tube [25]. Notably, a combination of tomosynthesis and digital mammography increases the brightness of invasive cancers while at the same time decreasing the likelihood of false-positive data [24]. Tomosynthesis has been applied to several clinical tasks, including dental imaging, angiography, breast imaging, bone imaging, and chest imaging [23]. In breast cancer, tomosynthesis increases the sensitivity of mammography, which could enhance the early detection of breast cancer due to the improved lesion margin conspicuity [25]. This is very beneficial to breast cancer patients, especially those with radiographically dense breasts. However, Poplack et al. [26] showed that breast tomosynthesis has a comparable or superior image when compared with diagnostic film-screen mammography in 89% of recruited subjects. More recently, this was supported by another study where one-view stand-alone digital breast tomosynthesis (DBT) detected more breast cancer than digital mammogram (DM) [27]. This suggests that the use of one-view DBT alone could be feasible in breast cancer screening. Although the acquisition procedures of tomosynthesis mimic standard mammography, the X-ray tube of tomosynthesis takes several low-dose exposures as it travels within a limited arc of motion unlike conventional mammography [26]. Sechopoulos [28] has written an excellent review of all aspects of tomosynthesis, including doses and reconstruction processes. When the overall dose used for visualization is constant, the quality of the image improves with a wider angular range [29]. However, the quality of image degenerates once the maximum is attained at a particular number of projections.

2.3. Ultrasound Imaging

Ultrasound (US) imaging diagnostics, otherwise known as sonography or ultrasound scanning, is a painless and safe approach. US makes use of 1 to 10 MHz sound waves to produce pictures that reveal the movement and structure of the breast, and other soft tissue [30,31]. It can also reveal the movements of blood and other materials within the blood vessels and body [31]. It is a cross-sectional technique that uses a small probe, known as a transducer, and gel that is directly placed on the breast/skin; it displays the tissues without overlap [31–33]. The high-frequency soundwaves travel from the probe via the gel into the body, and the probe receives the sounds that bounce back, which in turn produces an image on a computer. This type of imaging technique does not make use of radiation because it captures images in real-time [31–33].

In recent times, the development of high-resolution US technique has greatly improved the diagnosis of breast cancer because, in the past, US was thought to only be suitable for the diagnosis of cysts [34,35]. It has been shown to enhance the differential diagnosis of both benign and malignant lesions during guided interventional and local preoperative staging diagnosis. Due to the higher sensitivity of this type of imaging technique, it has been adopted as a complementary technique to mammography with limited sensitivity to identify early, node-negative cancer in dense breasts [36,37].

However, the use of US imaging techniques is diminishing due to the time and skill required to detect small tumors with hand-held imaging, and non-palpable cancers. The implementation of this imaging technique in breast cancer diagnostics has been hampered by limited numbers of qualified personnel and lack of uniformity in the results; this has caused low specificity that can lead to the generation of high numbers of false-positive results [38]. This assertion is corroborated by findings of some previous studies which revealed that US can identify and detect the presence of carcinoma in dense breasts. Some other studies have shown low detection of cancerous cells in dense breasts, but have proposed the addition of this imaging method to negate mammography which seems to have limited cost-efficiency and is controversial for women with dense breasts without any other major risk factors. In addition, due to the high scattering ability of the soundwaves at bone and air interfaces, various parts of the body are invisible, which limits the effectiveness of depth imaging in most organs to about 10 cm [39,40].

2.4. Dedicated Breast Computed Tomography

Dedicated breast computed tomography (DBCT) is a recently used and fastest-growing imaging technique that allows for true isotropic and provides three-dimensional (3D) information which can be reconstructed or rebuilt into several imaging planes. Although DBCT is comparable to breast magnetic resonance imaging (MRI), the process involved can be carried out without breast compression, and is not limited by breast implants or the density of the breast [41–43]. The radiation dose in this type of imaging technique is similar to that of a conventional two-view mammogram [42]. Boone et al. [44] investigated the feasibility of low dose radiation on the image quality of DBCT. The findings from their average glandular dose for 80-kVp breast CT study, when compared to two-view mammography, revealed that the breast CT dose for thicker breasts is approximately one-third lower than that of two-view mammography. For a typical breast of 5 cm 50% glandular, it was discovered that the maximum dose of mammography in 1 mm^3 voxel is far greater (20.0 mGy) than that of breast CT with 5.4 mGy. It was further stated that the CT images for 8 cm cadaveric breasts have an average glandular dose of 6.32 mGy, which is superior to the estimated dose of 5.06 mGy for the craniocaudal view, with an average glandular dose of 10.1 mGy for standard two-view mammography of the same specimen [44]. The invention, improvement, and development of DBCT with dedicated scanners with novel technology has been documented in the literature by Sarno et al. [45]. Studies further reported the development of low radiation dose scanners with improved spatial resolution and rapid image acquisition times, which is aimed at addressing the issue of imaging dense breasts and painful breast compression [41–43].

Kuzmiak et al. [42] investigated the confidence of radiology experts in the characterization of suspicious breast lesions with a DBCT system compared with the conventional diagnostics of two-dimensional (2D) digital mammography in terms of overall lesion visibility and dose. It was discovered that DBCT is superior in the characterization of the masses and radiologists' visualizations, although it is inferior to calcifications when diagnostic mammography is used. It was further averred that the DBCT application could help eliminate the 2D mammography drawback of overlapping tissue. Their study concluded that the technical challenges in breast imaging remain, but 3D DBCT could have a promising clinical application in breast cancer diagnosis or screening, however, this needs further investigation.

In 2008, Lindfors et al. [41] carried out a comparative study between the DBCT and screen-films mammograms where it was discovered, in the study of the selected group of women, that the visualization of breast lesions with both the DBCT and screen-film mammography is approximately the same. Although, DBCT was reported to be superior in the visualization of the masses, while in the imaging of microcalcification lesions screen-film mammography shows to be better. It was further deduced in their study that women are more comfortable with DBCT screening when compared to screen-film mammography. Hence, it was assumed that DBCT is a potential technology and may be a promising clinical application in diagnostic and screening for breast cancer investigation. Additionally, it was further presumed that DBCT is more accessible and could be a replacement for breast MRI or act as a control technique for tumor ablation procedures or robotic breast biopsy, all of this calls for further studies.

Recently, Shah et al. [43] investigated the characterization of computed tomography (CT). Hounsfield units were used in clinical settings for the purpose of tissue differentiation in a reconstructed CT image in 3D acquisition trajectories on a DBCT system. It was depicted in their statistical study that the approach has a better performance in the saddle orbit, mostly when close to the chest and the nipple areas of dense breast. It was further discovered that the saddle orbit functions significantly well and provides a tighter distribution of Hounsfield unit values in the reconstructed volumes. In addition, the study demonstrated the significance of the application of 3D acquisition for breast CT trajectories and other uses through the establishment of the robustness in Hounsfield unit values in the large reconstructed volumes.

2.5. Magnetic Resonance Imaging

Since the beginning of the third millennium, magnetic resonance imaging (MRI) has developed into a paramount tool in breast cancer screening, diagnosing, staging, and follow-up [46]. This imaging tool has played a vital role in the screening of high-risk breast cancer patients. Breast MRI uses an intravenous contrast agent such as gadolinium, which allows for the visualization of lesions. The sensitivity of this tool in breast cancer has been documented to be over 90% while the specificity is still about 72%; hence, the distinction between benign and malignant lesions is still challenging [46]. Although mammography is the basic imaging tool for breast tumor identification, it has been indicated that MRI has a higher sensitivity for detection of breast cancer, and the breast density does not affect it [47]. In most cases, the sensitivity of mammography in the detection of multiple malignant foci is below 50%. It is important to note that breast MRI is not meant to replace mammography particularly in ductal carcinoma in situ, which is not detectable by MRI but rather by mammography [48]. The MRI screening in women with genetic susceptibility to breast cancer has proved to be beneficial [49,50]. In a prospective cohort study, the sensitivity of MRI in women with a high risk of breast cancer but who were asymptomatic was between 93–100%, the 10-year survival was 95.3% [50]. Similarly, the sensitivity of MRI in contralateral breast tumor detection was documented to be 91%, and specificity was 88% [51]. In women with a known BRCA1/2 mutation, MRI surveillance detected breast cancer at early stages; encouragingly, there was no distant recurrence after 8.4 years follow-up since diagnosis [52]. This tool can be used in identifying the size and degree of the tumor towards achieving better surgery procedures. Nevertheless, the use of MRI before surgery continues to be controversial with extensive variations in the outcome; however, it helps in planning conservation in patients that respond to chemotherapy where feasible [46]. Despite the high sensitivity of this imaging tool in breast cancer, the cost involved in MRI makes it difficult to be employed in the general population. Conclusively, the invention and development of new imaging techniques such as diffusion-weighted imaging offer an added advantage in breast cancer management.

2.6. Diffusion-Weighted Imaging

Since the early years of the 21st century, diffusion-weighted imaging (DWI) has been at the forefront of cancer imaging attaining widespread recognition due to its ability in the diagnosis of stroke [53,54]. DWI is a noninvasive MRI technique that relies on the principle of random molecular motion of free water in tissues (Brownian movement). With the development of stronger diffusion gradients and application in whole-body imaging, DWI has attracted attention in oncology [55]. In breast cancer, Sinha et al. [56] demonstrated that DWI is reliable in a clinical setting with an echo-planar sequence and possesses potential in breast lesion characterization as either benign or malignant using apparent diffusion coefficient (ADC) values. Generally, breast lesions classified as malignant have a high-cellular level with limited water diffusion and lower ADC values when compared to benign lesions [57]. An earlier clinical study that recruited women with breast lesions stated that ADC values and the tumor biological aggressiveness correlate; hence, ADC is a promising factor in the evaluation and analysis of the degree of the malignancy [58]. In most clinical settings, DWI is interpreted in combination with dynamic contrast-enhanced (DCE)-MRI to increase the specificity. However, more recently, lesions in the breast (31 = malignant; 13 = benign) were analyzed using quantitative diffusion-weighted sequence on 3T MRI with b-values of 500 and 1000 s/mm^2 [59]. The ADC cut-off value for benign and malignant lesions was set to 1.21×10^{-3} mm^2/s for b = 500 s/mm^2 and 1.22×10^{-3} mm^2/s for b = 1000 s/mm^2, respectively. The sensitivity of DCE-MRI was 100% with a specificity of 66.7%, when DCE-MRI was combined with b = 1000 s/mm^2, 100% specificity was attained and sensitivity of 90.6%; there was no significant difference between the ADC and prognostic factors [59]. Non-contrast (NC)-MRI can be an alternative for DCE-MRI for breast cancer diagnosis, though its inferior lesion conspicuity and lower inter-reader agreement should be considered [60]. This study and many more have documented explanatory results for DWI as a tool for diagnosing breast lesion and aids the orthodox breast MRI procedures. Several pitfalls, which include but are not limited to motion artifacts, ADC value accuracy, image quality, and signal-to-noise ratio, are associated with DWI [61,62]. These challenges are bothersome and lay emphasis on the need to incorporate computer science into breast cancer diagnosis, for example, robotics could significantly decrease time in DWI MRI and create improved breast cancer detection.

2.7. Computed Tomography

CT scan is a method that exposes the pictures of cross-sections or 2D slices of the body's organs via a connected computer [63,64]. The use of a contrast solution (iodine), injected into the body via the arm, dramatically improves and aids in the visualization of the cancerous cells in organs. In 2003, the use of CT for breast cancer imaging was proposed by Suga et al. [65], after a surgical issue in patients, to obtain interstitial lymphography that can map and present sentinel lymph nodes of the breast. The use of CT in breast cancer has some advantages, which includes patient comfort and fast scanning time. However, CT has not been widely used in breast cancers due to the risks involved in radiation exposure and poor quality of the image produced.

Due to the dynamic technique of CT, it can be used in the detection and characterization of breast tumors, investigation of neoadjuvant chemotherapy effects, and local staging of cancerous cells in the breast. In 2015, Foo et al. [66] employed this imaging scan method to evaluate the staging of cancer cells in newly diagnosed breast cancer patients that are in a locally advanced stage. It was revealed that a limited number of patients involved in this study had some pelvic significance with relation to a patient who had peritoneal cancer with widespread metastasis, and a patient with a presumed gene carrier of a concurrent primary ovarian malignancy. It was further stated that 50% of all pelvic results required additional radiological examinations.

Although the CT scan technique in breast cancer examinations may not replace the conventional mammography routine, based on improvements carried out in some studies [67,68], it can be used to overcome several limitations associated with mammography such as detection of cancers in premenopausal, dysplastic, and dense breasts. The mean glandular dose of 8.2 ± 1.2 mGy has also been documented for different types of breast shapes and sizes [69]. As documented by Park et al. [68], in prone positions, low-dose perfusion CT is possible for imaging with regards to the quantification of tumor vascularity and radiation doses. CT can be used in the detection of unsuspected very small cancers in the breast that cannot be identified or seen by physical examinations or conventional mammography. It is useful in definitive diagnostic evaluation in a situation where physical examinations and mammography are inconclusive, and it can also be helpful in recognition of precancerous and high-risk lesions. More so, CT can be used in the discrimination of tumor tissue from normal tissue in breast cancer patients without the use of a contrast medium.

2.8. Near-Infrared (NIR) Fluorescence

During human surgery, X-ray fluoroscopy and ultrasound have been used widely. However, during X-ray fluoroscopy, patients and caregivers are exposed to ionizing radiation; in an ultrasound, only a thin surgical field-of-view is seen and requires direct contact with tissue, in this case, breast. Interestingly, none of the methods can be amended by target contrast agents to guide imaging during oncologic surgery due to the number of procedures required [70,71]. Thus, near-infrared (NIR) light, with a wavelength range of about 700 to 900 nm, has offered diverse significant advantages over some widely used tools including relatively high penetration of photon in and out of living tissue (breast) due to the reduction in the rate of absorbance and scatter. Owing to lower tissue autofluorescence, NIR has a higher signal-to-background ratio [71,72]. This technique has a great potential to interrogate deep tissues (breast) for molecular-based imaging. The NIR light is visible to the human eyes when conjugated with NIR excitable fluorophore or dyes. These are chemical compounds which convert light generated from one NIR wavelength into the NIR light of diverse wavelength. It has been recommended that the mapping of sentinel lymph nodes (SLN) is a standard approach for the management of breast cancer and care staging of the axilla [71].

NIR fluorescence imaging, which uses indocyanine green (ICG), has been shown to improve the procedure of the SLN mapping by facilitating percutaneous incisions and identifying the intraoperative ability of lymphatic channels and SLNs [71,72]. The safety and accuracy of NIR fluorescence imaging applications for identifying SLNs in patients suffering from breast cancer were demonstrated by Verbeek et al. [73]. The use of the Mini-FLARE camera system and 1.6 mL of 0.5 mM ICG showed the excellent identification of the SLN in patients with breast cancer. Although, the technique which should be used as the gold standard in future analyses, was raised as a question [73]. In a similar study by Mieog et al. [74], the clinical translation of a novel NIR fluorescence imaging system and the optimal ratio of ICG to the human serum albumin (HSA) dose for mapping of SLN in breast cancer was described. It was stated that 400 and 800 μM is the optimal dose of the injection ratio of ICG:HSA and this can be chosen based on the preferences of local preparation. For instance, a dose of 500 μM was depicted to be the most convenient in the United States due to the minimal requirement in the manipulation of albumin volumes. Other studies that have employed this approach in mapping SLNs in breast cancer patients include Sevick-Muraca et al. [75] which demonstrated the prospective feasibility in the use of the minimal dose of ICG in noninvasive optical imaging of lymph nodes in the breast cancer patients undergoing SLNs mapping. In 2008, Altınoğlu et al. [76]. demonstrated the synthesis and bioresorbable use of calcium phosphate nanoparticles (CPNPs) which incorporated the molecule of the NIR emitted fluorophore and ICG. In their study, the in vivo and ex vivo studies demonstrated the potentiality of the NIR CPNPs in diagnostic imaging of early breast solid tumors. Although, the result from their ex situ imaging of deep tissue showed that the depths of NIR CPNPs in porcine muscle tissue is 3 cm. Poellinger et al. [77] employed the use of NIR fluorescence imaging with the late and early enhancement of ICG, which corresponds to extravascular and vascular phases of contrast agent enhancement to distinguish between malignant and benign breast lesions as well as to detect breast cancer. Ke et al. [78] assessed the specificity of continuous-wave NIR fluorescence imaging by an intensified charge-coupled device (CDD) camera on a novel epidermal growth factor (EGF)-Cy5.5 to detect EGF receptors in breast cancer xenografts.

2.9. Single-Photon Emission Computed Tomography

Single-photon emission computed tomography (SPECT) is a medical imaging tool based on tomographic reconstruction protocols and routinely used in a clinical decision in cancer [79], coronary artery disease, left ventricular dysfunction [80], and Parkinson disease [81]. In fact, it is the most used tool in myocardial ischemia assessment. SPECT aims at getting a perfect 3D radioactivity distribution resulting from the uptake of a radiotracer in humans. One or more photons are released in random directions when a SPECT radioisotope decays [82]. However, collimators are used to focus the angle of the emitted photons that reach the detector because conventional lenses cannot restrict high-energy photons, and only 0.02% of the decay events is measured [82]. SPECT, coupled with CT, can be used when conventional images are complex to interpret, for example, suspicion of contamination [83]. Clinically, SPECT/CT provides more value in anatomical localization of sentinel nodes. This highlights a relevant role for this tool in the surgical approach and may improve staging [84]. The sentinel lymph node biopsy is a well-known procedure used in evaluating the status of the axillary lymph node in patients with early stages of breast cancer [85]. Markedly, SPECT/CT improved visualization from 84% to 92% in patients, but it only showed sentinel nodes in 11 out of 22 breast cancer patients (50%) with non-visualization on planar imaging [84]. Similarly, Lerman et al. [86] documented that the addition of SPECT/CT to lymphoscintigraphy enhances sentinel node identification in breast cancer patients who are overweight. Notably, SPECT/CT identified hot nodes in 91% of patients and sentinel nodes in 29 of 49 patients (59%) who were negative on planar imaging (planar lymphoscintigraphy) [86]. Hence, this technique is of high relevance in overweight breast cancer patients because intraoperative techniques have failed in the identification of draining nodes. Another SPECT/CT evaluation study demonstrated a sentinel node in 91.1% of breast cancer patients, and localization was more precise on SPECT/CT fusion images than on the planar views [87]. Mann et al. [88] documented that the use of dedicated SPECT identifies regions of interest at a global lower-level threshold within dense breast tissue without any negative effects, which in turn betters patient care. Additionally, dedicated breast positron emission tomography (PET)/CT can accurately visualize uncompressed breast suspected lesions in 3D [89]. However, this scanner was unable to generate a full quantitative image. Recently, Tornai et al. [90] developed a fully 3D CT in a hybrid SPECT/CT breast imaging system that facilitated complex trajectories, which improved the quality of the image when compared with simple circular breast CT acquisitions. The SPECT-subsystem allows viewing of the chest wall for pendant breast imaging [90]. Recently, it was shown that the hybrid SPECT/CT provides precise anatomical data that enables clear assessment of patients contaminated with radionuclide during the procedure [83]. Such precise data can assist surgeons towards a better surgical plan. Non-visualization of sentinel nodes, unexpected lymphatic drainage, and complicated planar imaging interpretation are challenges faced by these imaging techniques. However, this can be amended by incorporating AI, such as deep learning and machine learning algorithms, with currently available breast cancer imaging tools. Overall, such combinations will improve breast cancer diagnosis, predict treatment outcome and ultimately, improve the patient quality of life. The dose in the dedicated SPECT-CT system using both the geometric and anthropomorphic phantoms showed that the average doses absorbed in 100% fibroglandular-equivalent was 4.5 ± 0.4 mGy, while 100% adipose-equivalent tissues was 3.8 ± 0.2 mGy. More so, the dose measured in a cadaver breast using a radiochromic film in the same study yielded an average dose of 4.3 ± 0.3 mGY and 4.2 ± 0.3 mGy along two orthogonal planes [91].

3. Computational Techniques Used in Breast Cancer Imaging Diagnostics

A correct diagnosis of mammograms containing malignant tumors is a complex task for even the most experienced medical practitioner. To circumvent this complexity, several computational models have been developed to assist medical practitioners to distinguish between benign and malignant breast tumors. The models described in this paper are based on machine learning, deep learning, and robotics which have been shown to be useful in breast cancer diagnosis. In this section, we present some studies that have applied these models.

3.1. Machine Learning Algorithms

Several machine learning algorithms have been proposed for the detection and diagnosis of breast cancer. Despite this, the development of new algorithms and models for this purpose is still an active research area, especially in the detection of abnormalities in mammograms. In the following, we review machine learning models that have been used in diagnosing this type of cancer, such as artificial neural network (ANN) and support vector machine (SVM).

3.1.1. Support Vector Machines

SVMs are supervised learning models that aim at formulating a computationally effective approach of learning to separate hyperplanes in high-dimensional feature space [92]. It has been used and proven to be an efficient learning technique for several real-world problems such as image recognition [93], bioinformatics [94], and classification problems [95], among others. SVMs are one of the earliest machine learning techniques used for cancer diagnosis. Acharya et al. [96] focused on detecting breast abnormalities or cancer automatically by using infrared imaging. The approach used texture features and SVMs to detect breast cancer based on thermography. Texture features were obtained from a run-length matrix and co-occurrence matrix from 25 cancerous and 25 normal infra-red breast images. These features were then fed to an SVM for automatic classification and detection of malignant and normal breast conditions. A comparison of SVMs based classifiers with ANNs and Bayesian classifiers for the prognosis and diagnosis of breast cancer was done in Maglogiannis et al. [97]. The implementation of the comparison was performed on the Wisconsin prognostic breast cancer and the Wisconsin diagnostic breast cancer datasets. The expected result of the implementation was to predict a class that corresponds to a likely tumor recurrence in four-time intervals. The result also shows that SVM outperforms the other classifiers. Huang et al. [98] used SVM to evaluate several pathologically proven breast tumors. The study presented a computer-aided diagnosis (CAD) system with textural features for classifying malignant and benign breast tumors on medical ultrasound systems. The aim of the CAD is to assist medical practitioners and radiologists in identifying lesions and also to differentiate malignant lesions from benign lesions on the basis of medical images. The proposed SVM technique was able to identify solid breast nodules at very high accuracy. Recently, Wang et al. [7] proposed an approach to solving the limitations of machine learning models' performance in diagnosing breast cancer. The approach was based on an SVM-based ensemble learning algorithm; this approach reduces the diagnosis variance and increases diagnosis accuracy. In doing this, 12 different SVMs were hybrid using the proposed weight area under the receiver operating characteristics curve ensemble (WAUCE) approach.

3.1.2. Artificial Neural Network

ANN is a computational-intelligent model that uses different optimization tools to learn from the data available in the past and use that prior training to identify or predict new patterns or to classify new data. Several research works have applied ANN for medical purposes [99], such as cancer treatments [100]. The Memetic Pareto ANN (MPANN) approach was proposed by Abbass [101]. The approach was based on a pareto-differential evolution algorithm. This algorithm was augmented with a local search for the prediction and diagnosis of breast cancer. Tourassi et al. [102] proposed a new approach for breast cancer diagnosis based on the constraint satisfaction neural network (CSNN) technique using mammographic and breast cancer patient history findings. The main advantage of this technique is that it has a non-hierarchical architecture and flexibility that allows it to work as a predictive tool and as an analysis or data mining tool to discover the knowledge of association rules among clinical diagnosis and historical findings. In this work, the authors used two different datasets of breast cancer, each containing 250 patient cases. The CSNN was first used to train the first 250 datasets and the other 250 datasets were used to test the predictive strength of the CSNN. The result of the analysis was done based on the kind of mammographic lesions seen in each patient. The result of this study shows that CSNN is a very efficient CAD tool for predicting and diagnosing breast cancer from mammographic and historical findings. A study by Janghel et al. [103] implemented a model using ANN to assist medical practitioners in diagnosing breast cancer. The model has four phases, namely radial basis function networks (RBFN), back propagation algorithm (BPA), competitive learning network (CLN), and learning vector quantization (LVQ). The dataset used in this study consisted of 55 malignant cases and 184 benign cases. The result of the experiment showed that the LVQ output was the best result during testing then CLN, BPA, and RBFN in order. Figure 1 presents a simple ANN diagnosis for breast cancer.

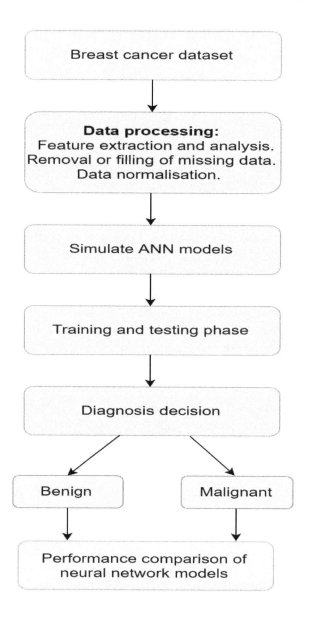

Figure 1. A simple artificial neural network (ANN) method on breast cancer [103].

Other works in the literature used data mining methods in diagnosing breast cancer [104,105]. Data mining is the process of extracting useful data from a larger set of raw data using one or more software. Çakır et al. [106] used Weka, a data mining tool to analyze 462 breast cancer patients data obtained from the Ankara Oncology Hospital. Classification algorithms are applied to each of the datasets and the outputs of the classification were compared to find the most effective treatment method. This work assists oncology doctors to suggest the best treatment method for a patient. Şahan et al. [107] proposed a hybrid system of a fuzzy-artificial immune system with the k-nearest neighbor (KNN) algorithm. This method was used to solve diagnosis problems through classifying the Wisconsin breast cancer dataset (WBCD). The system has a high classification accuracy on large datasets and can be used for any type of breast cancer diagnosis. Additionally, it can be used for other medical condition diagnoses. The Table 1 below presents an overview of machine learning (ML) techniques in breast cancer diagnosis that are explained in this section. The evaluation results presented in the table are the 50–50% training–test partition for the reference with three different training-test partitions.

Table 1. An overview of machine learning (ML) techniques in breast cancer diagnosis.

Reference	Computation Technique	Scope	Evaluation Results	Datasets
Acharya et al. [96]	Texture features + SVM	Breast cancer detection using thermal imaging	Accuracy = 88.10%, specificity = 90.48%, sensitivity = 85.71%	25 normal and 25 cancerous collected from Singapore General Hospital, Singapore
Maglogiannis et al. [97]	SVM	Diagnosis and prognosis	Accuracy = 96.91%, specificity = 97.67%, Sensitivity = 97.84%	Wisconsin prognostic breast cancer (WPBC)
Huang et al. [98]	SVM	Classifying benign and malignant	Accuracy = 94.4%, specificity = 94.4%, Sensitivity = 94.3%	250 images of benign breast tumors from 215 patients and carcinomas from 35 patients.
Wang et al. [7]	SVM	Reduce the diagnosis variance and increase the diagnostic accuracy of breast cancer	Variance = 97.89%, increase in accuracy by 33.34%	Wisconsin Breast Cancer, Wisconsin Diagnostic Breast Cancer, and the U.S. National Cancer Institute's Surveillance, Epidemiology, and End Results (SEER) program
Abbass [101]	EANN	Diagnosis	Average accuracy = 0.981 ± 0.005	Wisconsin
Bhardwaj et al. [108]	Genetically optimized neural network	Classification	Accuracy of 98.24%, 99.63% and 100% for 50–50, 60–40, 70–30 training–testing partition, respectively	WBCD
Tourassi et al. [102]	CSNN	Diagnosis	CSNN ROC area index = 0.84 ± 0.02	500 private images
Çakır et al. [106]	Weka	Treatment methods	Accuracy = 92%	462 patients data
Karabatak [109]	Weighted Naïve Bayesian	Detection	Sensitivity = 99.11%, specificity = 98.25%, accuracy = 98.54%	WBCD
Şahan et al. [107]	Fuzzy + KNN	Diagnosis	Accuracy = 99.14%	WBCD
Bagui et al. [110]	Rank nearest neighbor	Diagnosis	Accuracy = 98.1%	WBCD
Chen et al. [111]	Rough set_SVM	Distinguishing benign breast tumour from malignant one	Accuracy = 99.41%, Sensitivity = 100%, specificity = 100%	WBCD
Polat et al. [112]	Least square SVM	Classification	Accuracy = 94.87%, Sensitivity = 96.42%, specificity = 95.86%	WBCD

3.2. Deep Learning

In recent years, deep learning has set an exciting trend in the fields of machine learning and AI [113]. Deep learning techniques utilize computational models, composed of multiple processing layers that are used to learn data representations and applied to many real-world applications. These applications range from image recognition, object detection, power systems, breast cancer detection, speech recognition to drug discovery and genomics, etc. [114–117]. In the following sections, deep learning models for breast cancer diagnosis are presented.

3.2.1. Convolutional Neural Network

The convolutional neural network (CNN), often called ConvNet, is a type of deep learning model that has become dominant for many computer vision tasks, ranging from image classification, object tracking and detection to semantic segmentation [118,119]. CNN was designed to adaptively learn hierarchies of features, usually from low-level to high-level patterns [120]. Indolia et al. [121] explained that the CNN overcomes limitations as seen in traditional machine learning approaches; it has shown to be widely used for solving complex problems, especially in the medical imaging domain. Recent studies have adopted the CNN model for effective breast cancer diagnosis [122–124]. An example of CNN segmentation tasks for breast cancer diagnosis is presented in Figure 2.

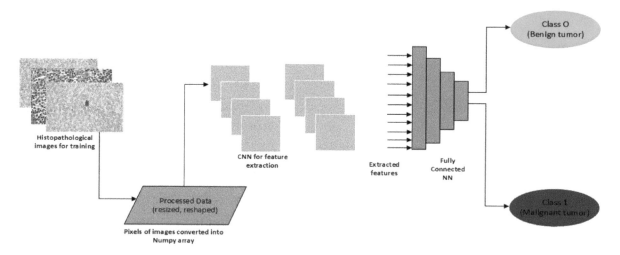

Figure 2. A convolutional neural network (CNN)-based approach for screening mammography [125].

For an improved diagnosis, Tan et al. [126] developed an imaging system called breast cancer detection using convolutional neural networks (BCDCNN) aimed at assisting medical practitioners to classify mammographic images into malignant or benign. The results showed that the BCDCNN system improved the accuracy of the classification tasks on the mini-Mammographic Image Analysis Society (mini-MIAS) database. Amit et al. [122] proposed an approach for dynamic contrast-enhanced (DCE) imaging that uses the CNN to correctly classify medical images and a pre-trained classifier to extract features in the images. The study showed that CNN outperformed the pre-trained classifier and accuracy improved significantly. In another study, Byra et al. [127] described a CAD approach that uses the Nakagami imaging method to train a CNN model, aimed at breast cancer diagnosis. The study was tested on 458 RF data matrices of breast lesions. The study showed that better area under the curve (AUC) results that amounts to 0.912 were obtained. Gao et al. [128] extended the use of CNN using the INbreast dataset to overcome the challenges faced with the contrast-enhanced digital mammography (CEDM), which is prone to a high false-positive rate. CNN was effective at differentiating benign cases from malignant lesions, which is the main challenge faced with a breast cancer diagnosis.

In a similar study, Wang et al. [129] explored a CAD method that utilizes feature fusion with CNN using a private dataset. The method uses CNN for feature extraction based on several image sub-regions. After the feature extraction tasks, the images were then classified into benign or malignant.

The study concluded that this task outperformed other existing methods. Murtaza et al. [124] applied the use of CNN on the BreakHis dataset to improve the detection of breast cancer. The study reported a high accuracy with the use of the CNN model. Other interesting areas of application of CNN to breast cancer diagnosis are found in the following references [126,130–136].

3.2.2. Generative Adversarial Networks

The advent of generative adversarial networks (GANs) by Goodfellow [137] has opened a new area of research within the image segmentation domain. According to Kazeminia et al. [138], GANs have been shown to generate realistic-looking images in the large, unlabelled corpus. One of the many challenges faced within the CV and medical image analysis (MIA) community is the heavy reliance on labelled training data, which can be a major limitation [7]. The communities have recognized the potential of GANs and have eagerly investigated in its efficacy to tackle many problems. Recently, a good deal of research has leveraged the use of GANs for image-to-image translation [139,140]. GANs have found many applications in generative modelling and distribution learning [139]. Furthermore, GANs unique generation and identification network is increasingly used for image segmentation and has achieved good results. GANs create outputs using its discriminator and generator [141]. Figure 3 shows the structure of GANs.

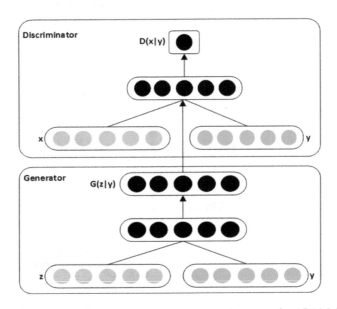

Figure 3. Structure of a generative adversarial networks (GANs) [142].

Shams et al. [143] developed DiaGRAM (deep GenerRAtive multi-task), which is based on GANs and CNN in a mammography study to detect early signs of breast cancer. The study concluded that feature learning with GANs led to high classification performance and an effective end-to-end scheme. A study by Singh et al. [144] applied GANs to segment mammographic images from regions of interests (ROIs) with varying length and sizes. GANs helped eliminate issues of overfitting on the datasets (INbreast and digital database for screening mammography (DDSM)) and showed effectiveness in the screening of cases. Wu et al. [145] addressed the issue of limited data and class imbalance for breast cancer classification using GANs. The classification performance of GANs was compared with other augmentation methods. The results showed that GANs improved the classification task. Guan et al. [146] applied GANs to generate synthetic images from a digital database for screening mammography. The authors opined that GANs performed better in augmenting the training dataset, which was useful for the study. Together, we have discussed the CNN and GANs approaches to breast cancer detection. Most of the works presented in this section are summarised in Table 2. In the table, we present the deep learning techniques, and scope of work that are used for breast cancer diagnosis. In addition, the performance metrics for each technique and the type of dataset used were presented.

Table 2. Summary of deep learning models in breast cancer diagnosis.

Reference	Deep Learning Technique	Scope	Evaluation Results	Datasets
Tan et al. [126]	CNN	Classification	Accuracy = 82%	mini-Mammographic Image Analysis Society (mini-MIAS)
Amit et al. [122]	CNN	Classification	Accuracy = 83%, Area under the curve = 0.91	ED (MRI)
Byra et al. [127]	CNN	Classification	Accuracy = 83%, Area under the curve = 0.912	ED (US, Nakagami)
Gao et al. [128]	CNN	Classification	Accuracy = 90% Area under the curve = 0.92	INbreast
Wang et al. [129]	CNN	Classification	Accuracy = 76.5%	Private
Tan et al. [126]	CNN	Classification	Accuracy = 95%, Area under the curve = 0.97	BreakHis
Litjens et al. [130]	CNN	Classification	Area under the curve = 0.99	Private
Araújo et al. [132]	CNN	Classification	Accuracy = 77.8% (four classes), Accuracy = 83.3% (two classes)	BICBH
Ragab et al. [135]	CNN with SVM	Feature extraction	Accuracy = 73%, Area under the curve = 0.94	Digital Database for Screening Mammography (DDSM), CBIS-DDSM
Acharya et al. [136]	CNN with K-means	Feature extraction	Accuracy = 97%	Private
Karthik et al. [147]	DNN	Classification	Accuracy = 98%	WBC
Yu et al. [134]	DNN + CNN	Classification	Accuracy = 81%, Area under the curve = 0.88	BCDR
Sun et al. [131]	CNN	Classification	Accuracy = 82.43%, Area under the curve = 0.8818	ED(Mg)
Hadad et al. [148]	CNN	Classification	Accuracy = 94%, Area under the curve = 0.98	ED(Mg, MRI)
Nahid et al. [123]	CNN	Classification	Accuracy = 91%	BreakHis
Shams et al. [143]	GANs	Classification	Area under the curve = 0.88, Area under the curve = 0.925	DDSM, INbreast
Singh et al. [144]	GANs + CNN	Classification	Accuracy = 72%	DDSM and Private
Wu et al. [149]	GANs	Classification	Accuracy = 89%	DDSM
Guan et al. [146]	GANs	Classification	Accuracy = 79.8%	DDSM

3.3. Robotics

With the improvements in medical robots' accuracy, robots in healthcare now assist by relieving medical practitioners from their routine tasks and also make medical procedures less costly and safer for patients [129]. These could be the reasons research into creating robots to detect and diagnose breast cancer in patients have been gaining popularity in the last decade. Robotics as a branch of AI, is developed based on some machine learning algorithms [129,150]. Such algorithms include but are not limited to reinforcement learning and deep reinforcement learning [150].

3.3.1. Reinforcement Learning

Reinforcement learning is an approach to machine learning that involves computational learning by interaction. It involves learning about what to do and how to map situations to actions to maximize a numerical solution. Unlike other machine learning approaches, reinforcement learning does not directly demonstrate how to perform a task but works through the problem on its own [129,150].

Examples of systems that are built based on the unsupervised learning approach of reinforcement learning are self-driving cars, a program playing chess (e.g., Alphago), etc. These systems interact with their environment, such that, when they complete a task successfully, they receive a reward state. Such tasks could be driving to a destination safely or winning a game. On the other hand, when the system does not complete a task successfully, they receive a penalty for performing incorrectly. Such a task could also be going off the road or being checkmated [150].

These systems, over time, make decisions to maximize their reward and minimize their penalty using dynamic programming. The advantage of this approach to AI is that it allows an AI program to learn without a programmer spelling out how a system should perform the task; this type of approach is popularly called unsupervised learning [150].

3.3.2. Robotic Tools for Breast Cancer Diagnosis

In the research reported by Kato et al. [151], a robotic system called WAPRO-4 was developed for the automatic palpation of breast cancer. The study aimed at palpating and diagnosing breast cancer without the assistance of medical personnel. The major objective was to aid the early detection of breast cancer. Additionally, WAPRO-4 consists of three parts which include the measuring instrument, the locomotion unit, and the microcomputer system [151]. The WAPRO-4 was constructed to detect tumors while ignoring breathing and the configuration of the chest wall. Kobayashi et al. [152] developed a palpation-based needle insertion method for diagnostic biopsy and treatment of breast cancer. The system locates cancerous tissues from force information and reduces tissue during needle insertion. Kobayashi et al. [152] compared the palpation-based needle insertion approach to the normal needle insertion approach using a numerical simulation of a breast tissue model. The outcome showed that palpation-based needle insertion had a smaller error which suggests that the procedure could be a safe and effective alternative [152].

Larson et al. [153] developed a robotic device to perform minimally invasive breast interventions with real-time MRI guidance for the early diagnosis and treatment of breast cancer. In this work, five computer-controlled degrees of freedom were used to perform minimally invasive interventions inside a closed MRI scanner. According to Larson et al. [153], the intervention consists of a biopsy of the suspicious lesion for diagnosis, which involves the therapies to destroy or remove malignant tissue in the breast. As a result, the procedure includes conditioning of the breast along with a prescribed orientation, the definition of an insertion vector by its height and pitch angle, and insertion into the breast. The entire device is made of materials compatible with an MRI machine, avoiding artefacts and distortion of the local magnetic field. This device was built to be remotely controlled via a graphical user interface.

Meanwhile, automated detection of breast lesions from DCE-MRI volumes was implemented based on deep reinforcement learning [154]. The method significantly reduces the inference time for lesion detection compared to an exhaustive search, while retaining state-of-the-art accuracy. The authors demonstrated their results on a dataset containing 117 DCE-MRI volumes, validating runtime and accuracy of lesion detection [154,155].

Moreover, Tsekos et al. [155] implemented a robotic device with haptic, tactile, and ultrasound capabilities, that can acquire and render the information of breast pathology remotely. In this work, the device is designed to screen for breast cancer by examination for the patient in a remote area without convenient access to medical personnel. The device was said to be more accurate than human medical personnel [155]. Further, a robotic based device designed to assist medical personnel in placing the instrument on the tumor location and automatically acquiring tumor images in real-time was implemented in [153,156]. This device has the potential to increase targeting accuracy while reducing the level of skill required to perform minimally invasive breast interventional procedures.

4. Conclusions

Breast cancer has shown to be one of the leading causes of female mortality in the world. Recent studies have shown that early diagnosis is the first step towards a successful treatment, which can help save many lives. This review presented a brief overview of past and present conventional diagnostics approaches as well as recent computational techniques that have contributed immensely to the diagnosis of breast cancer. Articles on breast cancer classification published from 2006 to 2020 were extensively reviewed. In total, 55 were carefully reviewed from different academic repositories. Several criteria were used for the review, such as conventional diagnostics approaches, the computational technique used, scope, evaluation results, and different types of datasets were used for these studies. We noticed that researchers preferred publicly available datasets over exclusive ones. For example, WBC and DDSM were seen to be popular among researchers. For computational approaches, we reviewed three areas: Machine learning, deep learning, and robotics. Out of these approaches, the deep learning techniques appear to be increasingly popular for most researchers. Among these techniques, we noticed that CNN was a popular choice, used for classification. Currently, GANs have shown to be a promising deep learning algorithm for breast cancer diagnosis due to its ability to give convincingly good results. Performance metrics such as AUC, accuracy, sensitivity, specificity, and measure were used for evaluating deep learning approaches.

Finally, this review provides a roadmap for future conversations about building better techniques for early detection, which could help save millions of lives. We believe that this comprehensive review will offer a better understanding of the breast cancer classification domain and provide valuable insights to researchers in this field.

Author Contributions: K.A., G.O., B.O., T.A.A., and R.T.A. conceived the idea; K.A., G.O., B.O., T.A.A., A.O.F., A.K., and R.T.A. designed and wrote the manuscript. All authors have read and agreed to the published version of the manuscript.

References

1.　Adekiya, T.A.; Aruleba, R.T.; Khanyile, S.; Masamba, P.; Oyinloye, B.E.; Kappo, A.P. Structural analysis and epitope prediction of MHC class-1-chain related protein-a for cancer vaccine development. *Vaccines* **2018**, *6*, 1. [CrossRef]

2.　Aruleba, R.T.; Adekiya, T.A.; Oyinloye, B.E.; Kappo, A.P. Structural studies of predicted ligand binding sites and molecular docking analysis of Slc2a4 as a therapeutic target for the treatment of cancer. *Int. J. Mol. Sci.* **2018**, *19*, 386. [CrossRef]

3.　Oyinloye, B.E.; Adekiya, T.A.; Aruleba, R.T.; Ojo, O.A.; Ajiboye, B.O. Structure-Based Docking Studies of GLUT4 Towards Exploring Selected Phytochemicals from Solanum xanthocarpum as a Therapeutic Target for the Treatment of Cancer. *Curr. Drug Discov. Technol.* **2019**, *16*, 406–416. [CrossRef]

4.　Shapiro, C.L. Cancer survivorship. *N. Engl. J. Med.* **2018**, *379*, 2438–2450. [CrossRef]

5.　Akram, M.; Iqbal, M.; Daniyal, M.; Khan, A.U. Awareness and current knowledge of breast cancer. *Biol. Res.* **2017**, *50*, 33. [CrossRef]

6.　Singh, S.K.; Singh, S.; Lillard, J.W., Jr.; Singh, R. Drug delivery approaches for breast cancer. *Int. J. Nanomed.* **2017**, *12*, 6205. [CrossRef]

7.　Wang, H.; Zheng, B.; Yoon, S.W.; Ko, H.S. A support vector machine-based ensemble algorithm for breast cancer diagnosis. *Eur. J. Oper. Res.* **2018**, *267*, 687–699. [CrossRef]

8.　Dande, P.; Samant, P. Acquaintance to artificial neural networks and use of artificial intelligence as a diagnostic tool for tuberculosis: A review. *Tuberculosis* **2018**, *108*, 1–9. [CrossRef]

9.　Lengauer, T.; Sing, T. Bioinformatics-assisted anti-HIV therapy. *Nat. Rev. Genet.* **2006**, *4*, 790–797. [CrossRef]

10. Vaishya, R.; Javaid, M.; Khan, I.H.; Haleem, A. Artificial Intelligence (AI) applications for COVID-19 pandemic. *Diabet. Metab. Syndr. Clin. Res. Rev.* **2020**, *14*, 337–339. [CrossRef]

11. Nover, A.B.; Jagtap, S.; Anjum, W.; Yegingil, H.; Shih, W.Y.; Shih, W.-H.; Brooks, A.D. Modern breast cancer detection: A technological review. *Int. J. Biomed. Imaging* **2009**, *2009*, 1–14. [CrossRef] [PubMed]

12. Kolb, T.M.; Lichy, J.; Newhouse, J.H. Comparison of the performance of screening mammography, physical examination, and breast US and evaluation of factors that influence them: An analysis of 27825 patient evaluations. *Radiology* **2002**, *225*, 165–175. [CrossRef] [PubMed]

13. Nelson, H.D.; Tyne, K.; Naik, A.; Bougatsos, C.; Chan, B.K.; Humphrey, L. Screening for breast cancer: An update for the US Preventive Services Task Force. *Ann. Intern. Med.* **2009**, *151*, 727–737. [CrossRef] [PubMed]

14. Bagni, B.; Franceschetto, A.; Casolo, A.; De Santis, M.; Bagni, I.; Pansini, F.; Di Leo, C. Scintimammography with 99mTc-MIBI and magnetic resonance imaging in the evaluation of breast cancer. *Eur. J. Nucl. Med. Mol. Imaging* **2003**, *30*, 1383–1388. [CrossRef]

15. Lladó, X.; Oliver, A.; Freixenet, J.; Martí, R.; Martí, J. A textural approach for mass false positive reduction in mammography. *Comput. Med. Imaging Graph.* **2009**, *33*, 415–422. [CrossRef] [PubMed]

16. Aiken, L.S.; West, S.G.; Woodward, C.K.; Reno, R.R. Health beliefs and compliance with mammography-screening recommendations in asymptomatic women. *Health Psychol.* **1994**, *13*, 122. [CrossRef]

17. Kennedy, D.A.; Lee, T.; Seely, D. A comparative review of thermography as a breast cancer screening technique. *Integr. Cancer Ther.* **2009**, *8*, 9–16. [CrossRef]

18. Schillaci, O.; Buscombe, J.R. Breast scintigraphy today: Indications and limitations. *Eur. J. Nucl. Med. Mol. Imaging* **2004**, *31*, S35–S45. [CrossRef]

19. Cherel, P.; Hagay, C.; Benaim, B.; De Maulmont, C.; Engerand, S.; Langer, A.; Talma, V. Mammographic evaluation of dense breasts: Techniques and limits. *J. Radiol.* **2008**, *89*, 1156. [CrossRef]

20. Mori, M.; Akashi-Tanaka, S.; Suzuki, S.; Daniels, M.I.; Watanabe, C.; Hirose, M.; Nakamura, S. Diagnostic accuracy of contrast-enhanced spectral mammography in comparison to conventional full-field digital mammography in a population of women with dense breasts. *Breast Cancer* **2017**, *24*, 104–110. [CrossRef]

21. Jung, J.I.; Kim, H.H.; Park, S.H.; Song, S.W.; Chung, M.H.; Kim, H.S.; Kim, K.J.; Ahn, M.I.; Seo, S.B.; Hahn, S.T. Thoracic manifestations of breast cancer and its therapy. *Radiographics* **2004**, *24*, 1269–1285. [CrossRef] [PubMed]

22. Savaridas, S.L.; Spratt, J.D.; Cox, J. Incidence and potential significance of internal mammary lymphadenopathy on computed tomography in patients with a diagnosis of primary breast cancer. *Breast Cancer Basic Clin. Res.* **2015**, *9*. [CrossRef] [PubMed]

23. Dobbins, J.T. Tomosynthesis imaging: At a translational crossroads. *Med. Phys.* **2009**, *36*, 1956–1967. [CrossRef] [PubMed]

24. Friedewald, S.M.; Rafferty, E.A.; Rose, S.L.; Durand, M.A.; Plecha, D.M.; Greenberg, J.S.; Hayes, M.K.; Copit, D.S.; Carlson, K.L.; Cink, T.M. Breast cancer screening using tomosynthesis in combination with digital mammography. *JAMA* **2014**, *311*, 2499–2507. [CrossRef] [PubMed]

25. Niklason, L.T.; Christian, B.T.; Niklason, L.E.; Kopans, D.B.; Castleberry, D.E.; Opsahl-Ong, B.; Landberg, C.E.; Slanetz, P.J.; Giardino, A.A.; Moore, R. Digital tomosynthesis in breast imaging. *Radiology* **1997**, *205*, 399–406. [CrossRef] [PubMed]

26. Poplack, S.P.; Tosteson, T.D.; Kogel, C.A.; Nagy, H.M. Digital breast tomosynthesis: Initial experience in 98 women with abnormal digital screening mammography. *Am. J. Roentgenol.* **2007**, *189*, 616–623. [CrossRef] [PubMed]

27. Lång, K.; Andersson, I.; Rosso, A.; Tingberg, A.; Timberg, P.; Zackrisson, S. Performance of one-view breast tomosynthesis as a stand-alone breast cancer screening modality: Results from the Malmö Breast Tomosynthesis Screening Trial, a population-based study. *Eur. Radiol.* **2016**, *26*, 184–190. [CrossRef]

28. Sechopoulos, I. A review of breast tomosynthesis. Part I. The image acquisition process. *Med. Phys.* **2013**, *40*, 014301. [CrossRef]

29. Van de Sompel, D.; Brady, M.; Boone, J. Task-based performance analysis of FBP, SART and ML for digital breast tomosynthesis using signal CNR and Channelised Hotelling Observers. *Med. Image Anal.* **2011**, *15*, 53–70. [CrossRef]

30. O'Brien, W.D., Jr. Ultrasound–biophysics mechanisms. *Prog. Biophys. Mol. Biol.* **2007**, *93*, 212–255.

31. Mason, T.J. Therapeutic ultrasound an overview. *Ultrason. Sonochem.* **2011**, *18*, 847–852. [CrossRef]

32. Dewall, R.J. Ultrasound elastography: Principles, techniques, and clinical applications. *Crit. Rev. Biomed. Eng.* **2013**, *41*, 1–19. [CrossRef] [PubMed]

33. Guo, R.; Lu, G.; Qin, B.; Fei, B. Ultrasound Imaging Technologies for Breast Cancer Detection and Management: A Review. *Ultrasound Med. Biol.* **2018**, *44*, 37–70. [CrossRef]

34. Thornton, G.D.; McPhail, M.J.W.; Nayagam, S.; Hewitt, M.J.; Vlavianos, P.; Monahan, K.J. Endoscopic ultrasound guided fine needle aspiration for the diagnosis of pancreatic cystic neoplasms: A meta-analysis. *Pancreatology* **2013**, *13*, 48–57. [CrossRef]

35. Liu, R.; Adler, D.G. Duplication cysts: Diagnosis, management, and the role of endoscopic ultrasound. *Endosc. Ultrasound* **2014**, *3*, 152–160. [CrossRef]

36. Park, M.K.; Jo, J.; Kwon, H.; Cho, J.H.; Oh, J.Y.; Noh, M.H.; Nam, K.J. Usefulness of acoustic radiation force impulse elastography in the differential diagnosis of benign and malignant solid pancreatic lesions. *Ultrasonography* **2014**, *33*, 26. [CrossRef] [PubMed]

37. Xie, X.-H.; Xu, H.-X.; Xie, X.-Y.; Lu, M.-D.; Kuang, M.; Xu, Z.-F.; Liu, G.-J.; Wang, Z.; Liang, J.-Y.; Chen, L.-D. Differential diagnosis between benign and malignant gallbladder diseases with real-time contrast-enhanced ultrasound. *Eur. Radiol.* **2010**, *20*, 239–248. [CrossRef] [PubMed]

38. Masroor, I.; Afzal, S.; Suffian, S.N. Imaging guided breast interventions. *J. Coll. Physicians Surg. Pak.* **2016**, *26*, 521–526.

39. Giuliano, V.; Giuliano, C. Improved breast cancer detection in asymptomatic women using 3D-automated breast ultrasound in mammographically dense breasts. *Clin. Imaging* **2013**, *37*, 480–486. [CrossRef]

40. Bachawal, S.V.; Jensen, K.C.; Lutz, A.M.; Gambhir, S.S.; Tranquart, F.; Tian, L.; Willmann, J.K. Earlier detection of breast cancer with ultrasound molecular imaging in a transgenic mouse model. *Cancer Res.* **2013**, *73*, 1689–1698. [CrossRef]

41. Lindfors, K.K.; Boone, J.M.; Nelson, T.R.; Yang, K.; Kwan, A.L.; Miller, D.F. Dedicated breast CT: Initial clinical experience. *Radiology* **2008**, *246*, 725–733. [CrossRef]

42. Kuzmiak, C.M.; Cole, E.B.; Zeng, D.; Tuttle, L.A.; Steed, D.; Pisano, E.D. Dedicated three-dimensional breast computed tomography: Lesion characteristic perception by radiologists. *J. Clin. Imaging Sci.* **2016**, *6*, 14. [CrossRef]

43. Shah, J.P.; Mann, S.D.; McKinley, R.L.; Tornai, M.P. Characterization of CT Hounsfield units for 3D acquisition trajectories on a dedicated breast CT system. *J. X-ray Sci. Technol.* **2018**, *26*, 535–551. [CrossRef]

44. Boone, J.M.; Nelson, T.R.; Lindfors, K.K.; Seibert, J.A. Dedicated breast CT: Radiation dose and image quality evaluation. *Radiology* **2001**, *221*, 657–667. [CrossRef]

45. Sarno, A.; Mettivier, G.; Russo, P. Dedicated breast computed tomography: Basic aspects. *Med. Phys.* **2015**, *42*, 2786–2804. [CrossRef]

46. Radhakrishna, S.; Agarwal, S.; Parikh, P.M.; Kaur, K.; Panwar, S.; Sharma, S.; Dey, A.; Saxena, K.; Chandra, M.; Sud, S. Role of magnetic resonance imaging in breast cancer management. *South Asian J. Cancer* **2018**, *7*, 69–71. [CrossRef]

47. Sardanelli, F.; Giuseppetti, G.M.; Panizza, P.; Bazzocchi, M.; Fausto, A.; Simonetti, G.; Lattanzio, V.; Del Maschio, A. Sensitivity of MRI versus mammography for detecting foci of multifocal, multicentric breast cancer in fatty and dense breasts using the whole-breast pathologic examination as a gold standard. *Am. J. Roentgenol.* **2004**, *183*, 1149–1157. [CrossRef]

48. Lee, C.H.; Dershaw, D.D.; Kopans, D.; Evans, P.; Monsees, B.; Monticciolo, D.; Brenner, R.J.; Bassett, L.; Berg, W.; Feig, S. Breast cancer screening with imaging: Recommendations from the Society of Breast Imaging and the ACR on the use of mammography, breast MRI, breast ultrasound, and other technologies for the detection of clinically occult breast cancer. *J. Am. Coll. Radiol.* **2010**, *7*, 18–27. [CrossRef]

49. Morrow, M.; Waters, J.; Morris, E. MRI for breast cancer screening, diagnosis, and treatment. *Lancet* **2011**, *378*, 1804–1811. [CrossRef]

50. Gareth, E.D.; Nisha, K.; Yit, L.; Soujanye, G.; Emma, H.; Massat, N.J.; Maxwell, A.J.; Sarah, I.; Rosalind, E.; Leach, M.O. MRI breast screening in high-risk women: Cancer detection and survival analysis. *Breast Cancer Res. Treat.* **2014**, *145*, 663–672. [CrossRef]

51. Lehman, C.D.; Gatsonis, C.; Kuhl, C.K.; Hendrick, R.E.; Pisano, E.D.; Hanna, L.; Peacock, S.; Smazal, S.F.; Maki, D.D.; Julian, T.B. MRI evaluation of the contralateral breast in women with recently diagnosed breast cancer. *N. Engl. J. Med.* **2007**, *356*, 1295–1303. [CrossRef] [PubMed]

52. Passaperuma, K.; Warner, E.; Causer, P.; Hill, K.; Messner, S.; Wong, J.; Jong, R.; Wright, F.; Yaffe, M.; Ramsay, E. Long-term results of screening with magnetic resonance imaging in women with BRCA mutations. *Br. J. Cancer* **2012**, *107*, 24–30. [CrossRef] [PubMed]

53. Bang, O.Y.; Li, W. Applications of diffusion-weighted imaging in diagnosis, evaluation, and treatment of acute ischemic stroke. *Precis. Future Med.* **2019**, *3*, 69–76. [CrossRef]

54. Chung, J.W.; Park, S.H.; Kim, N.; Kim, W.J.; Park, J.H.; Ko, Y.; Yang, M.H.; Jang, M.S.; Han, M.K.; Jung, C. Trial of ORG 10172 in Acute Stroke Treatment (TOAST) classification and vascular territory of ischemic stroke lesions diagnosed by diffusion-weighted imaging. *J. Am. Heart Assoc.* **2014**, *3*, e001119. [CrossRef] [PubMed]

55. Malayeri, A.A.; El Khouli, R.H.; Zaheer, A.; Jacobs, M.A.; Corona-Villalobos, C.P.; Kamel, I.R.; Macura, K.J. Principles and applications of diffusion-weighted imaging in cancer detection, staging, and treatment follow-up. *Radiographics* **2011**, *31*, 1773–1791. [CrossRef] [PubMed]

56. Sinha, S.; Lucas-Quesada, F.A.; Sinha, U.; De Bruhl, N.; Bassett, L.W. In vivo diffusion-weighted MRI of the breast: Potential for lesion characterization. *J. Magn. Reson. Imaging* **2002**, *15*, 693–704. [CrossRef]

57. Menezes, G.L.; Knuttel, F.M.; Stehouwer, B.L.; Pijnappel, R.M.; van den Bosch, M.A. Magnetic resonance imaging in breast cancer: A literature review and future perspectives. *World J. Clin. Oncol.* **2014**, *5*, 61. [CrossRef]

58. Costantini, M.; Belli, P.; Rinaldi, P.; Bufi, E.; Giardina, G.; Franceschini, G.; Petrone, G.; Bonomo, L. Diffusion-weighted imaging in breast cancer: Relationship between apparent diffusion coefficient and tumour aggressiveness. *Clin. Radiol.* **2010**, *65*, 1005–1012. [CrossRef]

59. Tan, S.; Rahmat, K.; Rozalli, F.; Mohd-Shah, M.; Aziz, Y.; Yip, C.; Vijayananthan, A.; Ng, K. Differentiation between benign and malignant breast lesions using quantitative diffusion-weighted sequence on 3 T MRI. *Clin. Radiol.* **2014**, *69*, 63–71. [CrossRef]

60. Baltzer, P.A.; Bickel, H.; Spick, C.; Wengert, G.; Woitek, R.; Kapetas, P.; Clauser, P.; Helbich, T.H.; Pinker, K. Potential of noncontrast magnetic resonance imaging with diffusion-weighted imaging in characterization of breast lesions: Intraindividual comparison with dynamic contrast-enhanced magnetic resonance imaging. *Investig. Radiol.* **2018**, *53*, 229–235. [CrossRef]

61. Chilla, G.S.; Tan, C.H.; Xu, C.; Poh, C.L. Diffusion weighted magnetic resonance imaging and its recent trend—A survey. *Quant. Imaging Med. Surg.* **2015**, *5*, 407. [PubMed]

62. Baliyan, V.; Das, C.J.; Sharma, R.; Gupta, A.K. Diffusion weighted imaging: Technique and applications. *World J. Radiol.* **2016**, *8*, 785. [CrossRef] [PubMed]

63. Scarfe, W.C.; Li, Z.; Aboelmaaty, W.; Scott, S.; Farman, A. Maxillofacial cone beam computed tomography: Essence, elements and steps to interpretation. *Aust. Dent. J.* **2012**, *57*, 46–60. [CrossRef] [PubMed]

64. Sun, W.; Lal, P. Recent development on computer aided tissue engineering—A review. *Comput. Methods Programs Biomed.* **2002**, *67*, 85–103. [CrossRef]

65. Suga, K.; Yuan, Y.; Ogasawara, N.; Okada, M.; Matsunaga, N. Localization of breast sentinel lymph nodes by MR lymphography with a conventional gadolinium contrast agent: Preliminary observations in dongs and humans. *Acta Radiol.* **2003**, *44*, 35–42. [CrossRef] [PubMed]

66. Foo, S.Y.; Gray, K. Computed tomography (CT) staging in breast cancer. *Clin. Radiol.* **2015**, *70*, S13. [CrossRef]

67. Okamura, Y.; Yoshizawa, N.; Yamaguchi, M.; Kashiwakura, I. Application of dual-energy computed tomography for breast cancer diagnosis. *Int. J. Med. Phys. Clin. Eng. Radiat. Oncol.* **2016**, *5*, 288–297. [CrossRef]

68. Park, E.K.; Seo, B.K.; Kwon, M.; Cho, K.R.; Woo, O.H.; Song, S.E.; Cha, J.; Lee, H.Y. Low-dose perfusion computed tomography for breast cancer to quantify tumor vascularity: Correlation with prognostic biomarkers. *Investig. Radiol.* **2019**, *54*, 273–281. [CrossRef] [PubMed]

69. Shah, J.P.; Mann, S.D.; McKinley, R.L.; Tornai, M.P. Three dimensional dose distribution comparison of simple and complex acquisition trajectories in dedicated breast CT. *Med. Phys.* **2015**, *42*, 4497–4510. [CrossRef]

70. Hawrysz, D.J.; Sevick-Muraca, E.M. Developments toward diagnostic breast cancer imaging using near-infrared optical measurements and fluorescent contrast agents1. *Neoplasia* **2000**, *2*, 388–417. [CrossRef]

71. Troyan, S.L.; Kianzad, V.; Gibbs-Strauss, S.L.; Gioux, S.; Matsui, A.; Oketokoun, R.; Ngo, L.; Khamene, A.; Azar, F.; Frangioni, J.V. The FLARE™ intraoperative near-infrared fluorescence imaging system: A first-in-human clinical trial in breast cancer sentinel lymph node mapping. *Ann. Surg. Oncol.* **2009**, *16*, 2943–2952. [CrossRef] [PubMed]

72.   Tagaya, N.; Yamazaki, R.; Nakagawa, A.; Abe, A.; Hamada, K.; Kubota, K.; Oyama, T. Intraoperative identification of sentinel lymph nodes by near-infrared fluorescence imaging in patients with breast cancer. *Am. J. Surg.* **2008**, *195*, 850–853. [CrossRef] [PubMed]

73.   Verbeek, F.P.; Troyan, S.L.; Mieog, J.S.D.; Liefers, G.-J.; Moffitt, L.A.; Rosenberg, M.; Hirshfield-Bartek, J.; Gioux, S.; van de Velde, C.J.; Vahrmeijer, A.L. Near-infrared fluorescence sentinel lymph node mapping in breast cancer: A multicenter experience. *Breast Cancer Res. Treat.* **2014**, *143*, 333–342. [CrossRef] [PubMed]

74.   Mieog, J.S.D.; Troyan, S.L.; Hutteman, M.; Donohoe, K.J.; Van Der Vorst, J.R.; Stockdale, A.; Liefers, G.-J.; Choi, H.S.; Gibbs-Strauss, S.L.; Putter, H. Toward optimization of imaging system and lymphatic tracer for near-infrared fluorescent sentinel lymph node mapping in breast cancer. *Ann. Surg. Oncol.* **2011**, *18*, 2483–2491. [CrossRef] [PubMed]

75.   Sevick-Muraca, E.M.; Sharma, R.; Rasmussen, J.C.; Marshall, M.V.; Wendt, J.A.; Pham, H.Q.; Bonefas, E.; Houston, J.P.; Sampath, L.; Adams, K.E. Imaging of lymph flow in breast cancer patients after microdose administration of a near-infrared fluorophore: Feasibility study. *Radiology* **2008**, *246*, 734–741. [CrossRef]

76.   Altınoğlu, E.I.; Russin, T.J.; Kaiser, J.M.; Barth, B.M.; Eklund, P.C.; Kester, M.; Adair, J.H. Near-infrared emitting fluorophore-doped calcium phosphate nanoparticles for in vivo imaging of human breast cancer. *ACS Nano* **2008**, *2*, 2075–2084. [CrossRef] [PubMed]

77.   Poellinger, A.; Burock, S.; Grosenick, D.; Hagen, A.; Lüdemann, L.; Diekmann, F.; Engelken, F.; Macdonald, R.; Rinneberg, H.; Schlag, P.-M. Breast cancer: Early-and late-fluorescence near-infrared imaging with indocyanine green—A preliminary study. *Radiology* **2011**, *258*, 409–416. [CrossRef]

78.   Ke, S.; Wen, X.; Gurfinkel, M.; Charnsangavej, C.; Wallace, S.; Sevick-Muraca, E.M.; Li, C. Near-infrared optical imaging of epidermal growth factor receptor in breast cancer xenografts. *Cancer Res.* **2003**, *63*, 7870–7875.

79.   Vallabhajosula, S.; Polack, B.D.; Babich, J.W. Molecular Imaging of Prostate Cancer: Radiopharmaceuticals for Positron Emission Tomography (PET) and Single-Photon Emission Computed Tomography (SPECT). In *Precision Molecular Pathology of Prostate Cancer*; Springer: Berlin/Heidelberg, Germany, 2018; pp. 475–501.

80.   Pellikka, P.A.; She, L.; Holly, T.A.; Lin, G.; Varadarajan, P.; Pai, R.G.; Bonow, R.O.; Pohost, G.M.; Panza, J.A.; Berman, D.S. Variability in ejection fraction measured by echocardiography, gated single-photon emission computed tomography, and cardiac magnetic resonance in patients with coronary artery disease and left ventricular dysfunction. *JAMA Netw. Open* **2018**, *1*, e181456. [CrossRef]

81.   Noyce, A.J.; Dickson, J.; Rees, R.N.; Bestwick, J.P.; Isaias, I.U.; Politis, M.; Giovannoni, G.; Warner, T.T.; Lees, A.J.; Schrag, A. Dopamine reuptake transporter-single-photon emission computed tomography and transcranial sonography as imaging markers of prediagnostic Parkinson's disease. *Mov. Disord.* **2018**, *33*, 478–482. [CrossRef]

82.   Frangioni, J.V. New technologies for human cancer imaging. *J. Clin. Oncol.* **2008**, *26*, 4012. [CrossRef] [PubMed]

83.   Koizumi, M.; Koyama, M. Comparison between single photon emission computed tomography with computed tomography and planar scintigraphy in sentinel node biopsy in breast cancer patients. *Ann. Nucl. Med.* **2019**, *33*, 160–168. [CrossRef] [PubMed]

84.   Van der Ploeg, I.M.; Nieweg, O.E.; Kroon, B.B.; Rutgers, E.J.; Baas-Vrancken Peeters, M.J.; Vogel, W.V.; Hoefnagel, C.A.; Olmos, R.A. The yield of SPECT/CT for anatomical lymphatic mapping in patients with breast cancer. *Eur. J. Nucl. Med. Mol. Imaging* **2009**, *36*, 903–909. [CrossRef] [PubMed]

85.   Maza, S.; Valencia, R.; Geworski, L.; Zander, A.; Guski, H.; Winzer, K.J.; Munz, D.L. Peritumoural versus subareolar administration of technetium-99m nanocolloid for sentinel lymph node detection in breast cancer: Preliminary results of a prospective intra-individual comparative study. *Eur. J. Nucl. Med. Mol. Imaging* **2003**, *30*, 651–656. [CrossRef] [PubMed]

86.   Lerman, H.; Lievshitz, G.; Zak, O.; Metser, U.; Schneebaum, S.; Even-Sapir, E. Improved sentinel node identification by SPECT/CT in overweight patients with breast cancer. *J. Nucl. Med.* **2007**, *48*, 201–206.

87.   Pecking, A.P.; Wartski, W.; Cluzan, R.; Bellet, D.; Albérini, J. SPECT–CT fusion imaging radionuclide lymphoscintigraphy: Potential for limb lymphedema assessment and sentinel node detection in breast cancer. In *Cancer Metastasis and the Lymphovascular System: Basis for Rational Therapy*; Springer: Berlin/Heidelberg, Germany, 2007; pp. 79–84.

88.   Mann, S.D.; Perez, K.L.; McCracken, E.K.; Shah, J.P.; Wong, T.Z.; Tornai, M.P. Initial in vivo quantification of Tc-99m sestamibi uptake as a function of tissue type in healthy breasts using dedicated breast SPECT-CT. *J. Oncol.* **2012**, *2012*, 1–7. [CrossRef]

89. Bowen, S.L.; Wu, Y.; Chaudhari, A.J.; Fu, L.; Packard, N.J.; Burkett, G.W.; Yang, K.; Lindfors, K.K.; Shelton, D.K.; Hagge, R. Initial characterization of a dedicated breast PET/CT scanner during human imaging. *J. Nucl. Med.* **2009**, *50*, 1401–1408. [CrossRef]

90. Tornai, M.P.; Shah, J.P.; Mann, S.D.; McKinley, R.L. Development of Fully-3D CT in a Hybrid SPECT-CT Breast Imaging System. In Proceedings of the 13th International Workshop on Breast Imaging, Malmo, Sweden, 19–22 June 2016; pp. 567–575.

91. Crotty, D.J.; Brady, S.L.; Jackson, D.V.C.; Toncheva, G.I.; Anderson, C.E.; Yoshizumi, T.T.; Tornai, M.P. Evaluation of the absorbed dose to the breast using radiochromic film in a dedicated CT mammotomography system employing a quasi-monochromatic X-ray beam. *Med. Phys.* **2011**, *38*, 3232–3245. [CrossRef]

92. Suthaharan, S. Machine learning models and algorithms for big data classification. *Integr. Ser. Inf. Syst.* **2016**, *36*, 1–12.

93. Tsai, H.-H.; Chang, Y.-C. Facial expression recognition using a combination of multiple facial features and support vector machine. *Soft Comput.* **2018**, *22*, 4389–4405. [CrossRef]

94. Manavalan, B.; Shin, T.H.; Lee, G. PVP-SVM: Sequence-based prediction of phage virion proteins using a support vector machine. *Front. Microbiol.* **2018**, *9*, 476. [CrossRef]

95. Chen, S.; Wu, X.; Zhang, R. A novel twin support vector machine for binary classification problems. *Neural Process. Lett.* **2016**, *44*, 795–811. [CrossRef]

96. Acharya, U.R.; Ng, E.Y.-K.; Tan, J.-H.; Sree, S.V. Thermography based breast cancer detection using texture features and support vector machine. *J. Med. Syst.* **2012**, *36*, 1503–1510. [CrossRef]

97. Maglogiannis, I.; Zafiropoulos, E.; Anagnostopoulos, I. An intelligent system for automated breast cancer diagnosis and prognosis using SVM based classifiers. *Appl. Intell.* **2009**, *30*, 24–36. [CrossRef]

98. Huang, Y.-L.; Wang, K.-L.; Chen, D.-R. Diagnosis of breast tumors with ultrasonic texture analysis using support vector machines. *Neural Comput. Appl.* **2006**, *15*, 164–169. [CrossRef]

99. Abu-Elanien, A.E.; Salama, M.; Ibrahim, M. Determination of transformer health condition using artificial neural networks. In Proceedings of the 19th International Symposium on Innovations in Intelligent Systems and Applications, Warsaw, Poland, 28–30 June 2011; pp. 1–5.

100. Lisboa, P.J.; Taktak, A.F. The use of artificial neural networks in decision support in cancer: A systematic review. *Neural Netw.* **2006**, *19*, 408–415. [CrossRef] [PubMed]

101. Abbass, H.A. An evolutionary artificial neural networks approach for breast cancer diagnosis. *Artif. Intell. Med.* **2002**, *25*, 265–281. [CrossRef]

102. Tourassi, G.D.; Markey, M.K.; Lo, J.Y.; Floyd, C.E., Jr. A neural network approach to breast cancer diagnosis as a constraint satisfaction problem. *Med. Phys.* **2001**, *28*, 804–811. [CrossRef] [PubMed]

103. Janghel, R.; Shukla, A.; Tiwari, R.; Kala, R. Breast cancer diagnosis using artificial neural network models. In Proceedings of the 3rd International Conference on Information Sciences and Interaction Sciences, Chengdu, China, 23–25 June 2010; pp. 89–94.

104. Delen, D.; Walker, G.; Kadam, A. Predicting breast cancer survivability: A comparison of three data mining methods. *Artif. Intell. Med.* **2005**, *34*, 113–127. [CrossRef]

105. Sarvestani, A.S.; Safavi, A.; Parandeh, N.; Salehi, M. Predicting breast cancer survivability using data mining techniques. In Proceedings of the 2nd International Conference on Software Technology and Engineering, San Juan, PR, USA, 3–5 October 2010; p. V2-227.

106. Çakır, A.; Demirel, B. A software tool for determination of breast cancer treatment methods using data mining approach. *J. Med. Syst.* **2011**, *35*, 1503–1511. [CrossRef]

107. Şahan, S.; Polat, K.; Kodaz, H.; Güneş, S. A new hybrid method based on fuzzy-artificial immune system and k-nn algorithm for breast cancer diagnosis. *Comput. Biol. Med.* **2007**, *37*, 415–423. [CrossRef] [PubMed]

108. Bhardwaj, A.; Tiwari, A. Breast cancer diagnosis using genetically optimized neural network model. *Expert Syst. Appl.* **2015**, *42*, 4611–4620. [CrossRef]

109. Karabatak, M. A new classifier for breast cancer detection based on Naïve Bayesian. *Measurement* **2015**, *72*, 32–36. [CrossRef]

110. Bagui, S.C.; Bagui, S.; Pal, K.; Pal, N.R. Breast cancer detection using rank nearest neighbor classification rules. *Pattern Recognit.* **2003**, *36*, 25–34. [CrossRef]

111. Chen, H.-L.; Yang, B.; Liu, J.; Liu, D.-Y. A support vector machine classifier with rough set-based feature selection for breast cancer diagnosis. *Expert Syst. Appl.* **2011**, *38*, 9014–9022. [CrossRef]

112. Polat, K.; Güneş, S. Breast cancer diagnosis using least square support vector machine. *Digit. Signal Process.* **2007**, *17*, 694–701. [CrossRef]

113. Le Cun, Y.; Bengio, Y.; Hinton, G. Deep learning. *Nature* **2015**, *521*, 436–444. [CrossRef]

114. Zhao, R.; Yan, R.; Chen, Z.; Mao, K.; Wang, P.; Gao, R.X. Deep learning and its applications to machine health monitoring. *Mech. Syst. Signal Process.* **2019**, *115*, 213–237. [CrossRef]

115. Zou, J.; Huss, M.; Abid, A.; Mohammadi, P.; Torkamani, A.; Telenti, A. A primer on deep learning in genomics. *Nat. Genet.* **2019**, *51*, 12–18. [CrossRef]

116. Lee, S.M.; Seo, J.B.; Yun, J.; Cho, Y.-H.; Vogel-Claussen, J.; Schiebler, M.L.; Gefter, W.B.; Van Beek, E.J.; Goo, J.M.; Lee, K.S. Deep Learning Applications in Chest Radiography and Computed Tomography. *J. Thorac. Imaging* **2019**, *34*, 75–85. [CrossRef]

117. Mishra, S.; Glaws, A.; Palanisamy, P. Predictive Analytics in Future Power Systems: A Panorama and State-Of-The-Art of Deep Learning Applications. In *Optimization, Learning, and Control for Interdependent Complex Networks*; Springer: Berlin/Heidelberg, Germany, 2020; pp. 147–182.

118. Kalchbrenner, N.; Grefenstette, E.; Blunsom, P. A convolutional neural network for modelling sentences. *arXiv* **2014**, arXiv:1404.2188.

119. Cong, I.; Choi, S.; Lukin, M.D. Quantum convolutional neural networks. *Nat. Phys.* **2019**, *15*, 1273–1278. [CrossRef]

120. Coley, C.W.; Jin, W.; Rogers, L.; Jamison, T.F.; Jaakkola, T.S.; Green, W.H.; Barzilay, R.; Jensen, K.F. A graph-convolutional neural network model for the prediction of chemical reactivity. *Chem. Sci.* **2019**, *10*, 370–377. [CrossRef] [PubMed]

121. Indolia, S.; Goswami, A.K.; Mishra, S.; Asopa, P. Conceptual understanding of convolutional neural network-a deep learning approach. *Procedia Comput. Sci.* **2018**, *132*, 679–688. [CrossRef]

122. Amit, G.; Ben-Ari, R.; Hadad, O.; Monovich, E.; Granot, N.; Hashoul, S. Classification of breast MRI lesions using small-size training sets: Comparison of deep learning approaches. In Proceedings of the Medical Imaging: Computer-Aided Diagnosis Conference, Orlando, FL, USA, 11–16 February 2017; p. 101341H.

123. Nahid, A.-A.; Mehrabi, M.A.; Kong, Y. Histopathological breast cancer image classification by deep neural network techniques guided by local clustering. *BioMed Res. Int.* **2018**. [CrossRef] [PubMed]

124. Murtaza, G.; Shuib, L.; Mujtaba, G.; Raza, G. Breast cancer multi-classification through deep neural network and hierarchical classification approach. *Multimed. Tools Appl.* **2019**. [CrossRef]

125. Dabeer, S.; Khan, M.M.; Islam, S. Cancer diagnosis in histopathological image: CNN based approach. *Inform. Med. Unlocked* **2019**, *16*, 100231. [CrossRef]

126. Tan, Y.; Sim, K.; Ting, F. Breast cancer detection using convolutional neural networks for mammogram imaging system. In Proceedings of the 27th International Conference on Robotics, Automation and Sciences (ICORAS), Melaka, Malaysia, 27–29 November 2017; pp. 1–5.

127. Byra, M.; Piotrzkowska-Wróblewska, H.; Dobruch-Sobczak, K.; Nowicki, A. Combining Nakagami imaging and convolutional neural network for breast lesion classification. In Proceedings of the 2017 IEEE International Ultrasonics Symposium (IUS), Washington, DC, USA, 6–9 September 2017; pp. 1–4.

128. Gao, F.; Wu, T.; Li, J.; Zheng, B.; Ruan, L.; Shang, D.; Patel, B. SD-CNN: A shallow-deep CNN for improved breast cancer diagnosis. *Comput. Med. Imaging Graph.* **2018**, *70*, 53–62. [CrossRef]

129. Wang, Z.; Li, M.; Wang, H.; Jiang, H.; Yao, Y.; Zhang, H.; Xin, J. Breast cancer detection using extreme learning machine based on feature fusion with CNN deep features. *IEEE Access* **2019**, *7*, 105146–105158. [CrossRef]

130. Litjens, G.; Sánchez, C.I.; Timofeeva, N.; Hermsen, M.; Nagtegaal, I.; Kovacs, I.; Hulsbergen-Van De Kaa, C.; Bult, P.; Van Ginneken, B.; Van Der Laak, J. Deep learning as a tool for increased accuracy and efficiency of histopathological diagnosis. *Sci. Rep.* **2016**, *6*, 26286. [CrossRef]

131. Sun, W.; Tseng, T.-L.B.; Zhang, J.; Qian, W. Enhancing deep convolutional neural network scheme for breast cancer diagnosis with unlabeled data. *Comput. Med. Imaging Graph.* **2017**, *57*, 4–9. [CrossRef] [PubMed]

132. Araújo, T.; Aresta, G.; Castro, E.; Rouco, J.; Aguiar, P.; Eloy, C.; Polónia, A.; Campilho, A. Classification of breast cancer histology images using convolutional neural networks. *PLoS ONE* **2017**, *12*, e0177544. [CrossRef] [PubMed]

133. Hernández-Julio, Y.F.; Prieto-Guevara, M.J.; Nieto-Bernal, W.; Meriño-Fuentes, I.; Guerrero-Avendaño, A. Framework for the development of data-driven Mamdani-type fuzzy clinical decision support systems. *Diagnostics* **2019**, *9*, 52. [CrossRef] [PubMed]

134. Yu, S.; Liu, L.; Wang, Z.; Dai, G.; Xie, Y. Transferring deep neural networks for the differentiation of mammographic breast lesions. *Sci. China Technol. Sci.* **2019**, *62*, 441–447. [CrossRef]

135. Ragab, D.A.; Sharkas, M.; Marshall, S.; Ren, J. Breast cancer detection using deep convolutional neural networks and support vector machines. *PeerJ* **2019**, *7*, e6201. [CrossRef]

136. Acharya, S.; Alsadoon, A.; Prasad, P.; Abdullah, S.; Deva, A. Deep convolutional network for breast cancer classification: Enhanced loss function (ELF). *J. Supercomput.* **2020**. [CrossRef]

137. Goodfellow, I.J. On distinguishability criteria for estimating generative models. *arXiv* **2014**, arXiv:1412.6515.

138. Kazeminia, S.; Baur, C.; Kuijper, A.; van Ginneken, B.; Navab, N.; Albarqouni, S.; Mukhopadhyay, A. GANs for medical image analysis. *Artif. Intell. Med.* **2020**. [CrossRef]

139. Odena, A.; Olah, C.; Shlens, J. Conditional image synthesis with auxiliary classifier gans. In Proceedings of the 34th International Conference on Machine Learning (ICML), Sydney, Australia, 6–11 August 2017; pp. 2642–2651.

140. Son, J.; Park, S.J.; Jung, K.-H. Retinal vessel segmentation in fundoscopic images with generative adversarial networks. *arXiv* **2017**, arXiv:1706.09318.

141. Pan, Z.; Yu, W.; Yi, X.; Khan, A.; Yuan, F.; Zheng, Y. Recent progress on generative adversarial networks (GANs): A survey. *IEEE Access* **2019**, *7*, 36322–36333. [CrossRef]

142. Mirza, M.; Osindero, S. Conditional generative adversarial nets. *arXiv* **2014**, arXiv:1411.1784.

143. Shams, S.; Platania, R.; Zhang, J.; Kim, J.; Lee, K.; Park, S.-J. Deep generative breast cancer screening and diagnosis. In Proceedings of the 21st International Conference on Medical Image Computing and Computer-Assisted Intervention, Granada, Spain, 16–20 September 2018; pp. 859–867.

144. Singh, V.K.; Romani, S.; Rashwan, H.A.; Akram, F.; Pandey, N.; Sarker, M.M.K.; Abdulwahab, S.; Torrents-Barrena, J.; Saleh, A.; Arquez, M. Conditional generative adversarial and convolutional networks for X-ray breast mass segmentation and shape classification. In Proceedings of the 21st International Conference on Medical Image Computing and Computer-Assisted Intervention, Granada, Spain, 16–20 September 2018; pp. 833–840.

145. Wu, E.; Wu, K.; Cox, D.; Lotter, W. Conditional infilling GANs for data augmentation in mammogram classification. In *Image Analysis for Moving Organ, Breast, and Thoracic Images*; Springer: Berlin/Heidelberg, Germany, 2018; pp. 98–106.

146. Guan, S.; Loew, M. Breast cancer detection using synthetic mammograms from generative adversarial networks in convolutional neural networks. *J. Med. Imaging* **2019**, *6*, 031411. [CrossRef] [PubMed]

147. Karthik, S.; Perumal, R.S.; Mouli, P.C. Breast cancer classification using deep neural networks. In *Knowledge Computing and Its Applications*; Springer: Berlin/Heidelberg, Germany, 2018; pp. 227–241.

148. Hadad, O.; Bakalo, R.; Ben-Ari, R.; Hashoul, S.; Amit, G. Classification of breast lesions using cross-modal deep learning. In Proceedings of the IEEE 14th International Symposium on Biomedical Imaging (ISBI 2017), Melbourne, Australia, 18–21 April 2017; pp. 109–112.

149. Wu, E.; Wu, K.; Lotter, W. Synthesizing lesions using contextual GANs improves breast cancer classification on mammograms. *arXiv* **2020**, arXiv:2006.00086.

150. Sutton, S.R.; Barto, G.A. Reinforcement Learning: An Introduction. In *A Bradford Book*; The MIT Press: Cambridge, MA, USA, 2015.

151. Kato, I.; Koganezawa, K.; Takanishi, A. Automatic breast cancer palpation robot: WAPRO-4. *Adv. Robot.* **1988**, *3*, 251–261. [CrossRef]

152. Kobayashi, Y.; Suzuki, M.; Kato, A.; Konishi, K.; Hashizume, M.; Fujie, M.G. A robotic palpation-based needle insertion method for diagnostic biopsy and treatment of breast cancer. In Proceedings of the IEEE/RSJ International Conference on Intelligent Robots and Systems, St Louis, MO, USA, 11–15 October 2009; pp. 5534–5539.

153. Larson, B.T.; Tsekos, N.V.; Erdman, A.G. A robotic device for minimally invasive breast interventions with real-time MRI guidance. In Proceedings of the Third IEEE Symposium on Bioinformatics and Bioengineering, Bethesda, MD, USA, 10–12 March 2003; pp. 190–197.

154. Maicas, G.; Carneiro, G.; Bradley, A.P.; Nascimento, J.C.; Reid, I. Deep reinforcement learning for active breast lesion detection from DCE-MRI. In Proceedings of the 20th International Conference on Medical Image Computing and Computer-Assisted Intervention, Quebec City, QC, Canada, 10–14 September 2017; pp. 665–673.

155. Tsekos, N.V.; Shudy, J.; Yacoub, E.; Tsekos, P.V.; Koutlas, I.G. Development of a robotic device for MRI-guided interventions in the breast. In Proceedings of the 2nd Annual IEEE International Symposium on Bioinformatics and Bioengineering (BIBE 2001), Bethesda, MD, USA, 4–6 November 2001; pp. 201–208.

156. Mallapragada, V.; Sarkar, N.; Podder, T.K. Toward a robot-assisted breast intervention system. *IEEE/ASME Trans. Mechatron.* **2010**, *16*, 1011–1020. [CrossRef]

2

Parallel Classification Pipelines for Skin Cancer Detection Exploiting Hyperspectral Imaging on Hybrid Systems

Emanuele Torti [1,*], Raquel Leon [2], Marco La Salvia [1], Giordana Florimbi [1], Beatriz Martinez-Vega [2], Himar Fabelo [2], Samuel Ortega [2], Gustavo M. Callicó [2,*] and Francesco Leporati [1]

1   Department of Electrical, Computer and Biomedical Engineering, University of Pavia, 27100 Pavia, Italy; marco.lasalvia01@universitadipavia.it (M.L.S.); giordana.florimbi01@universitadipavia.it (G.F.); leporati@unipv.it (F.L.)
2   Institute for Applied Microelectronics (IUMA), University of Las Palmas de Gran Canaria (ULPGC), 35017 Las Palmas de Gran Canaria, Spain; slmartin@iuma.ulpgc.es (R.L.); bmartinez@iuma.ulpgc.es (B.M.-V.); hfabelo@iuma.ulpgc.es (H.F.); sortega@iuma.ulpgc.es (S.O.)
*   Correspondence: emanuele.torti@unipv.it (E.T.); gustavo@iuma.ulpgc.es (G.M.C.)

Abstract: The early detection of skin cancer is of crucial importance to plan an effective therapy to treat the lesion. In routine medical practice, the diagnosis is based on the visual inspection of the lesion and it relies on the dermatologists' expertise. After a first examination, the dermatologist may require a biopsy to confirm if the lesion is malignant or not. This methodology suffers from false positives and negatives issues, leading to unnecessary surgical procedures. Hyperspectral imaging is gaining relevance in this medical field since it is a non-invasive and non-ionizing technique, capable of providing higher accuracy than traditional imaging methods. Therefore, the development of an automatic classification system based on hyperspectral images could improve the medical practice to distinguish pigmented skin lesions from malignant, benign, and atypical lesions. Additionally, the system can assist general practitioners in first aid care to prevent noncritical lesions from reaching dermatologists, thereby alleviating the workload of medical specialists. In this paper is presented a parallel pipeline for skin cancer detection that exploits hyperspectral imaging. The computational times of the serial processing have been reduced by adopting multicore and many-core technologies, such as OpenMP and CUDA paradigms. Different parallel approaches have been combined, leading to the development of fifteen classification pipeline versions. Experimental results using in-vivo hyperspectral images show that a hybrid parallel approach is capable of classifying an image of 50 × 50 pixels with 125 bands in less than 1 s.

Keywords: real-time systems; graphic processing units; multicore CPU; cancer detection; hyperspectral imaging

1. Introduction

Hyperspectral imaging (HSI) is a form of imaging spectroscopy that produces three-dimensional images whose pixels are characterized by the spectral information of the acquired scene. This cube contains the reflectance values of the acquired image, i.e., the fraction of incident electromagnetic radiation that is reflected upon a surface. Each material presents a specific variation of reflectance values with respect to wavelengths. This variation is called spectral signature and it is unique for each type of material, allowing precise discrimination [1]. Hyperspectral image classification systems aim at recognizing the material contained in every pixel in the scene. The classification is performed adopting several supervised and unsupervised algorithms, whose elaboration could be computationally intensive. This is a critical issue since most of the applications require a response in a short processing time or even in real-time. Therefore, the scientific community have proposed several works exploiting parallel technologies for HSI classification [2].

HS images were created mainly for military purposes in the remote-sensing field [3]. Since then, they have become very useful in different areas, such as in geology [4], archaeology [5], or food inspection [6], among others [7]. HSI were used only by few companies and research institutes since the HS cameras and the computational systems were very expensive. The recent technological advances have facilitated the use of the HS images in other fields, such as medicine [8,9] and, in particular, cancer detection [8–11]. The reason why this technique is exploited, especially in cancer detection, is that HSI is a non-invasive, non-contact and non-ionizing method, capable of obtaining both spatial and spectral information from the scene. Moreover, the biochemical and morphological changes associated with lesions modify the optical characteristics of a tissue, such as absorption, scattering or fluorescence. These variations provide valuable diagnostic information useful in the diagnosis and detection phases [12–16]. In such a context, it is of crucial importance to achieve a fast or near real-time response. In order to reduce the processing time, modern systems adopt a simultaneous elaboration of the pixels of the image, when allowed by the algorithm. Therefore, the use of parallel technologies is suitable for a pixel-wise classification, where each processing core is in charge of elaborating a single pixel or a group of pixels. The state of the art relies on hybrid systems including multicore and many-core devices. The choice of hybrid systems is justified by the features of the processing chains that typically include algorithms with different levels of complexity [17–20]. The key idea is that each algorithm is managed by the device that best meets the processing constraints. The output of these classification systems is a thematic map, where a color is assigned to each pixel representing a specific tissue type or condition.

Skin cancer is one of the most common forms of cancer in the world and can be categorized as non-melanoma skin cancer (NMSC) and melanoma. NMSC was the 5th most common form of cancer worldwide in 2018, while melanoma was the 21st [21]. Pigmented skin lesions (PSLs) are caused by an extreme progression of melanocytes and can be classified as benign or malignant [22]. Atypical moles, also known as dysplastic nevi, are benign PSLs and are associated with an increased risk of evolving to melanoma [23]. Previous works in skin cancer detection have applied machine learning approaches to identify PSL using HS in-vivo skin cancer data [24]. In [25], the authors used a genetic algorithm to optimize the supervised machine learning algorithms for the identification of four types of PSLs: nevus, BCC (basal cell carcinoma), melanoma, and others (other types of PSLs not included in the remaining classes). A HS dermatologic classification system based on a combination of unsupervised and supervised algorithms was proposed to discriminate between malignant and benign PSLs [26]. Other commercial systems, such as SIAscope/SIAscopy [27] or MelaFind [28], use multispectral images to detect only melanoma lesion, limiting the identification of other malignant PSL that should be analyzed.

This work presents a parallel implementation of a HS dermatologic classification framework based on K-means and SVM (support vector machines) algorithms and snapshot HS cameras with the goal of achieving an automatic in-situ PSL identification. In our previous works, we described the HS in-situ acquisition system and performed an initial study to validate the hypothesis that HSI can be used to differentiate between PSLs through pixel-wise supervised classification [25]. However, in [26], we developed a complete classification framework for processing the HS data to differentiate between malignant and benign PSLs, but without considering the implementation and parallelization of the proposed algorithm. This manuscript presents a variation of the classification framework aiming to differentiate between malignant, benign, and atypical PSLs as well as an exhaustive study of the implementation and parallelization of such algorithm to obtain real-time performance. This real-time diagnosis could assist dermatologists in the discrimination of PSLs during clinical routing practice, providing more diagnostic information regarding non-melanoma skin cancer than other commercial systems that only discriminate between melanoma and non-melanoma [27,28].

The paper is organized as follows. In Section 2, the hyperspectral skin cancer database and the classification framework are described. Section 3 presents the parallel implementations based on multicore CPU and many-core graphical processing unit (GPU) technologies. Then, the experimental results are reported and discussed in Section 4. Finally, Section 5 discusses some conclusions regarding the research presented.

2. Materials and Methods

2.1. Hyperspectral Skin Cancer Database

The HS dermatologic acquisition system developed in [25] was used to create the HS in-vivo skin cancer dataset employed in this work. The system is based on a snapshot HS camera (Cubert UHD 185, Cubert GmbH, Ulm, Germany) coupled to a Cinegon 1.9/10 (Schneider Optics Inc., Hauppauge, NY, USA) lens with a F-number of 1.9 and a focal length of 10.4 nm. The illumination system (Dolan-Jenner, Boxborough, MA, USA) employs a 150 W QTH (Quartz-Tungsten Halogen) lamp coupled to a fiber optic ring light guide to obtain cold light emission. This ring light is attached to the HS camera through a customized 3D printed dermoscopic contact structure. The resulting HS image contains 125 spectral bands covering the visual and near-infrared (VNIR) spectral range from 450 to 950 nm, having a spatial resolution of 50×50 pixels (pixel size of 240×240 µm).

The HS skin cancer database is composed of 76 HS images obtained from 61 subjects with different PSLs located in different parts of the body. The HS images were labeled using a labeling tool [29] based on the SAM (spectral angle mapper) algorithm to create a labeled dataset. This tool allows to manually select a reference pixel and label the most similar pixels according to the spectral angle metric. The data were labeled in three different classes: benign, malignant, and atypical. The HS labeled dataset was partitioned into training, validation, and test set. Validation and test set were composed by 9 HS images.

2.2. Hyperspectral Dermatologic Classification Framework

The HS dermatologic classification framework is composed of three main steps: HS data pre-processing, automatic PSL segmentation, and supervised classification. Figure 1 shows a block diagram of this framework. The first step consists in performing the pre-processing chain to homogenize the incoming raw HS image captured by the HS dermatologic acquisition system. After performing the pre-processing, the resulting image is automatically segmented, where the normal skin and PSL pixels are discriminated. This discrimination is performed using a spectral signature reference library, composed of three spectral signatures of benign, malignant and atypical PSL (in blue, red and black colors respectively in Figure 1) and three skin spectral signatures (in green color in Figure 1). To obtain the spectral reference from the PSL class, the average of the labeled spectral signatures was computed using the training set and from the skin class, the normal skin data were divided into three groups using the K-means clustering algorithm, where the number of clusters employed was selected after evaluating the results using the Silhouette [30], Calinski Harabasz [31], and Davies Bouldin [32] methods. These normal skin spectral signatures correspond with the centroids obtained with the K-means algorithm. Split the normal class into three groups allows having a variety of different skin types. These skin differences are particularly highlighted in the NIR region. Finally, the pixels previously identified as lesion are classified by a supervised classifier, providing the class results, i.e., benign, malignant, and atypical.

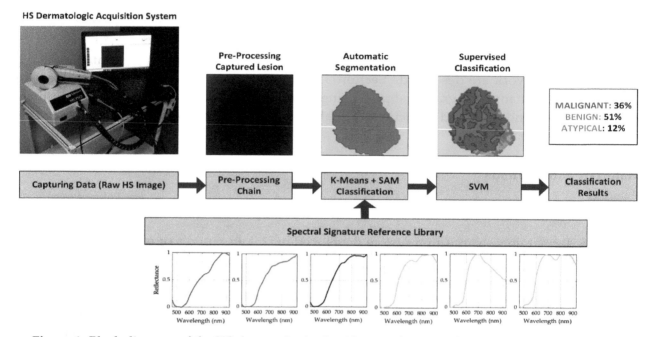

Figure 1. Block diagram of the HS dermatologic classification framework (pre-processing, automatic segmentation, and supervised classification) and HS dermatologic acquisition system. HS dermatologic acquisition system is composed by: HS snapshot camera; QTH (Quartz-Tungsten Halogen) source light; Fiber optic ring light guide; Skin contact part attached to the ring light; Laptop with the acquisition software installed. Spectral signature reference library is composed of six spectral signatures: benign, malignant, and atypical pigmented skin lesion spectral signatures in blue, red, and black colors respectively, and three different skin spectral signatures in green color.

2.2.1. Pre-Processing Chain

The HS data captured by the HS dermatologic acquisition system were pre-processed to homogenize the spectral signatures among the different patients. The pre-processing chain consists of four stages: calibration, extreme bands removal, noise filtering and normalization. The pseudo-code of the pre-processing chain is shown in Algorithm 1, where Y indicates a HS image with n pixels and b bands.

In Algorithm 1, lines from 3 to 7 perform the calibration stage. The raw HS image (Y) is calibrated employing a white reference image (W_{ref}), captured using a white reference tile able to reflect the 99% of the incident light, and a dark reference image (D_{ref}) obtained by having the light turned off and the camera shutter closed. Both images, W_{ref} and D_{ref} were obtained before the data acquisition using the same illumination conditions. The resulting calibrated image ($Y_{calibrated}$) is obtained following the equation shown in line 5.

After the calibration stage, the first 4 bands and the last 5 bands are removed due to the HS sensor low response. This extreme bands removal is performed in line 9 and the final spectral signature consists of 116 bands. Moreover, the HS data is filtered using a smooth filter to reduce the spectral noise in the remaining spectral bands. For each i-th iteration of the for loop in line 11, the smooth filter is applied to a pixel of the HS image with its respective 116 spectral bands. This filter is based on a moving average filter and requires that the first and last elements of the vector must not change. Line 12 contains the loop declaration where N is the value of the neighbors previously chosen. For this application, N is set to 5.

Finally, a normalization process between 0 and 1 is applied to each pixel with the goal of homogenizing its amplitude. Lines from 21 to 26 perform the normalization process where the resulting normalized image is obtained following equation shown in line 24.

Algorithm 1. Pre-processing chain.

Input: $Y \rightarrow$ Hyperspectral image with n pixels and b bands
$D_{ref} \rightarrow$ Dark reference
$W_{ref} \rightarrow$ White reference
$N \rightarrow$ number of neighbours

1.   Hyperspectral image Y acquisition
2.   *Stage 1.1: Image calibration*
3.   **for** $i = 0$ to $n\text{-}1$ **do:**
4.   **for** $j = 0$ to $b\text{-}1$ **do:**
5. $Y_{calibrated}(i, j) = \frac{Y(i,j) - D_{ref}}{W_{ref} - D_{ref}};$
6.   **end**
7.   **end**
8.   *Stage 1.2: Extreme bands removal*
9.   Remove the first 4 and last 5 noisy bands
10. *Stage 1.3: Smooth filtering*
11. **for** $i = 0$ to $n\text{-}1$ **do:**
12. **for** $j = 1$ to $b\text{-}N\text{-}1$ **do:**
13. $sum = 0;$
14. **for** $x = 0$ to $b\text{-}1$ **do:**
15. $sum + = Y_{calibrated}(i, j + x);$
16. **end**
17. $Y_{calibrated}(i, j) = sum/b;$
18. **end**
19. **end**
20. *Stage 1.4: Normalization*
21. **for** $i = 0$ to $n\text{-}1$ **do:**
22. Find the *max* and *min* values over the bands
23. **for** $j = 0$ to $b\text{-}1$ **do:**
24. $Y_{calibrated}(i, j) = \frac{Y_{calibrated}(i,j) - min}{max - min};$
25. **end**
26. **end**

Output: $Y_{calibrated}(i, j)$

2.2.2. Automatic PSL Segmentation

The pre-processed HS image is divided into normal skin and PSL using an automatic segmentation method based on K-means and SAM algorithms. The first step consists of performing the segmentation using the K-means algorithm to divide the HS images into k different clusters. The k value was previously selected after employing a clustering evaluation method [26]. The optimal k value for this application is three. After performing the segmentation into three clusters, a two-class segmentation map is generated to identify normal skin and PSL. This map is generated using the SAM algorithm, which compares the centroid from each cluster with a spectral signature reference library. The most similar spectral signature to each centroid is assigned to a certain class (PSL or normal skin). The library is obtained by computing the average of the labeled spectral signatures using the training set and the normal skin data were divided into three groups, allowing to have a variety of different skin types. Finally, the library contains six different spectral signatures: three from PSL (malignant, benign, and atypical lesions in Figure 1, represented in red, blue, and black colors, respectively) and three from normal skin (in green color in Figure 1).

The pseudo-code of the automatic segmentation is shown in Algorithm 2, where the number of clusters is determined by k, the threshold error by *threshold* and the maximum number of iterations by *MAX_ITER*. Line 2 performs the initialization of the *actual_centroids* variable to select the centroids used by the K-means algorithm. This variable is initialized with k different HS pixels randomly chosen from the input image Y. The *error* variable in line 3 is calculated as the average of the absolute values of the difference between centroids. This parameter is used as a constraint for the convergence of the algorithm. The main loop of the algorithm from line 6 to 13 computes the distances between a certain pixel and the centroids with an iterative procedure. The distance is computed using the Euclidean metric where each pixel of the HS image is assigned to a certain cluster when the minimum distance is reached. The use of *actual_centroids* and *previous_centroids* variables allows to analyze the variation from the previous iteration. This loop finishes when the error becomes lower than the established threshold or after a maximum number of iterations.

Algorithm 2. Automatic segmentation.

Input: *Y, k, threshold, MAX_ITER, HUGE_VAL*

1.   *Stage 2.1: K-means initialization*
2.   Randomly choose k pixels as *actual_centroids*
3.   *error = HUGE_VAL;*
4.   *iter = 0;*
5.   *Stage 2.2: K-means clustering*
6.   **while** *error < threshold* && *iter < MAX_ITER* **do**:
7.   Compute the distance between pixels and centroids
8.   Clusters update
9.   *previous_centroids = actual_centroids;*
10. Update *actual_centroids*
11. Compute error between *actual_centroids* and *previous_centroids*
12. *iter + +;*
13. **end**
14. **for** $i = 0$ to k-1 **do**:
15. **for** $j = 0$ to n_{ref}-1 **do**:
16. *dist(j)* = compute SAM between *actual_centroids(i)* and *ref(j)*
17. **end**
18. h = find the index of the minimum value of *dist*
19. Assign to the i-th cluster the same class as *ref(h)*
20. **end**

Output: PSL pixels

When the *while* loop finishes, the segmented output image is made of different clusters. To identify which cluster belongs to each class (normal skin or PSL), the spectral signature reference library is compared with each cluster using the SAM algorithm. Lines from 14 to 20 correspond to this procedure (similarity evaluation) where the six reference spectral signatures are compared with each cluster and assigned when the SAM result reached the minimum value.

2.2.3. Supervised Classification

The pixels identified as PSL by the automatic segmentation were classified using a supervised algorithm. the support vector machine (SVM) algorithm was selected to perform the classification because it has been commonly used for HS data classification in medical applications [8]. The goal of the SVM algorithm is to find the best hyperplane to separate different data and compute the probability to belong to each class of study [33]. Different kernel functions can be used to achieve the best result and each kernel function has different hyperparameters that can be tuned to obtain the optimal configuration.

In this study, the Sigmoid kernel was selected after comparing the performance results with the Linear and Radial Basis Function (RBF) kernels with the optimal hyperparameters (as it will be presented in Section 4.1). Algorithm 3 shows the pseudo-code of the supervised classification where *pix_no_skin* contains the lesion pixels obtained in the output of the previous algorithm.

Algorithm 3. Supervised classification.

Input: pix_no_skin, $n_{\mathrm{pix\_no\_skin}}$, $class$, n_{sv}, sv, $epsilon$

1.   *Stage 3.1: SVM data preparation*
2.   **for** i = 0 to $n_{pix\_no\_skin}$-1 **do**:
3.   *Stage 3.2: SVM distance computation*
4.   **for** j = 0 to n_{sv}-1 **do**:
5. $prod = sv(j) * pix\_no\_skin(i)$;
6. $dist(j) = \tan\mathrm{h}(slope * prod + intercept)$
7.   **end**
8.   *Stage 3.3: SVM binary classification*
9.   **for** j = 0 to *class*-2 **do**:
10. **for** z = j to *class*-1 **do**:
11. Solve binary classification problem between class j and class z
12. **end**
13. **end**
14. *Stage 3.4: SVM multiclass probability*
15. $Pc1 = \ldots = Pcclass = \frac{1}{class}$;
16. Computing the matrix Qp using the binary probabilities
17. **for** z = 0 to *class*-1 **do**:
18. **for** *iter* = 0 to 99 **do**:
19. **if** Pc_z – Pc_z_prev < epsilon **do**:
20. **break;**
21. **end**
22. Update multiclass probability of the i-th pixel to belong to class z
23. **end**
24. **end**
25. Compute class with maximum probability for the i-th pixel
26. **end**
27. Update similarity evaluation labels with SVM results

Output: Probabilities class.

The pseudo-code of the SVM classification algorithm is characterized by four main phases: data preparation, distance computation, binary classification, and multiclass probability. The probability is computed with an iterative procedure in the *for* loop from line 2 to 26, where the probability of the i-th pixel to belong to a certain class is obtained. To evaluate this probability, it is necessary to calculate the distance using the Sigmoid kernel. In line 5, the pixel is multiplied by a support vector and in line 6 the distance is computed using the parameters of the sigmoid kernel: *slope* and *intercept*. The next stage, from line 9 to 13, performs the binary classification on the basis of probability of a certain pixel to belong to the two classes under study. Finally, the multiclass probability is performed from line 15 to 24, using the probabilities obtained in the previous stage. Line 15 initializes the class probabilities and the matrix Qp is computed using the binary probabilities. In an iterative procedure, the pixel probability of belonging to a class is refined. This process ends when the value of the previous iteration is under a certain threshold, or if the number of iterations reaches 100. When one of these two conditions takes place, the multiclass probabilities of the pixel are computed.

The HS dermatologic classification framework features high computational complexity on serial systems, thus preventing real-time processing. Therefore, the exploration of parallel architectures is mandatory to provide an efficient instrument for the clinical practice.

3. Parallel Classification Pipelines

In order to reduce the processing time of the serial classification pipeline, different parallel strategies targeting multicore and many-core technologies have been explored. The first step has been the classification framework (pre-processing, K-means, and SVM) development in C language. This serial code represents a basis for the parallel versions that are successively developed integrating the OpenMP and the CUDA frameworks for the multicore and many-core philosophy, respectively. Several parallel classification pipelines have been developed, where, for each algorithm, an OpenMP or CUDA version is included to determine the best solution to be considered in the final classification system.

3.1. Parallel Pre-Processing Versions

As already discussed, the pre-processing chain consists of four steps: calibration, extreme bands removal, filtering, and normalization. Two parallel versions of this algorithm (multicore and many-core) have been developed and, in both cases, a pixel-wise parallelization is carried out. A serial code profiling has shown that the most time-consuming phases are filtering and normalization. Therefore, only these two steps are parallelized. Each thread performs the filtering and normalization of a single HS pixel. These two steps are included in a *for* loop that iterates over the number of pixels. The iterations are elaborated simultaneously since the *pragma omp parallel for* directive has been introduced before the loop. Moreover, the loop variable is declared as private, while the HS image is shared among all the threads.

The same parallelization strategy has been adopted in the CUDA version development. After the image calibration and the bands removal, data are allocated and transferred to the device global memory. Among the transferred data, there are the reduced image and an array storing groups of five contiguous bands for each pixel. This array is used in the smooth filtering step to avoid data overwrite during the moving average computation. The filtering is performed by a kernel through a grid containing a number of threads equal to the number of pixels. The grid includes blocks of 32 threads. This number has been chosen according to the warp definition given by NVIDIA. If the number of pixels is not an integer multiple of 32, the last block will contain some threads that are not related to a pixel. In this case, these threads do not perform any computation. It is worth noticing that these inactive threads do not slow down the computation because their number is negligible compared to the total number of pixels. Another kernel, with the same grid and block parameters, computes the maximum and minimum values of each pixel across the bands. These values are then used in the normalization step, performed by a further kernel. The normalized image overwrites the original one, which is initially transferred to the device global memory. The result of the pre-processing is transferred back to the host memory only if the K-means is performed using a serial or an OpenMP processing. Otherwise, the normalized image is left in the device memory to be used by the CUDA version of the K-means. The flowchart of the CUDA pre-processing is shown in Figure 2.

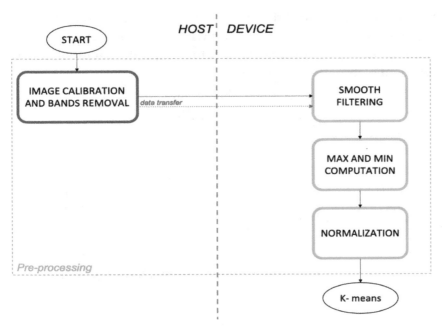

Figure 2. Flowchart of the pre-processing CUDA version.

3.2. Parallel K-Means Versions

The most time-consuming part of this algorithm is the distance computation between each pixel and each centroid. It should be emphasized that this computation must be performed a number of times equal to the number of pixels by the number of clusters. Since the other operations have a negligible computational cost when performed on a serial processor, only the distance computation has been pixel-wise parallelized using OpenMP. Also, in this case, the *pragma omp parallel for* has been introduced before the *for* loop iterating over the pixels. Again, the loop variables are declared private and the HS image is shared. Moreover, also the centroids are shared among the pixels.

In the parallel CUDA version, a different strategy has been adopted. In this case, all the steps have been performed on the device to minimize data transfers between host and device memories. The flowchart of this parallel version is shown in Figure 3. The flow starts on the host, where the indexes for the centroid's initialization are generated. These indexes are used to identify which pixels are selected to define the initial centroids. Then, these values are transferred to the device. It must be noticed that if the pre-processing has been performed on the device, the image is already stored in the GPU global memory. Otherwise, it is also transferred from the host.

The first task performed by the GPU is the centroid initialization, which consists of copying the values of the selected pixels into the centroids. This step is elaborated by a kernel, whose threads number is equal to the cluster number. The error computation is split between device and host. At first, a kernel computes the difference between the actual and the previous centroids (initialized to zero). Then, the *cublasSasum* function is used to sum the absolute values of these differences. This function directly transfers the output on the host, where the division by the number of clusters is performed using a serial thread. At this point, the iterative K-means process starts on the host. The next steps are repeated until the error converges to a fixed threshold or the maximum number of iterations is reached. In this iterative part, the first step concerns the distance computation performed on the device by a kernel, whose number of threads is equal to the number of pixels. In particular, each thread simultaneously computes the distance between the pixels and the centroids. Then, the clusters and the centroids are updated with two different kernels. The former provides a pixel-wise parallelization since each thread finds the nearest centroids for the assigned pixel. The latter includes a number of threads equal to the number of clusters to perform the update. At this point, the error is evaluated as already explained. Once the condition of the *while* loop is false, the flow continues with the similarity evaluation step, which assigns a biological meaning to each cluster (PSL or normal skin). In this phase, the difference among the centroids and the six reference spectral signatures are computed. All the elements belonging to the same cluster are labelled with the class of the reference spectral signature with the minimum distance. It is worth noticing that this computation involves a restricted number of data, allowing its efficient elaboration on the host.

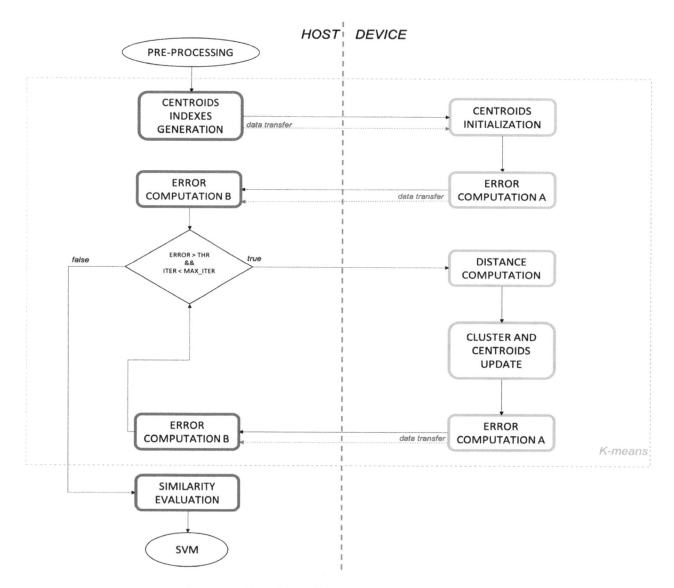

Figure 3. Flowchart of the K-means CUDA version.

3.3. Parallel Support Vector Machine Versions

As introduced before, the SVM algorithm is composed of three main steps: distance and non-linear function evaluation, binary classification, and multiclass probabilities computation. The first phase is the most time-consuming part, and for this reason, an OpenMP parallelization of this routine has been developed. It must be considered that only a subset of the original HS image is sent to the SVM algorithm as input. The SVM training has generated a model with 9242 support vectors, which is higher than the number of pixels of each image. For this reason, the *for* loop that iterates over the support vectors to improve the performance has been parallelized. In particular, each thread performs the dot product between the assigned support vector and the pixel. Then, it applies the hyperbolic tangent to the product result, after considering the slope and intercept values. In this case, the shared variables are the pixels to be classified and the support vectors. The private variables are the *for* loops indexes.

When considering the CUDA parallelization, three different versions have been developed to find the most efficient one. The first and second CUDA versions flowchart is shown in Figure 4.

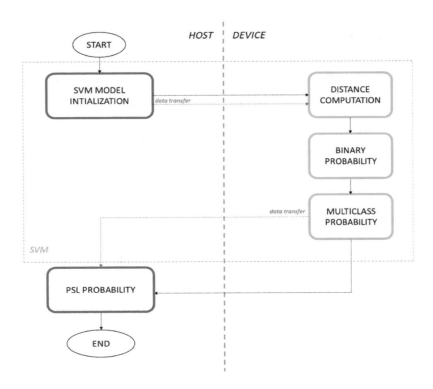

Figure 4. Flowchart of the first and second CUDA SVM versions.

The flow starts on the host, where the SVM model parameters and the pixels to be classified are transferred to the device memory. Here, a kernel called *distance computation* is performed, where the dot product between support vectors and pixels is computed. Moreover, the hyperbolic tangent is evaluated. In this kernel, the number of threads is equal to the number of the support vectors for the same reason explained in the OpenMP version. Again, each block contains 32 threads. The binary probability is computed in another kernel, whose grid dimension represents the difference between the first and second SVM CUDA versions. In the first case, the number of threads is equal to the number of support vectors, while in the second case, the kernel is processed by a single thread. The main reason for this choice is that the binary probability computation is a very efficient task to be processed in serial. The idea is to reproduce a serial processing on the device (avoiding a further memory transfer) even if the GPU working frequency is lower than the CPU one.

The last kernel computes the multiclass probabilities. In this case, the number of threads is equal to the number of classes: each thread evaluates the probability of a pixel to belong to that class. Then, the *cublasIsamax* function determines the class with the highest probability for each pixel. This function also transfers the output (i.e., the pixel labels) to the host, where the percentage of pixels classified to each PSL class is shown (*PSL probability*).

Concerning the third CUDA version, it is again based on the consideration that the binary classification performs very efficiently on serial processors. Therefore, this computation has been moved to the host side to evaluate if it is better to transfer back data, performing the elaboration on the host, or if a serial kernel is the best solution. The flowchart of this version is shown in Figure 5, where it is possible to see that, after the distance computation, there are data transfer to the host to allow the binary computation on the CPU. In particular, for each pixel, an array with a number of elements equal to the number of support vector is transferred to the host. The binary probability computation result is then transferred back to the device. This result has a dimension equal to the number of pixels by the number of binary classification problems. The kernels related to the distance computation and the evaluation of multiclass probabilities are not changed compared to the previous CUDA versions. Moreover, in this case, the SVM result will be the output of the system, indicating the user the percentage of pixels classified to each class.

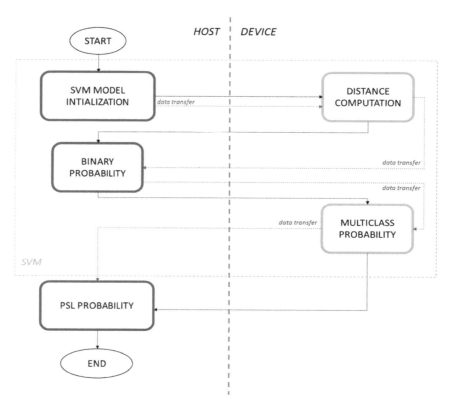

Figure 5. Flowchart of the third CUDA SVM version.

3.4. Complete Classification System

After the single algorithm parallelization, several complete system versions have been developed, integrating the serial, multicore and many-core codes. Table 1 presents fifteen versions developed in this work. In this integration, the basic idea is to find the best configuration in terms of processing time. Analyzing the single algorithms profiling, it can be concluded that all the pre-processing versions provide equivalent performance. For this reason, all the versions for the final configuration have been evaluated. In particular, even if the CUDA performance is similar to the serial one, it was decided to quantify if an initial data transfer can give benefits to the subsequent steps of the processing chain. In fact, concerning the K-means clustering, only the CUDA version has been included in the different complete systems, since it largely outperforms the serial and OpenMP processing. Thus, the speedup of the multicore and many-core K-means versions, compared to the serial processing, are about 1.5× and 6×, respectively. It is worth noticing that the similarity evaluation is always performed on the host. This is because it is part of the final output that is always managed by a CPU. Finally, all the SVM versions are considered in the integration for the final system. It has been also developed a configuration (not included in Table 1) that considers all the serial versions and that is used as a reference to compute the final speedup.

Considering the first ten versions (Figure 6a), the pre-processing is managed by the CPU since in the V1-V5 and in the V6-V10 versions, the serial (yellow box in Figure 6a) and OpenMP (orange box in Figure 6a) codes are included, respectively. In all these cases, the pre-processed image is transferred to the device before the K-means execution. On the other hand, in V11-V15 (Figure 6b), after the calibration and bands removal (*pre-processing A* in Figure 6b), the image is transferred to the GPU for the next pre-processing steps (*pre-processing B* in Figure 6b). As already mentioned, the K-means is performed on the device and its output is transferred to the host to elaborate the similarity evaluation. On the base of the considered SVM version, its parameters are transferred on the GPU (violet boxes in Figure 6a,b) or kept on the host memory for a serial or OpenMP elaboration (yellow and orange boxes in Figure 6a,b). At the end, if the SVM is performed on the GPU, the final result is transferred to the host to generate the final segmentation map.

Table 1. Different versions of the classification framework, integrating the serial (S), OpenMP (O), and CUDA (C) codes of the single algorithms. C1, C2, and C3 refer to the three SVM CUDA versions.

	Pre-Processing			K-Means		SVM			
	S	O	C	C	S	O	C1	C2	C3
V1	×			×	×				
V2	×			×		×			
V3	×			×			×		
V4	×			×				×	
V5	×			×					×
V6		×		×	×				
V7		×		×		×			
V8		×		×			×		
V9		×		×				×	
V10		×		×					×
V11			×	×	×				
V12			×	×		×			
V13			×	×			×		
V14			×	×				×	
V15			×	×					×

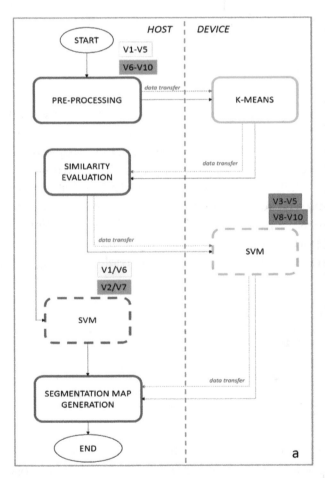 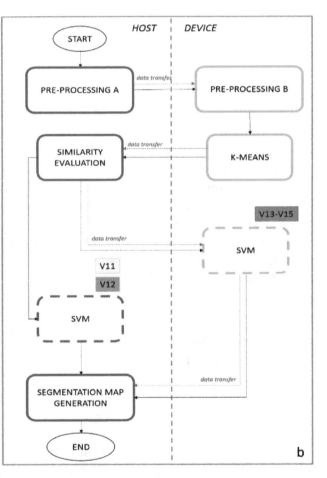

Figure 6. (a) Flowchart of the first ten versions (V1–V10). (b) Flowchart of the last five versions (V11–V15). The dashed boxes indicate that there is the possibility to perform the algorithm on the host or on the device. The yellow boxes refer to the serial processing, the orange boxes refer to the OpenMP processing, and the violet boxes refer to the CUDA processing. The notation "*Vi-Vj*" indicates all the versions from *Vi* to *Vj*.

4. Experimental Results and Discussion

4.1. Skin Cancer Classification Performance

In order to find the optimal configuration of the SVM, the hyperparameters for each type of kernel were adjusted using a genetic algorithm (GA) [26]. The methodology proposed was a patient stratified assignment where the labeled data was divided into three independent sets: test, validation, and training. A custom figure of merit (*FoM*) was conceived to evaluate the GA performance. This *FoM* is based on the accuracy per class (*ACC*) results to find the most balanced accuracy results for each class, where i and j are the indices of the classes that are being computed and n is the number of classes, as it can be seen in Equation (1). Finally, to evaluate the results obtained for the optimized classifier, the false negative rate per class (*FNRc*) was computed. *FNRc* reveals the misclassifications produced by the classifier and discovers which classes were misclassified. Equation (2) shows the mathematical expression of the *FNRc*, where FN_i is the number of false negatives in the *i-th* class and P is the total number of positive samples.

$$FoM = \frac{1}{2} \cdot \left(\sum_{\substack{i,j \\ i < j}}^{n} \frac{ACC_i + ACC_j}{|ACC_i - ACC_j| + 1} \right) \cdot \binom{n}{2}^{-1} \tag{1}$$

$$FNRc = \frac{FN_i}{P} \tag{2}$$

Table 2 shows the *FoM* results and the values of the optimized hyperparameters obtained with the GA algorithm for each kernel classifier. The obtained results show the SVM Sigmoid algorithm achieved the best *FoM* (60.67%), followed by the SVM Linear and the RBF (38.82% and 29.98%, respectively). Additionally, random forest (RF) [34] and artificial neural network (ANN) [35] classifiers were tested, achieving very low *FoM* performance, 27.25% and 33.55%, respectively. The MATLAB® Machine Learning and Deep Learning ToolBox™ were employed to implement the RF and ANN classifiers using as hyperparameters $nTress = 2431$ and $neurons_{per\ layer} = [1; 255; 3; 184]$. In both classifiers the hyperparameters used were the optimal ones after performing an automatic optimization procedure using a Genetic Algorithm. Considering these results, the SVM with Sigmoid kernel was selected for the HS dermatologic classification framework.

Table 2. Validation Classification Results.

Classifier	Hyperparameters	*FoM* (%)
SVM Linear	$C = -21.56$	38.82
SVM RBF	$C = 9.85; \gamma = 4.83$	29.98
SVM Sigmoid	$C = 1.54; s = -20.79; cf = -1.97$	60.67

C: Cost; γ: Gamma; cf: Intercept Constant; s: Slope.

Figure 7a illustrates the *FNRc* results for each validation HS image, where it is possible to observe that images *P15_C1*, *P15_C2*, *P20_C2* and *P113_C1* present an accurate identification of the diagnosed PSL, while images *P96_C1* and *P99_C1* have some pixels that were misclassified but clearly reveal the correct diagnosis. On the contrary, images *P60_C1*, *P60_C2* and *P68_C1* misclassified more than 50% of the labeled pixels. Image *P68_C1* classified 58.2% and 9.9% of the pixels as benign and atypical classes, respectively, being a malignant PSL. In summary, six out of nine images of the validation set were correctly diagnosed with the proposed classification framework based on the optimized SVM Sigmoid classifier. Figure 8a shows the qualitative classification maps obtained for the validation set where green color indicates the skin pixels, while red, orange, and blue colors represent the pixels classified as malignant, atypical, and benign PSLs, respectively. These results also include the detailed percentage of pixels classified as each PSL in each HS cube.

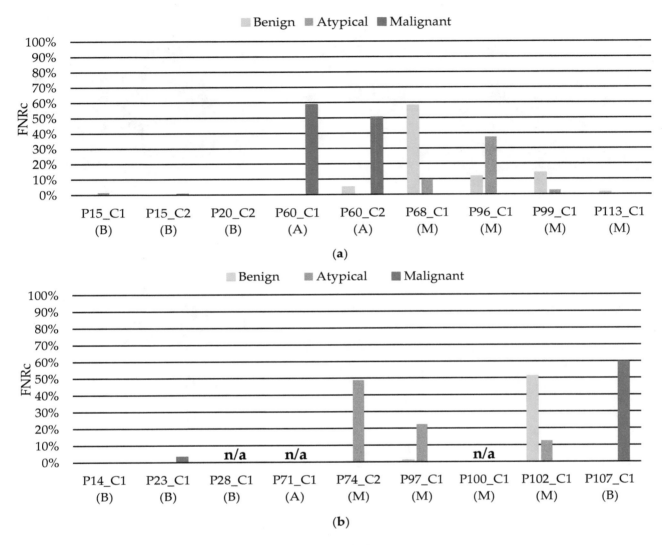

Figure 7. Classification FNRc results per each HS image obtained with the SVM Sigmoid classifier. (a) Validation classification results. (b) Test classification results. Below each patient ID, the correct diagnosis of the PSL is presented. B: Benign; A: Atypical; M: Malignant.

In order to assess the results obtained with the SVM Sigmoid classifier optimized with the validation set, the classifier was evaluated on the test set. Figure 7b shows the *FNRc* results of each HS test image. On the one hand, in the images *P28_C1, P71_C1,* and *P100_C1*, no pixels were identified as PSL by the segmentation stage and the classification stage could not provide the results. The lack of identification of PSL pixels in such cases occurs because the PSL spectral signatures of these HS images were highly similar to the normal skin references employed in the K-means segmentation [26]. This can be appreciated in the gray scale images of the PSLs presented in Figure 8b, where the PSL pixels of such images are quite similar to the skin pixels. These results could indicate the necessity of increasing the HS skin database for including high inter-patient variability of data. On the other hand, the PSL images *P14_C1, P23_C1,* and *P97_C1* were correctly identified, having in the latter one only 22.3% of pixels misclassified as atypical class. In the case of image *P74_C1*, 48.7% of the pixels were misclassified as atypical class, but the remaining 51.3% were correctly identified as malignant PSL. In the remaining images (*P102_C1,* and *P107_C1)* the misclassifications values were above 50%. *P102_C1* misclassified 51% and 12.5% of pixels as benign and atypical classes, respectively, being a malignant PSL. Finally, in *P107_C1*, 59.6% of pixels were classified as malignant class, being a benign PSL. Figure 8b shows the classification maps of the test set.

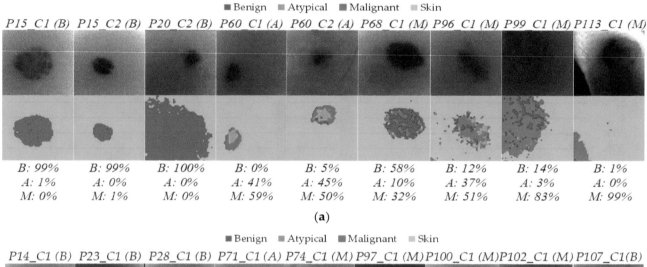

(a)

(b)

Figure 8. Qualitative classification results of each HS image. (**a**) Validation set. (**b**) Test set. On the right side of each patient ID, the correct diagnosis of the PSL is presented between brackets (B: Benign; A: Atypical; M: Malignant). The first row shows the grayscale image, while the second row shows the classification map, where skin, malignant, benign, and atypical pixels are represented in green, red, blue, and orange colors, respectively. Below the classification map, the percentages of PSL pixels classified to each class are detailed.

Figure 9 shows the processing time of the complete HS dermatologic classification framework using the test set implemented in MATLAB®. These data were obtained using an Intel i7-4790K with a working frequency of 4.00 GHz and a RAM of 8 GB.

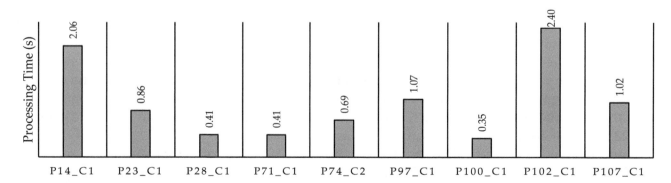

Figure 9. Processing time (in seconds) of the MATLAB execution for each HS image.

4.2. Real-Time Elaboration

The acquisition system, shown in Figure 1, takes ~1 s to capture an image with 50×50 pixels and 125 bands. As can be seen from the results in Section 4.1, the MATLAB implementation cannot always guarantee real-time processing. For this reason, parallel computing has been exploited to provide a real-time compliant solution. As a first step, the C serial code development provides a basis for the parallel implementation and ensures the same classification results as MATLAB. Intending to find the most efficient solution, several parallel versions presented in Section 3 have been developed, exploiting OpenMP API and CUDA framework. Moreover, different hardware devices to identify the system that best meets the processing constraints have been evaluated. Specifically, two systems have been considered: the first is a desktop PC (Test System 1-TS1) equipped with an Intel i9-9900X CPU, working at 3.5 GHz and with 128 GB of RAM. The system is also equipped with a NVIDIA RTX 2080 GPU (Turing architecture), with 2944 cores, working at 1.71 GHz and with 8 GB of RAM. The second system (Test System 2-TS2) is equipped with an Intel i7-3770 CPU, working at 3.4 GHz, with 8 GB of RAM and connected to a NVIDIA Tesla K40 GPU (Kepler architecture). This device has 2880 cores, 12 GB of RAM and its working frequency is 875 MHz.

All the code versions have been developed using Microsoft Visual Studio 2019, under Microsoft Windows 10. For all the versions, suitable compiler options have been set to generate an executable code optimized for processing speed. Moreover, the versions elaborated by a GPU also include the compute capability option (3.5 and 7.5 for Kepler and Turing architectures, respectively).

The processing times have been measured as the mean of five different executions. It is worth noticing that for the GPU versions also the data transfer time has been considered. Figure 10 shows the processing times for the described test systems using each HS image of the test set. As can be seen from these processing times, not all the versions are real-time compliant. An exhaustive discussion of the obtained results is given in the next section.

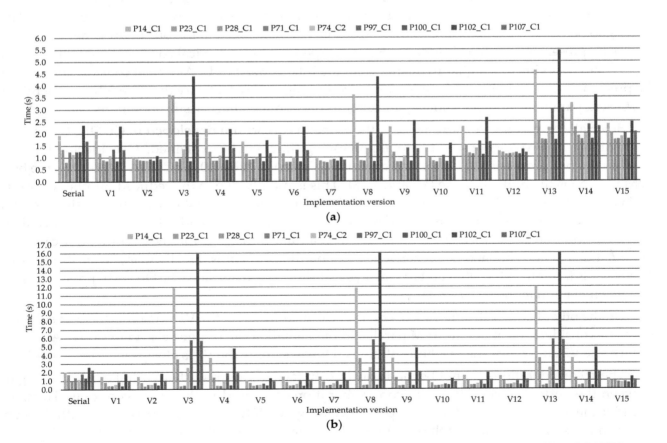

Figure 10. Processing times (in seconds) of the serial and parallel versions using the (a) TS1 and (b) TS2.

4.3. Comparison and Discussion

In the previous paragraphs, the processing chain that has been validated in MATLAB has been described. In many cases, this version is not real-time compliant, even if it exploits automatic code parallelization. In fact, some elaborations take more than one or two seconds to classify the image (Figure 9). In Figure 10, it is possible to observe that even writing the serial code in C language is not enough to achieve a real-time processing even if, in this version, memory management and mathematical operations have been optimized by hand. This version has only been developed as a basis for the parallel implementations.

Concerning the parallel processing times, the first consideration that can be made is that the results vary not only among the different versions, but also considering different images within the same implementation. In fact, since all the images have the same dimensions, this variability depends on two main factors: the former is that the number of the K-means iterations depends on the random initialization; the latter is the number of pixels to be classified by the SVM stage. Particularly, this last factor greatly changes among the images. As an example, considering the processing times of the images P28_C1, P71_C1, and P100_C1, they do not contain pixels labelled as PSL from the K-means stage and, therefore, no pixels are classified by the SVM. The elaboration of these images is real-time compliant considering both the test systems, except in the cases where the pre-processing is performed on the RTX 2080 GPU (V11-V15 on TS1). This is due to the low performance of the pre-processing on this specific GPU.

Concerning the pre-processing step of all the images, the OpenMP elaboration always outperforms the CUDA one on TS1. The same trend can be observed in most of the cases on TS2, where the multicore elaborations slightly outperform the CUDA ones. In the other cases, times are comparable. Analyzing these results in both the test systems, it can be verified that the OpenMP pre-processing version is the most efficient one (especially V7 and V10 in TS1 and TS2, respectively). It is possible to conclude that an efficient parallelization of the filtering and normalization steps adopting a multicore approach is preferable than transferring the image to perform the pre-processing on the device. The larger gap between the OpenMP-CUDA versions in TS1, compared to the one of the other system, is due to the presence of an Intel i9-9900X CPU, equipped with ten physical cores equivalent to twenty logical ones, working at a higher frequency than the Intel i7-3770 CPU. As a final consideration about the pre-processing, this phase features a lower computational complexity than the others. Therefore, its efficient parallelization does not significantly impact on the final classification time.

Since all the parallel versions include the K-means algorithm developed in CUDA, the impact of the different SVM versions on the total processing time will be explained. Considering the TS1, whether the pre-processing is elaborated exploiting OpenMP (V6-V10) or CUDA (V11-V15), the best SVM version is the multicore one (V7 and V12). This is mainly due to the reduced number of pixels to classify with the SVM (i.e., about 45% of the 2500 pixels in the worst case). The classification on the Intel i9 CPU, with twenty cores working at a high frequency, provides better performance than the elaboration on the device, which requires also a data transfer. Moreover, in this last case, the computational load is not enough to efficiently exploit the GPU cores. Finally, comparing V7 and V12, the former is faster than the latter and it is always real-time compliant since the OpenMP pre-processing is more efficient than the CUDA one.

On the other hand, if the pre-processing is performed in serial, the V2 version is the best solution. The same consideration about the SVM parallel implementation can be done also in this case. As a final remark, the V2 and V7 are the two best solutions. However, only the V7 is always real-time compliant.

These considerations cannot be made on TS2. In fact, in this case, there is not a significant gap between the performance of the multicore elaboration compared to the many-core one. Thus, let consider the versions with an OpenMP pre-processing (V6-V10): the implementation with the best performance is the one including the CUDA SVM with the binary probability computation on the host side (V10). Despite this, the elaboration times are not significantly lower than the V7 version, containing the OpenMP SVM. Moreover, if the V11-V15 versions are considered (CUDA pre-processing), the elaboration time of V12 (OpenMP SVM) and V15 (CUDA SVM, version 3) are comparable.

It is worth noticing that, considering both the test systems, the first and second SVM CUDA versions show the worst performance (V3-V4, V8-V9, V13-V14). Considering the SVM CUDA versions, the binary probability computation is the task that mostly impacts on the performance. As said in Section 3, the binary probability computation is a very efficient task to be processed in serial. Thus, the results demonstrate that it is convenient to perform this step on the host even if the number of data transfer is increased.

Comparing the performance of the two test systems and considering the images where the SVM is not performed (P28_C1, P71_C1, P100_C1), it should be emphasized that TS2 is always faster than TS1. The Tesla K40 GPU features a lower processing time on the K-means clustering than the RTX 2080 one. The former board does not manage the graphical context of the operating system and can use all the resources to perform the computation. The latter is a standard GPU that shares resources among the graphical context management and the computation.

Summarizing, the best solutions for this application are the V7 and V10 versions for the TS1 and TS2, respectively. Even if the V7 version (TS1) shows slightly lower performances than V10 (TS2), it is the only version that always meets the real-time constraint. This parallel framework can be included in the existing prototype for its use in the routine patient examination.

5. Conclusions

In this paper, a parallel classification framework based on HSI has been presented. This framework exploited the K-means and the SVM algorithms to perform an automatic in-situ PSL identification. The framework has been validated using an in-vivo dataset and the parameters of the algorithms have been tuned in MATLAB for a later implementation of the processing framework on high-performance computing platforms (multicore CPUs and GPUs).

To ensure a real-time classification, several parallel versions, exploiting multicore and many-core technologies have been developed. Firstly, OpenMP and CUDA parallel versions of the single algorithms have been developed, which were successively integrated to provide the full parallel classification pipeline. Tests have been conducted on two different systems, equipped with an Intel i9-9900X with an NVIDIA RTX 2080 GPU (TS1) and an Intel i7-3770 with an NVIDIA Tesla K40 GPU (TS2), respectively. The best solution performed the pre-processing and the SVM stages in OpenMP, while the K-means was executed in CUDA. This version, on the TS1, is always real-time compliant since it processed 50×50 pixels with 125 bands images in less than 1 s.

This preliminary study demonstrates the potential use of HSI technology to assist dermatologists in the discrimination of different types of PSLs. However, additional research must be carried out to validate and improve the results obtained before being used during clinical routine practice using a real-time and non-invasive handheld device. Particularly, a multicenter clinical trial whereby more patients and samples are included in the database will be necessary to further validate the proposed approach.

Author Contributions: Conceptualization, E.T., H.F., and M.L.S.; methodology, E.T., R.L., and G.F.; software, E.T., B.M.-V., R.L., M.L.S., and G.F.; validation, R.L., H.F., and S.O.; formal analysis, E.T. and M.L.S.; investigation, B.M.-V. and R.L.; data curation, B.M.-V. and R.L.; writing—original draft preparation, E.T., R.L., and G.F.; writing—review and editing, M.L.S., B.M.-V., H.F., S.O., G.M.C., and F.L.; supervision, G.M.C. and F.L.; project administration, G.M.C. and F.L.; funding acquisition, G.M.C. All authors have read and agreed to the published version of the manuscript.

References

1.   Kamruzzaman, M.; Sun, D.-W. Introduction to Hyperspectral Imaging Technology. In *Computer Vision Technology for Food Quality Evaluation*; Elsevier: Amsterdam, The Netherlands, 2016; pp. 111–139. ISBN 9780128022320.

2.   Torti, E.; Fontanella, A.; Plaza, A.; Plaza, J.; Leporati, F. Hyperspectral Image Classification Using Parallel Autoencoding Diabolo Networks on Multi-Core and Many-Core Architectures. *Electronics* **2018**, 411. [CrossRef]

3.   Shimoni, M.; Haelterman, R.; Perneel, C. Hypersectral imaging for military and security applications: Combining Myriad processing and sensing techniques. *IEEE Geosci. Remote Sens. Mag.* **2019**, *7*, 101–117. [CrossRef]

4.   Teke, M.; Deveci, H.S.; Haliloglu, O.; Gurbuz, S.Z.; Sakarya, U. A short survey of hyperspectral remote sensing applications in agriculture. In Proceedings of the 2013 6th International Conference on Recent Advances in Space Technologies (RAST), Instambul, Turkey, 12–14 June 2013; pp. 171–176.

5.   Legnaioli, S.; Lorenzetti, G.; Cavalcanti, G.H.; Grifoni, E.; Marras, L.; Tonazzini, A.; Salerno, E.; Pallecchi, P.; Giachi, G.; Palleschi, V. Recovery of archaeological wall paintings using novel multispectral imaging approaches. *Herit. Sci.* **2013**, *1*. [CrossRef]

6.   Lorente, D.; Aleixos, N.; Gomez-Sanchis, J.; Cubero, S.; Garcia-Navarrete, O.L.; Blasco, J.; Gómez-Sanchis, J.; Cubero, S.; Garc\'\ia-Navarrete, O.L.; Blasco, J. Recent Advances and Applications of Hyperspectral Imaging for Fruit and Vegetable Quality Assessment. *Food Bioprocess. Technol.* **2011**, *5*, 1121–1142. [CrossRef]

7.   Khan, M.J.; Khan, H.S.; Yousaf, A.; Khurshid, K.; Abbas, A. Modern Trends in Hyperspectral Image Analysis: A Review. *IEEE Access* **2018**, *6*, 14118–14129. [CrossRef]

8.   Lu, G.; Fei, B. Medical hyperspectral imaging: A review. *J. Biomed. Opt.* **2014**, *19*, 10901. [CrossRef]

9.   Ortega, S.; Halicek, M.; Fabelo, H.; Callico, G.M.; Fei, B. Hyperspectral and multispectral imaging in digital and computational pathology: A systematic review [Invited]. *Biomed. Opt. Express* **2020**, *11*, 3195. [CrossRef]

10. Halicek, M.; Fabelo, H.; Ortega, S.; Callico, G.M.; Fei, B. In-Vivo and Ex-Vivo Tissue Analysis through Hyperspectral Imaging Techniques: Revealing the Invisible Features of Cancer. *Cancers* **2019**, *11*, 756. [CrossRef] [PubMed]

11. Ortega, S.; Fabelo, H.; Iakovidis, D.; Koulaouzidis, A.; Callico, G.; Ortega, S.; Fabelo, H.; Iakovidis, D.K.; Koulaouzidis, A.; Callico, G.M. Use of Hyperspectral/Multispectral Imaging in Gastroenterology. Shedding Some–Different–Light into the Dark. *J. Clin. Med.* **2019**, *8*, 36. [CrossRef]

12. Panasyuk, S.V.; Yang, S.; Faller, D.V.; Ngo, D.; Lew, R.A.; Freeman, J.E.; Rogers, A.E. Medical hyperspectral imaging to facilitate residual tumor identification during surgery. *Cancer Biol. Ther.* **2007**, *6*, 439–446. [CrossRef] [PubMed]

13. Akbari, H.; Uto, K.; Kosugi, Y.; Kojima, K.; Tanaka, N. Cancer detection using infrared hyperspectral imaging. *Cancer Sci.* **2011**, *102*, 852–857. [CrossRef] [PubMed]

14. Akbari, H.; Halig, L.V.; Schuster, D.M.; Osunkoya, A.; Master, V.; Nieh, P.T.; Chen, G.Z.; Fei, B. Hyperspectral imaging and quantitative analysis for prostate cancer detection. *J. Biomed. Opt.* **2012**, *17*, 0760051. [CrossRef] [PubMed]

15. Liu, Z.; Wang, H.; Li, Q. Tongue tumor detection in medical hyperspectral images. *Sensors* **2011**, *12*, 162–174. [CrossRef] [PubMed]

16. Halicek, M.; Fabelo, H.; Ortega, S.; Little, J.V.; Wang, X.; Chen, A.Y.; Callico, G.M.; Myers, L.; Sumer, B.D.; Fei, B. Hyperspectral imaging for head and neck cancer detection: Specular glare and variance of the tumor margin in surgical specimens. *J. Med. Imaging* **2019**, *6*, 1. [CrossRef]

17. Florimbi, G.; Fabelo, H.; Torti, E.; Ortega, S.; Marrero-Martin, M.; Callico, G.M.; Danese, G.; Leporati, F. Towards Real-Time Computing of Intraoperative Hyperspectral Imaging for Brain Cancer Detection Using Multi-GPU Platforms. *IEEE Access* **2020**, *8*, 8485–8501. [CrossRef]

18. Lazcano, R.; Madronal, D.; Florimbi, G.; Sancho, J.; Sanchez, S.; Leon, R.; Fabelo, H.; Ortega, S.; Torti, E.; Salvador, R.; et al. Parallel Implementations Assessment of a Spatial-Spectral Classifier for Hyperspectral Clinical Applications. *IEEE Access* **2019**, *7*, 152316–152333. [CrossRef]

19. Torti, E.; Florimbi, G.; Castelli, F.; Ortega, S.; Fabelo, H.; Callicó, G.M.; Marrero-Martin, M.; Leporati, F.; Torti, E.; Florimbi, G.; et al. Parallel K-Means Clustering for Brain Cancer Detection Using Hyperspectral Images. *Electronics* **2018**, *7*, 283. [CrossRef]

20. Wu, Z.; Shi, L.; Li, J.; Wang, Q.; Sun, L.; Wei, Z.; Plaza, J.; Plaza, A. GPU Parallel Implementation of Spatially Adaptive Hyperspectral Image Classification. *IEEE J. Sel. Top. Appl. Earth Obs. Remote Sens.* **2018**, *11*, 1131–1143. [CrossRef]

21. Bray, F.; Ferlay, J.; Soerjomataram, I.; Siegel, R.L.; Torre, L.A.; Jemal, A. Global cancer statistics 2018: GLOBOCAN estimates of incidence and mortality worldwide for 36 cancers in 185 countries. *CA. Cancer J. Clin.* **2018**, *68*, 394–424. [CrossRef]

22. LeBoit, P.E.; Burg, G.; Weedon, D.; Sarasin, A. *Pathology and Genetics of Skin Tumours*; IARC: Lion, France, 2006; Volume 6.

23. Perkins, A.; Duffy, R.L. Atypical Moles: Diagnosis and Management. *Am. Fam. Phys.* **2015**, *91*, 762–767.

24. Johansen, T.H.; Møllersen, K.; Ortega, S.; Fabelo, H.; Garcia, A.; Callico, G.M.; Godtliebsen, F. Recent advances in hyperspectral imaging for melanoma detection. *Wiley Interdiscip. Rev. Comput. Stat.* **2019**, e1465. [CrossRef]

25. Fabelo, H.; Carretero, G.; Almeida, P.; Garcia, A.; Hernandez, J.A.; Godtliebsen, F.; Melian, V.; Martinez, B.; Beltran, P.; Ortega, S.; et al. Dermatologic Hyperspectral Imaging System for Skin Cancer Diagnosis Assistance. In Proceedings of the 2019 XXXIV Conference on Design of Circuits and Integrated Systems (DCIS), Bilbao, Spain, 20–22 November 2019; pp. 1–6.

26. Leon, R.; Martinez-Vega, B.; Fabelo, H.; Ortega, S.; Melian, V.; Castaño, I.; Carretero, G.; Almeida, P.; Garcia, A.; Quevedo, E.; et al. Non-Invasive Skin Cancer Diagnosis Using Hyperspectral Imaging for In-Situ Clinical Support. *J. Clin. Med.* **2020**, *9*, 1662. [CrossRef] [PubMed]

27. Moncrieff, M.; Cotton, S.; Claridge, E.; Hall, P. Spectrophotometric intracutaneous analysis: A new technique for imaging pigmented skin lesions. *Br. J. Dermatol.* **2002**, *146*, 448–457. [CrossRef] [PubMed]

28. Monheit, G.; Cognetta, A.B.; Ferris, L.; Rabinovitz, H.; Gross, K.; Martini, M.; Grichnik, J.M.; Mihm, M.; Prieto, V.G.; Googe, P.; et al. The performance of MelaFind: A prospective multicenter study. *Arch. Dermatol.* **2011**, *147*, 188–194. [CrossRef] [PubMed]

29. Fabelo, H.; Ortega, S.; Szolna, A.; Bulters, D.; Pineiro, J.F.; Kabwama, S.; J-O'Shanahan, A.; Bulstrode, H.; Bisshopp, S.; Kiran, B.R.; et al. In-Vivo Hyperspectral Human Brain Image Database for Brain Cancer Detection. *IEEE Access* **2019**, *7*, 39098–39116. [CrossRef]

30. Rousseeuw, P.J. Silhouettes: A graphical aid to the interpretation and validation of cluster analysis. *J. Comput. Appl. Math.* **1987**, *20*, 53–65. [CrossRef]

31. Caliñski, T.; Harabasz, J. A Dendrite Method Foe Cluster Analysis. *Commun. Stat.* **1974**, *3*, 1–27.

32. Davies, D.L.; Bouldin, D.W. A Cluster Separation Measure. *IEEE Trans. Pattern Anal. Mach. Intell.* **1979**, *PAMI-1*, 224–227. [CrossRef]

33. Wang, L.; Zhao, C. *Hyperspectral Image Processing*; Springer: Berlin, Germany, 2016; ISBN 978-3-662-47455-6.

34. Dietterich, T.G. Ensemble Methods in Machine Learning. In *Multiple Classifier Systems*; Springer Nature: Berlin, Germany, 2000; pp. 1–15.

35. Jahed Armaghani, D.; Hasanipanah, M.; Mahdiyar, A.; Abd Majid, M.Z.; Bakhshandeh Amnieh, H.; Tahir, M.M.D. Airblast prediction through a hybrid genetic algorithm-ANN model. *Neural Comput. Appl.* **2018**, *29*, 619–629. [CrossRef]

3

A Perspective on Ovarian Cancer Biomarkers: Past, Present and Yet-To-Come

Frederick R. Ueland

Department of Obstetrics and Gynecology, Division of Gynecologic Oncology and the Markey Cancer Center, University of Kentucky College of Medicine, Lexington, KY 40515, USA; fuela0@uky.edu

Academic Editor: Andreas Kjaer

Abstract: The history of biomarkers and ultrasonography dates back over more than 50 years. The present status of biomarkers used in the context of ovarian cancer is addressed. Attention is given to new interpretations of the etiology of ovarian cancer. Cancer antigen 125 (CA125) and multivariate index assays (Ova1, Risk of Ovarian Malignancy Algorithm, Overa) are biomarker-driven considerations that are presented. Integration of biomarkers into ovarian cancer diagnostics and screening are presented in conjunction with ultrasound. Consideration is given to the serial application of both biomarkers and ultrasound, as well as morphology-based indices. Attempts are made to foresee how individualized molecular signatures may be able to both provide an alert of the potential for ovarian cancer and to provide molecular treatments tailored to a personalized genetic signature. In the future, an annual pelvic ultrasound and a comprehensive serum biomarker screening/diagnostic panel may replace the much maligned bimanual examination as part of the annual gynecologic examination. Taken together, it is likely that a new medical specialty for screening and early diagnostics will emerge for physicians and epidemiologists, a field of study that is independent of patient gender, organ, or the subspecialties of today.

Perspective

Ghost of Christmas Yet-To-Come

Original illustration by John Leech, 1843

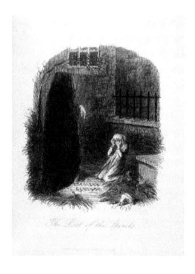

Keywords: biomarkers; ovarian tumor biomarkers; ultrasound; serial ultrasound; ovarian cancer

As one year closes and another begins, I find myself reflecting on ovarian cancer diagnostics. It is truly humbling how little we have accomplished in this field over the last half-century. All the while, the rest of the world has been busy. Since the first biomarker was reported, we have harnessed the atom and ushered in the Nuclear Age. Since the first *ovarian* biomarker was reported, we have invented the integrated circuit and spawned the dynamic Information Age. Yet, as gynecologic oncologists, we continue to struggle with the early identification of ovarian cancer and whether ovarian cancer actually begins in the ovary at all. The first serum biomarker for epithelial ovarian cancer was introduced in 1965 (carcinoembyonic antigen, CEA) [1]. This was a milestone in cancer diagnostics, as prior to this, oncologists were equipped with little to detect or monitor ovarian cancer. Keep in mind that this was when ultrasound was just emerging as a very rudimentary medical diagnostic instrument, and well before the advent of computed tomography (CT) or magnetic resonance imaging (MRI). Now some fifty years later, it is easy to ask, "Why haven't we done more?" Perhaps the recent focus on molecular-genetic technology and personalized cancer treatment will inspire a new Diagnostic Age in oncology. I am an optimist at heart, and am hopeful that our biomarker story will read somewhat like the Charles Dickens novella, A Christmas Carol, where the return of Jacob Marley's ghost 7 years after his death helps give clarity to the past, present, and yet-to-come.

First, it is important to clarify our diagnostic objective. My generation has believed, quite sensibly I think, that epithelial ovarian cancer arises from the ovary. Ovarian cancer has always utilized a taxonomy-based classification system first introduced in the 1930s, then validated by the World Health Organization's Classification in 1973, and propagated into modern day. The story was as follows: ovarian epithelial inclusion cysts are trapped beneath the surface epithelium of the ovary and eventually undergo malignant transformation giving rise to invasive cancer. It was all a little mysterious and the association with ovulation was difficult to validate, but "incessant ovulation" did appear to be a significant risk factor. Until recently, true fallopian tube cancers were very rare. The historic requirement for the diagnosis of a fallopian tube cancer included the following: (1) the main tumor is grossly in the fallopian tube; (2) microscopically, the mucosa is chiefly involved and has a papillary pattern; and (3) if the tubal wall is involved to a great extent, the transition between benign and malignant tubal epithelium should be demonstrated [2]. Truthfully, many serous "ovarian cancers" probably do begin elsewhere and metastasize to the ovary since ovarian stromal involvement is the principle requirement to categorize a malignancy as primary ovarian cancer. Since serous peritoneal, fallopian tube, and ovarian cancers are histologically and morphologically similar regardless of where they begin, and are treated alike, they have been collectively categorized as ovarian cancer. Today, our approach to treatment is based on this premise, specifically that all these cancers are lumped together as one. National collaborative group trials for ovarian cancer have typically studied all three malignancies together rather than individually, even non-serous cell types. And this was very sensible, since we thought of ovarian cancer in terms of its anatomic origin and combining made practical sense for clinical trial accrual. This dilemma is apropos given the current belief that the fallopian tube (serous tubal intraepithelial carcinoma, STIC) may be the primary culprit in the etiology of many serous cancers of the ovary [3]. It is very helpful to know what the target is, not just for purposes of tidiness and taxonomy, but also for understanding how to envision the next generation of diagnostic tests.

Kurman and coauthors recently described the need for a paradigm shift in our understanding of ovarian cancer [4]. Endometrial precursors are likely responsible for many of the Type I ovarian cancers as endometrioid and clear cell types originate ostensibly from endometriotic implants. These are typically indolent, low-grade malignancies, and endometrioid, transitional and clear cell cancers with distinct molecular markers: KRAS, BRAF, ERB-2, PTEN and others, but not TP-53. And most gastrointestinal-type tumors involving the ovary are also secondary malignancies, with primary mucinous ovarian cancers comprising only 3% of all epithelial ovarian cancers. Fallopian tube precursors are likely the cause of the more common Type II, high-grade serous ovarian cancers which are characterized by TP-53 mutations. In the end, stromal and germ cell tumors may be the only true anatomic ovarian malignancies. The challenge of course, is that all gynecologic cancers are not organ-specific, so our diagnostic and treatment strategies need to evolve.

1. Past

The biomarker past was an era of single-marker diagnostics. CEA was first described in 1965 as a serum biomarker for mucinous colon cancer, and in 1976 as a blood test for women with ovarian cancer [1,5]. At the time, this was a tremendous advance in science. Not long after, cancer antigen 125 (CA125) was announced as a serum biomarker specific for ovarian cancer [6] (Table 1). To move from an age of very limited imaging and diagnostics to an ovarian cancer blood test was transformational. In retrospect, it can be argued that CA125 has done little to improve ovarian cancer care. The Food and Drug Administration (FDA) never approved CA125 for preoperative use in the United States, but only for cancer surveillance for women with a known diagnosis of ovarian cancer. Ironically, the majority of CA125 tests ordered today are for the evaluation of an ovarian tumor prior to surgery. The use of serum CA125 has also never been associated with a survival benefit, whether utilized before or after diagnosis. This may be an indictment of the test itself, of the disease, the stage at diagnosis, treatment options, or a combination of these factors.

Table 1. Common serum biomarkers for ovarian cancer, year of publication or Food and Drug Administration (FDA) clearance. CEA, carcinoembyonic antigen; CA125, cancer antigen 125; ROMA, Risk of Ovarian Malignancy Algorithm; HE4, human epididymis protein 4; Ova1 and Overa are proprietary multivariate index assays, Vermillion, Inc.

Biomarker	Year
CEA	1965
CA125	1981
HE4	2008
Ova1	2009
ROMA	2010
Overa	2016

Although CA125 is the best-known serum ovarian cancer biomarker, it is not the only one: CEA (mucinous), LDH (dysgerminoma, mixed germ cell tumors), β-hCG (choriocarcinoma, mixed germ cell tumors), inhibin B (granulosa cell tumors), α-fetoprotein (yolk sac tumors, embryonal cell tumors), and HE4 are also available. In 2008, HE4 was cleared by the FDA for use in monitoring patients with a known diagnosis of ovarian cancer, able to detect recurrence of epithelial cancers 2 to 3 months in advance of CA125. Like CA125, it does not have a preoperative diagnostic indication from the FDA. CA125 is the most studied biomarker for serous epithelial cancer arising from the ovary, fallopian tube, or peritoneal cavity, but it is neither a sensitive nor particularly specific cancer marker. This may partly explain why its use has not translated into an improvement in patient survival. For 35 years, we have been trying to overcome this biomarker's inadequacy by combining it with other markers, combining it with imaging, or monitoring its behavior over time: all ultimately without epic success. Success, our patients have discovered, is identifying ovarian cancer in the earliest of stages where treatment can have a lasting impact on survival. Our understanding of protein biomarkers has improved recently as a result of advances in proteomic diagnostic technologies.

2. Present

In 2009, the FDA cleared the first preoperative serum biomarker test for ovarian cancer. After five years of diagnostic discovery and systematic clinical testing, a 5-protein biomarker panel named Ova1® became the first multivariate index assay (MIA) to gain clearance in the United States [7,8]. Ova1 combines the second generation CA125-II with other inflammatory and transport proteins (transferrin, β-2 microglobulin, apolipoprotein A-1, and transthyretin) into a test result of low or high risk for ovarian cancer. The following year, a two-protein test was FDA-cleared that combined CA125 and HE4 (Risk of Ovarian Malignancy Algorithm, ROMA®) for identical indications [9]. These MIA tests were a significant improvement for preoperative testing compared to single biomarker tests because of increased sensitivity (Table 2) [10]. Importantly, these tests are not true diagnostic tests, but rather triage or referral tests. When a woman is known to have an ovarian tumor that requires surgery, these tests are used to determine the likelihood of malignancy. A primary care provider can utilize the test to determine whether referral to a gynecologic oncologist is indicated. These tests have two critical requirements: (1) a mass has been confirmed on imaging, and (2) the ovarian tumor has already been determined to require surgery. Since the test itself is not used to determine whether or not surgery is necessary, it should result in minimal tangible harm. Nationwide, the majority of ovarian cancer surgeries are not initially performed by a gynecologic oncologist, so the hope is that the quality of patient care and cancer survival will improve over time as appropriate referrals are made. Provided that the two critical requirements are observed, this carefully considered strategy should prevent unnecessary surgery from a falsely positive biomarker test, an important consideration for the women, their doctors, and the FDA.

Table 2. Test performance for detecting ovarian cancer of all histologic types.

Biomarker	Sensitivity	Specificity
CA125 *,+,#	76%	94%
Ova1 *	94%	54%
ROMA ˆ	89%	83%
Overa *	91%	69%

* Studied in same patient population; + CA125-II assay (second generation); # CA125 not FDA-approved for preoperative use; ˆ Meta-analysis [11]

Multivariate index assays have continued to evolve. In 2016, the FDA cleared a new generation Ova1 test (Overa®) that essentially combines two MIA tests and maintains a high diagnostic sensitivity with improved specificity [12], Table 2. The individual markers are CA125-II, HE4, apolipoprotein A-1, follicle stimulating hormone, and transferrin. The preoperative indications are the same. Other panels will soon follow [13]. Naturally, there are always temptations to move a diagnostic test into a screening role, but without proper study, this is a premature and potentially harmful notion. Cancer screening and cancer diagnostics are vastly different challenges with regard to disease prevalence and endpoint objectives.

Ovarian biomarkers are not restricted to the blood. Ultrasound, like all imaging, is a biomarker of disease. Ultrasound has been widely studied in the United States and Europe as a screening tool and as a diagnostic adjunct. We are beginning to discover that ovarian ultrasound screening alone, or in combination with CA125, may have the potential to save lives [14,15]. Findings from the United Kingdom Collaborative Trial of Ovarian Cancer Screening (UKCTOCS) recently reported preliminary results of a shift to early stage disease and a reduction in cancer deaths on follow up to 14 years with multimodal ovarian cancer screening with serum CA125 interpreted using the Risk of Ovarian Cancer Algorithm (ROCA), transvaginal ultrasound, and clinical assessment. ROCA is an algorithm used to interpret longitudinal CA125 values for ovarian cancer screening. This story is far from over, but it is definitely premature to begin screening the general population off protocol. In fact, shortly following the UKCTOCS publication, the FDA, the American College of Obstetrics and Gynecology, and the Society of Gynecologic Oncology all made prompt safety statements announcing that ROCA is not an approved screening strategy and may trigger unnecessary surgical procedures.

How we combine biomarkers has a significant impact on their overall test performance. Tests can be combined in series or parallel. When combined in series (A, B and C, etc.), the statistical consequence is improved specificity at the expense of sensitivity. Conversely, tests combined in parallel (A or B or C, etc.) will result in improved sensitivity with a compromise in specificity. At the risk of oversimplification, the MIA tests are essentially combining individual biomarker tests in a parallel manner. Ova1 is a good example. Five biomarkers are applied in parallel in the same serum specimen with resultant high sensitivity (and high negative predictive value), making it an excellent triage test. If the test is low-risk, it is very unlikely to be malignant and the patient can have surgery without consulting a specialist. But the apparent drawback of this MIA strategy can be a modest specificity and ovarian tumors may have a high-risk test result even though cancer is not present. By requiring that a mass be confirmed on imaging prior to ordering Ova1, there is a mandate of sorts to combine an additional test (imaging) that localizes the problem to the ovary, improving both the sensitivity of finding an abnormality and the specificity that the problem arises from the ovary (though not that it is necessarily malignant).

Today, serum biomarkers alone are not enough. In developed countries, there is no practical way to divorce serum biomarkers from ovarian imaging since ultrasound and CT scan are ubiquitous tests available to nearly every woman. Ultrasound is far less expensive than a CT scan or MRI, but ultrasound findings are limited mainly to the pelvis. An ultrasound-based morphology scoring system is an effective and objective way to identify ovarian tumors at high-risk for malignancy. The International Ovarian Tumor Analysis group (IOTA) has a multifaceted algorithm that has been systematically evaluated in Europe to high acclaim [16]. There have also been attempts to simplify the IOTA algorithm [17,18], and IOTA has yet to be evaluated in the United States. Other morphology-based indices have been proposed and validated in the U.S. and abroad [19–21]. Moreover, much like longitudinal CA125 (ROCA), serial ultrasound offers improved diagnostic results over a single evaluation (Figure 1) [22,23]. Serial ultrasonography is a sensible approach because each tumor is evaluated both on its changing complexity and its physiologic evolution. There can be clinical reasons not to perform serial evaluations on women with ovarian tumors. First, the presentation may be so concerning for malignancy that prompt surgery is best. Second, the woman may be symptomatic from the tumor so delayed intervention is problematic. Third, the patient may be traveling a great distance or have other personal reasons why a delay in treatment is not feasible. In the absence of these issues, a thoughtful re-evaluation is a valuable diagnostic option, and the data support this concept for serum CA125 in ovarian cancer screening (ROCA) and serial ultrasound with a quantifiable morphology index score in ovarian diagnostics (and maybe screening). The coup de gras, given our present diagnostic capability, would be a combination of serial MIA biomarkers with serial ultrasound. This data has yet to be published.

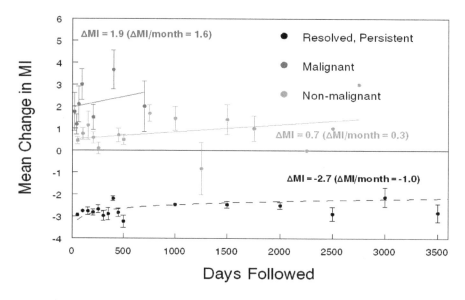

Figure 1. Results of serial ultrasound evaluation of ovarian tumors. MI, Morphology Index score, University of Kentucky (Lexington, KY, USA).

3. Yet-To-Come

Dickens was artful in his portrayal of Ebenezer Scrooge, allowing him to see his unflattering future through Marley's ghost of Christmas yet-to-come. Of course, after his apparitional vision on Christmas Eve, Scrooge awoke transformed. And transformation is what we need for ovarian cancer diagnostics. It is certainly possible that new innovations will give rise to novel diagnostic insights, just as cancer therapy is trending toward targeted, molecular-based treatment. Although personalized cancer treatment is still far from the standard of care, it does raise the question, "Can we pursue a similar evolution in ovarian cancer diagnostics?" After 50 years, it is regrettable that we are still searching for effective approaches to early cancer diagnosis, but we are. As we transition our thinking and our oncology research to a molecular genetic model, we will recognize that this will unite malignancies in a different way, based on common molecular footprints rather than on an anatomic location or a given oncology specialty.

In the near term, we will see new types of serum cancer biomarkers that outperform our current protein-based markers in both selectivity and accuracy. Nucleic acids are showing promise as a new group of serum markers, including free DNA, mRNA, microRNAs, and circulating tumor DNA (ctDNA) [24,25]. A thoughtful combination of protein and nucleic acid markers may permit a comprehensive screening and diagnostic panel that captures all gynecologic malignancies in one blood test. In the future, an annual pelvic ultrasound and a comprehensive serum biomarker screening/diagnostic panel may replace the much maligned bimanual examination as part of the annual gynecologic examination. If abnormal, repeat testing will provide a personalized, serial database that will recalculate the likelihood of malignancy based on the objective change over time in tumor morphology and physiology. As the diagnosis and treatment of cancer changes, so too must clinical trial design to accommodate the new era of multiple biomarkers and targeted, personalized therapies [26].

Beyond the near future, germ-line cancer testing will be initiated at birth as part of newborn screening. Today, we often recommend genetic cancer testing following a malignant diagnosis, which is helpful for their future screening and for their relatives, but it is obviously a little late to prevent their own cancer. The power of knowing individual genetic risk at birth is that it may potentially modify behavior in those found to have a germ-line mutation, which comprise 5%–10% of cancers, and permit selective screening algorithms that are customized to personal cancer risk. And periodic genomic screening throughout one's lifetime may help identify acquired mutations that predispose to specific cancers, heighten awareness, alter personal behavior, and dictate medical surveillance. The technology to sort, store and personalize this colossal amount of data is available today, a consequence of Moore's law whereby computer processing speeds and power have roughly doubled every two years beginning in the 1960s. Cancer testing will quickly move beyond organ and specialty-specific screening. Whole body scans and universal cancer panels will screen and monitor all cancers, solid and hematogenous. An asymptomatic patient may not even need to see a physician if the annual evaluation is normal. A new medical field for screening and early diagnostics will emerge for physicians and epidemiologists, a field of study that is independent of patient gender, organ, or the subspecialties of today.

To get there, we must agree to work with industry innovators in medicine, technology and finance to develop and fund novel strategies for diagnosis and screening. We must encourage the national collaborative groups and the National Cancer Institute's Clinical Trials Reporting Program to promote screening and diagnostic trials with as much vigor as the interventional treatment trials. Since the early detection of any cancer has the promise of shifting diagnosis to an earlier stage, cancer survival will improve. This approach could ultimately revolutionize how we provide care for our patients, and perhaps spare us yet another salvage chemotherapy trial for relapsed ovarian cancer.

So let us awake on a future Christmas morning with newfound clarity. Let us transform how we categorize ovarian cancer, how we identify ovarian cancer, how we treat ovarian cancer, and possibly how we screen for cancer in general. It did not take long for the Nuclear Age to change our worldview or for the Information Age to profoundly alter our daily lives; with any luck, it will not take long to revisit our approach to early diagnostics for ovarian cancer. If Ebenezer Scrooge can change his ways …

References

1. Gold, P.; Freedman, S. Demonstration of tumor-specific antigens in human colonic carcinomata by immunological tolerance and absorption techniques. *J. Exp. Med.* **1965**, *121*, 439–462. [CrossRef] [PubMed]

2. Hu, C.; Taymor, M.; Hertig, A. Primary carcinoma of the fallopian tube. *Am. J. Obstet. Gynecol.* **1950**, *59*, 58–67. [CrossRef]

3. Kindelberger, D.; Miron, L.; Hirsch, M.; Feltmate, C.; Medeiros, F.; Callahan, M.; Garner, E.; Gordon, R.; Birch, C.; Berkowitz, R.; et al. Intraepithelial carcinoma of the fimbria and pelvic serous carcinoma: Evidence for a causal relationship. *Am. J. Surg. Pathol.* **2007**, *2*, 161–169. [CrossRef] [PubMed]

4. Kurman, R.; Shih, I. Molecular pathogenesis and extraovarian origin of epithelial ovarian cancer—Shifting the paradigm. *Hum. Pathol.* **2011**, *7*, 918–931. [CrossRef] [PubMed]

5. Khoo, S.; MacKay, E. Carcinoembryonic antigen (CEA) in ovarian cancer: Factors influencing its incidence and changes which occur in response to cytotoxic drugs. *Br. J. Obstet. Gynaecol.* **1976**, *83*, 753–759. [CrossRef] [PubMed]

6. Bast, R.; Feeney, M.; Lazarus, H.; Nadler, L.; Knapp, R. Reactivity of a monoclonal antibody with human ovarian carcinoma. *J. Clin. Investig.* **1981**, *68*, 1331–1337. [CrossRef] [PubMed]

7. Ueland, F.; DeSimone, C.; Seamon, L.; Miller, R.; Goodrich, S.; Podzielinski, I.; Sokoll, L.; Smith, A.; van Nagell, J.R., Jr.; Zhang, Z. Effectiveness of a multivariate index assay in the preoperative assessment of ovarian tumors. *Obstet. Gynecol.* **2011**, *117*, 1289–1297. [CrossRef] [PubMed]

8. Zhang, Z.; Chan, D. The road from discovery to clinical diagnostics: Lessons learned from the first FDA-cleared in vitro diagnostic multivariate index assay of proteomic biomarkers. *Cancer Epidemiol. Biomark. Prev.* **2010**, *19*, 2995–2999. [CrossRef] [PubMed]

9. Moore, R.; Miller, M.; Disilvestro, P.; Landrum, L.; Gajewski, W.; Ball, J.; Skates, S. Evaluation of the diagnostic accuracy of the risk of ovarian malignancy algorithm in women with a pelvic mass. *Obstet. Gynecol.* **2011**, *118*, 280–288. [CrossRef] [PubMed]

10. Bristow, R.; Smith, A.; Zhang, Z.; Chan, D.; Crutcher, G.; Fung, E.; Munroe, D. Ovarian malignancy risk stratification of the adnexal mass using a multivariate index assay. *Gynecol. Oncol.* **2013**, *128*, 252–259. [CrossRef] [PubMed]

11. Li, F.; Tie, R.; Chang, K.; Wang, F.; Deng, S.; Lu, W.; Yu, L.; Chen, M. Does risk for ovarian malignancy algorithm excel human epididymis protein 4 and CA125 in predicting epithelial ovarian cancer: A meta-analysis. *BMC Cancer* **2012**, *12*, 258. [CrossRef] [PubMed]

12. Coleman, R.; Herzog, T.; Chan, D.; Munroe, D.; Pappas, T.; Smith, A.; Zhang, Z.; Wolf, J. Validation of a second-generation multivariate index assay for malignancy risk of adnexal masses. *Am. J. Obstet. Gynecol.* **2016**, *215*, 82.e1–82.e11. [CrossRef] [PubMed]

13. Simmons, A.; Clarke, C.; Badgwell, D.; Lu, Z.; Sokoll, L.; Lu, K.; Zhang, Z.; Bast, R.; Skates, S. Validation of a biomarker panel and longitudinal biomarker performance for early detection of ovarian cancer. *Int. J. Gynecol. Cancer* **2016**, *26*, 1070–1077. [CrossRef] [PubMed]

14. Jacobs, I.; Menon, U.; Ryan, A.; Maharaj, A.; Burnell, M.; Kalsi, J.; Amso, N.; Apostolidou, S.; Benjamin, E.; Cruickshank, D.; et al. Ovarian cancer screening and mortality in the UK Collaborative Trial of Ovarian Cancer Screeening (UKCTOCS): A randomized controlled trial. *Lancet* **2016**, *387*, 945–956. [CrossRef]

15. Ormsby, E.; Pavlik, E.; van Nagell, J. Ultrasound follow up of an adnexal mass has the potential to save lives. *Am. J. Obstet. Gynecol.* **2015**, *213*, 657–661. [CrossRef] [PubMed]

16. Timmerman, D.; van Calster, B.; Testa, A.; Guerriero, S.; Fischerova, D.; Lissoni, A.; van Holsbeke, C.; Fruscio, R.; Czekierdowski, A.; Jurkovic, D.; et al. Ovarian cancer prediction in adnexal masses using ultrasound-based logistic regression models: A temporal and external validation study by the IOTA group. *Ultrasound Obstet. Gynecol.* **2010**, *36*, 226–234. [CrossRef] [PubMed]

17. Timmerman, D.; Testa, A.; Bourne, T.; Ameye, L.; Jurkovic, D.; van Holsbeke, C.; Paladini, D.; van Calster, B.; Vergote, I.; van Huffel, S.; et al. Simple ultrasound-based rules for the diagnosis of ovarian cancer. *Ultrasound Obstet. Gynecol.* **2008**, *31*, 681–690. [CrossRef] [PubMed]

18. Van Caster, B.; van Hoorde, K.; Valentin, L.; Testa, A.; Fischerova, D.; van Holsbeke, C.; Savelli, L.; Franchi, D.; Epstein, E.; Kaijser, J.; et al. Evaluating the risk of ovarian cancer before surgery using the ADNEX model to differentiate between benign, borderline, early and advanced stage invasive, and secondary metastatic tumours: Prospective multicentre diagnostic study. *BMJ* **2014**, *349*, 1–14. [CrossRef] [PubMed]

19. Ueland, F.; DePriest, P.; Pavlik, E.; Kryscio, R.; van Nagell, J., Jr. Preoperative differentiation of malignant from benign ovarian tumors: The efficacy of morphology indexing and Doppler flow sonography. *Gynecol. Oncol.* **2003**, *91*, 46–50. [CrossRef]

20. Barnsfather, K.; Fitzpatrick, C.; Wilson, J.; Linn, C.; Brizendine, E.; Schilder, J. The Morphology Index: Predictive value of malignancy among clinicians at various levels of training. *Gynecol. Oncol.* **2012**, *127*, 94–97. [CrossRef] [PubMed]

21. Jeoung, H.; Choi, H.; Lim, Y.; Lee, M.; Kim, S.; Han, S.; Ahn, T.; Choi, S. The efficacy of sonographic morphology indexing and serum CA-125 for preoperative differentiation of malignant from benign ovarian tumors in patients after operation with ovarian tumors. *J. Gynecol. Oncol.* **2008**, *19*, 229–235. [CrossRef] [PubMed]

22. Elder, J.; Pavlik, E.; Long, A.; Miller, R.; DeSimone, C.; Hoff, J.; Ueland, W.; Kryscio, R.; van Nagell, J.; Ueland, F. Serial ultrasonographic evaluation of ovarian abnormalities with a morphology index. *Gynecol. Oncol.* **2014**, *135*, 8–12. [CrossRef] [PubMed]

23. Pavlik, E.; Ueland, F.; Miller, R.; Ubellacker, J.; DeSimone, C.; Elder, J.; Hoff, J.; Baldwin, L.; Kryscio, R.; van Nagell, J.R., Jr. Frequency and disposition of ovarian abnormalities followed with serial transvaginal sonography. *Obstet. Gynecol.* **2013**, *122*, 210–217. [CrossRef] [PubMed]

24. Schwarzenbach, H.; Hoon, D.; Pantel, K. Cell-free nucleic acids as biomarkers in cancer patients. *Nat. Rev. Cancer* **2011**, *11*, 426–437. [CrossRef] [PubMed]

25. Bettegowda, C.; Sausen, M.; Leary, R.; Kinde, I.; Wang, Y.; Agrawal, N.; Bartlett, B.; Wang, H.; Luber, B.; Alani, R.; et al. Detection of circulating tumor DNA in early- and late-stage human malignancies. *Sci. Transl. Med.* **2014**, *224*, 224ra24. [CrossRef] [PubMed]

26. Venook, A.; Arcila, M.; Benson, A.; Berry, D.; Camidge, D.; Carlson, R.; Choueiri, T.; Guild, V.; Kalemkerian, G.; Kurzrock, R.; et al. NCCN Work Group Report: Designing clinical trials in the era of multiple biomarkers and targeted therapies. *J. Natl. Compr. Cancer Netw.* **2014**, *12*, 1629–1649.

4

Circulating Tumor Cells and Metabolic Parameters in NSCLC Patients Treated with Checkpoint Inhibitors

Angelo Castello [1], Francesco Giuseppe Carbone [2], Sabrina Rossi [3], Simona Monterisi [4], Davide Federico [5], Luca Toschi [3] and Egesta Lopci [1,*]

[1] Nuclear Medicine, Humanitas Clinical and Research Center-IRCCS, 20089 Rozzano, Italy; angelo.castello@cancercenter.humanitas.it

[2] Anatomy and Histopathology, Santa Chiara Hospital, 38122 Trento, Italy; francesco.gcarbone@gmail.com

[3] Oncology and Hematology, Humanitas Clinical and Research Center-IRCCS, 20089 Rozzano, Italy; sabrina.rossi@cancercenter.humanitas.it (S.R.); luca.toschi@cancercenter.humanitas.it (L.T.)

[4] Immunology and Inflammation, Humanitas Clinical and Research Center-IRCCS, 20089 Rozzano, Italy; simonterisi@gmail.com

[5] Pathology, Humanitas Clinical and Research Center-IRCCS, 20089 Rozzano, Italy; davide.federico@humanitas.it

* Correspondence: egesta.lopci@gmail.com

Abstract: Circulating tumor cells (CTC) count and characterization have been associated with poor prognosis in recent studies. Our aim was to examine CTC count and its association with metabolic parameters and clinical outcomes in non-small cell lung carcinoma (NSCLC) patients treated with immune checkpoint inhibitors (ICI). For this prospective study, data from 35 patients (23 males, 12 females) were collected and analyzed. All patients underwent an 18F-fluorodeoxyglucose positron emission tomography/computed tomography (18F-FDG-PET/CT) scan and CTC detection through Isolation by Size of Tumor/Trophoblastic Cells (ISET) from peripheral blood samples obtained at baseline and 8 weeks after ICI initiation. Association of CTC count with clinical and metabolic characteristics was studied. Progression-free survival (PFS) and overall survival (OS) were analyzed using the Kaplan–Meier method and the log-rank test. Median follow-up was 13.2 months (range of 4.9–21.6). CTC were identified in 16 out of 35 patients (45.7%) at baseline and 10 out of 24 patients at 8 weeks (41.7%). Mean CTC numbers before and after 8 weeks were 15 ± 28 and 11 ± 19, respectively. Prior to ICI, the mean CTC number was significantly higher in treatment-naïve patients (34 ± 39 vs. 9 ± 21, $p = 0.004$). CTC count variation (ΔCTC) was significantly associated with tumor metabolic response set by European Organization for Research and Treatment of Cancer (EORTC) criteria ($p = 0.033$). At the first restaging, patients with a high tumor burden, that is, metabolic tumor volume (MTV) and total lesion glycolysis (TLG), had a higher CTC count ($p = 0.009$). The combination of mean CTC and median MTV at 8 weeks was associated with PFS ($p < 0.001$) and OS ($p = 0.024$). Multivariate analysis identified CTC count at 8 weeks as an independent predictor for PFS and OS, whereas ΔMTV and maximum standardized uptake value variation (ΔSUVmax) was predictive for PFS and OS, respectively. Our study confirmed that CTC number is modulated by previous treatments and correlates with metabolic response during ICI. Moreover, elevated CTC count, along with metabolic parameters, were found to be prognostic factors for PFS and OS.

Keywords: non-small-cell lung cancer; circulating tumor cells; PET/CT; immunotherapy; response to treatment

1. Introduction

The introduction of antibodies against programmed cell death protein-1 (PD-1) and its ligand (PD-L1), a crucial axis involved in the immune surveillance, has prompted encouraging results in the treatment of advanced non-small cell lung carcinoma (NSCLC), although only a minority of patients show clinical response [1]. As a consequence, there is a compelling need to understand the molecular basis of cancer growth and identify potential biomarkers of response, in order to better select patients who will benefit from such new agents.

In the last years, circulating tumor cells' (CTC) count and characterization have become of great interest in the scientific community [2,3]. Some studies have demonstrated that CTC enumeration is related to poor prognosis in different metastatic malignancies, including lung, breast, colorectal, prostate, and gastric cancer. Furthermore, molecular characterization of CTC might expand our knowledge on tumor heterogeneity, especially in patients for whom tissue biopsies are difficult to perform [4–8].

Molecular imaging, using 18F-fluorodeoxyglucose (18F-FDG) with positron emission tomography/computed tomography (PET/CT), is widely applied in oncology as a useful marker of tumor biology. Indeed, by differentiating higher versus less-active metabolic tumor tissues, semi-quantitative metabolic parameters can offer the possibility for non-invasive, in vivo tumor characterization and for correct evaluation of tumor response [9–11]. However, available studies analyzing the association between 18F-FDG PET/CT and CTC in NSCLC are limited to chemotherapy-naïve patients or those treated with "traditional" antitumor drugs [12–15].

On the basis of these premises, our aim was to examine CTC count in NSCLC patients treated with immune checkpoint inhibitors (ICI) and determine its relationship with metabolic parameters by 18F-FDG PET/CT and clinical outcomes.

2. Results

2.1. Patients' Characteristics

A total of 20 patients (57.1%) received nivolumab, 12 (34.3%) pembrolizumab, 2 patients (5.7%) had a combination of nivolumab and ipilimumab, and only 1 (2.9%) patient was treated with atezolizumab. The median number of immunotherapy cycles was 8 (range of 1–47). Median follow-up was 13.2 months (range of 4.9–21.6 months).

2.2. CTC and Clinic-Pathologic Features

CTC were identified (CTC ≥ 1) in 16 out of 35 patients (45.7%) at baseline prior to ICI therapy, and the CTC count ranged between 0 and 130 (mean ± standard deviation (SD), 15 ± 28). The minimum number of CTC detected was 5, in particular 8 patients had a CTC count between 5 and 20, whereas the other 8 patients had CTC from 25 to 130.

At the first restaging, peripheral blood samples were available for 24 patients because of progression of disease or a worsening of clinical conditions in the other cases. CTC were detected in 10 out of 24 patients (41.7%). The median number of CTC was 11 ± 19 in 10 mL of blood. CTC count ranged between 5 and 20 in six patients, and between 30 and 60 in the other four patients. In addition, we demonstrated a reduction of CTC in nine patients (37.5%), unchanged in eight patients (33.3%), and increased in seven patients (29.2%). Although a reduction in the mean number of CTC before and after 8 weeks of treatment was detected, this decrease was not statistically significant.

The association between CTC count and patient characteristics was explored, both before treatment and at the first restaging. There was a statistically significant association between CTC count and previous treatments. Of note, patients who underwent ICI as first-line treatment had a mean number of CTC at baseline higher than patients who started ICI after more lines of treatment (34 ± 39 vs. 9 ± 21, $p = 0.004$) (Figure 1A). Likewise, a trend was observed with high baseline CTC count and pembrolizumab ($p = 0.09$); indeed, the latter is often used in first-line settings. No further association was found between CTC counts, as well as the other clinical variables, such as age, gender, smoking history, and tumor type.

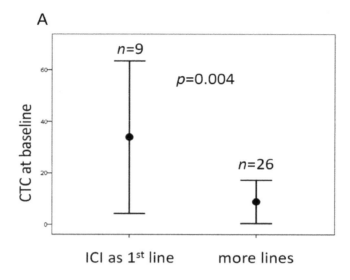

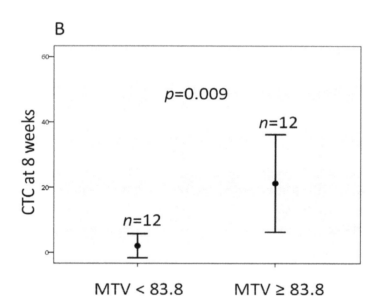

Figure 1. Association of circulating tumor cells (CTC) count with clinical-metabolic features. (**A**) Mean number of CTC at baseline according to the number of previous lines of treatment. (**B**) Mean number of CTC at the first restaging (about 8 weeks) and the median value of metabolic tumor volume (MTV).

2.3. Relationship of CTC and Tumor Response

Of the 35 patients enrolled, 31 patients underwent tumor assessment by computed tomography (CT), whereas 18F-FDG PET/CT scans were available from 28 patients at the first response assessment. According to Response Evaluation Criteria In Solid Tumors (RECIST) 1.1, partial response (PR) was observed in 6 patients, stable disease (SD) was observed in 12, and progressive disease (PD) in 13. We found that patients with PD showed a trend toward higher baseline CTC count (26 ± 36) compared with patients with partial response (14 ± 14) or stable disease (9 ± 26) ($p = 0.076$). There was no significant difference in the CTC count after 8 weeks among the three groups of response.

According to the European Organization for Research and Treatment of Cancer (EORTC) criteria, partial metabolic response (PMR), stable metabolic disease (SMD), and progressive metabolic disease (PMD) were observed in 10, 6, and 12 patients, respectively. There was no significant difference in the baseline CTC count, as well as after 8 weeks, among the three groups. However, considering CTC changes (ΔCTC) within individual patients, among the 24 patients that had their CTC analyzed after 8 weeks of treatment, we found that the increase of CTC count was associated with poor response to ICI by means 18F-FDG PET/CT, as PMD rates were significantly different between patients with CTC increase at 8 weeks and patients with stable or decreased number of CTC (71.4% vs. 28.6% vs. 0%, respectively, $p = 0.033$) (Table 1).

Table 1. Association between circulating tumor cells (CTC) count and response to immune checkpoint inhibitors (ICI).

Parameter	EORTC		
	CMR/PMR	**SMD**	**PMD**
Baseline CTC count			
CTC $\leq$ 15 ($n = 18$)	27.8% (5)	33.3% (6)	38.9% (7)
CTC > 15 ($n = 10$)	50% (5)	0% (0)	50% (5)
p-value	ns	ns	ns
ΔCTC count after 8 weeks			
decreased ($n = 9$)	66.7% (6)	11.1% (1)	22.2% (2)
stable ($n = 8$)	12.5% (1)	37.5% (3)	50% (4)
increased ($n = 7$)	0% (0)	28.6% (2)	71.4% (5)
p-value	ns	ns	0.033

CMR/PMR, complete metabolic response/partial metabolic response; SMD, stable metabolic disease; PMD, progressive metabolic disease. ns: not significant.

2.4. CTC and Semi-Quantitative 18F-FDG Parameters

The median maximum standardized uptake value (SUVmax), average SUV (SUVmean), metabolic tumor volume (MTV), and total lesion glycolysis (TLG) before the initiation of treatment were 13.5 (range of 4.9–35.7), 5.9 (3.2–9.8), 68 (8–1772), and 362.8 (31–2504), respectively. Median SUVmax, SUV mean, MTV, and TLG after 8 weeks were 12.1 (3.6–38.4), 5.6 (3–13.8), 83.8 (2.5–623.3), and 511.2 (7.6–4332.7), respectively. Median ΔSUVmax, ΔSUVmean, ΔTLG, and ΔMTV were −12.9% (−75.5–107.1%), −0.88% (−61.3–130%), 47.8% (−99.4–1295%), and 30.4% (−98–1245%). At baseline, the number of CTC did not correlate with metabolic parameters, and only a trend for SUVmax was observed ($p = 0.072$). Conversely, after 8 weeks of treatment, CTC count was significantly associated with metabolic volume, expressed by MTV and TLG. Indeed, patients with MTV and TLG above the median values had higher mean number of CTC than patients with low metabolic tumor burden (both MTV and TLG $p = 0.009$) (Figure 1B). No difference was found between CTC and percentage changes of metabolic parameters.

2.5. Relationship between CTC Count, 18F-FDG PET Parameters, and Survival

The median progression-free survival (PFS) and overall survival (OS) of patients with CTC counts $\leq$ 11 after 8 weeks were 6.5 months (range of 5.1–7.9 months) and 18 months (range of 12–24 months), respectively. The median PFS and OS of patients with CTC counts > 11 were 1.8 months (range of 1.7–1.8 months) and 4 months (range of 2.7–5.3 months), respectively. The differences in PFS and OS were both statistically significant ($p < 0.001$, $p = 0.019$ for PFS and OS, respectively) (Figure 2A,B).

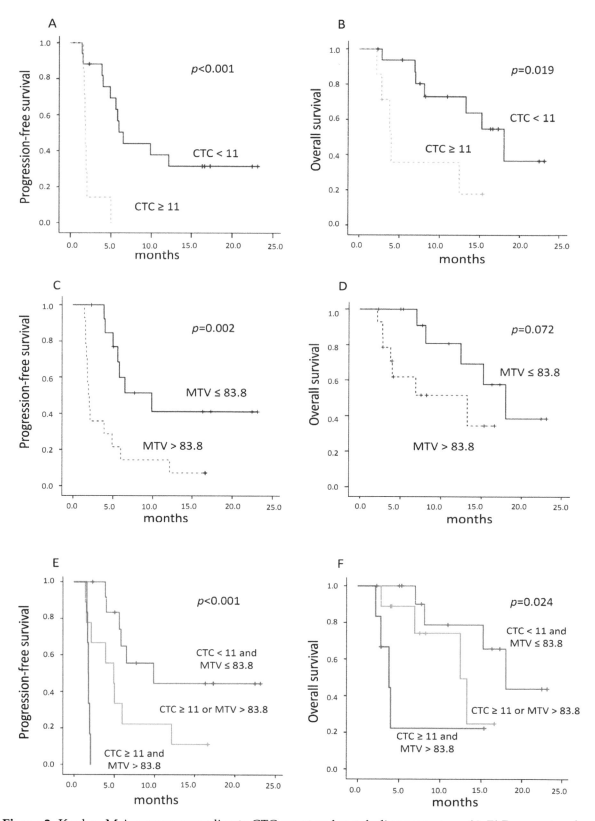

Figure 2. Kaplan–Meier curves according to CTC count and metabolic parameters. (**A,B**) Progression-free survival (PFS) and overall survival (OS) according to CTC count at 8 weeks, below or above the mean value. (**C,D**) PFS and OS of patients with MTV at 8 weeks greater or lower than median value. (**E,F**) PFS and OS according to the combination of mean number of CTC and median MTV after 8 weeks of treatment.

The median PFS and OS of patients with median MTV ≤ 83.8 were 9.9 months (range of 3.6–16.1 months) and 18 months (range of 12.6–23.4 months), respectively. The median PFS and OS of patients with median MTV > 83.8 were 1.9 months (range of 1.5–2.4 months) and 13.2 months (range of 2–24.5 months), respectively. The difference for PFS was statistically significant ($p = 0.002$), whereas for OS it showed only a trend ($p = 0.072$) (Figure 2C,D). Furthermore, we tested whether the combination of CTC count and MTV at 8 weeks could provide further discriminatory value in predicting clinical outcomes. Of note, all patients with MTV ≤ 83.8 and CTC ≤ 11 had the longest PFS and OS. Among patients with median MTV greater than 83.8, those with CTC count ≤ 11 were associated with longer PFS and OS than patients whose CTC were above the mean value (Figure 3E,F) ($p < 0.001$ and $p = 0.024$ for PFS and OS, respectively). Regarding percentage changes of metabolic parameters, we found that ΔMTV and ΔTLG were associated with PFS (both 9.9 vs. 2.1 months, $p = 0.010$ and $p = 0.009$, respectively), whereas ΔSUVmax was prognostic for OS (median not reached vs. 12.4 months, $p = 0.013$).

Finally, due to the low number of events, only three parameters were included in the multivariate Cox analysis. Of note, the number of CTC at the first restaging was confirmed as a predictive factor for PFS and OS, along with ΔMTV for PFS and ΔSUVmax for OS (Table 2).

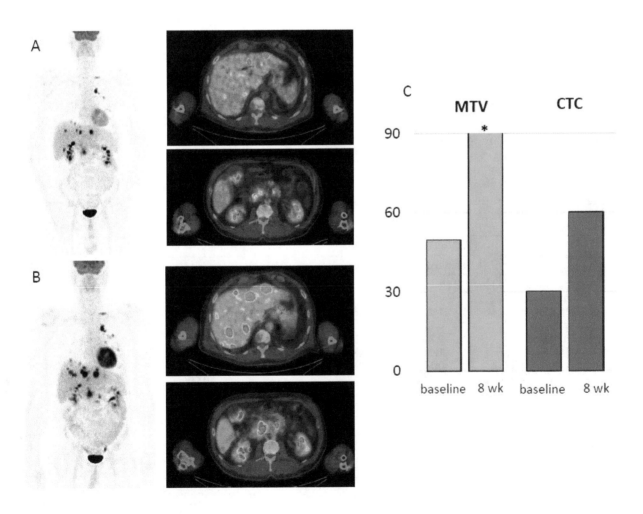

Figure 3. *Cont.*

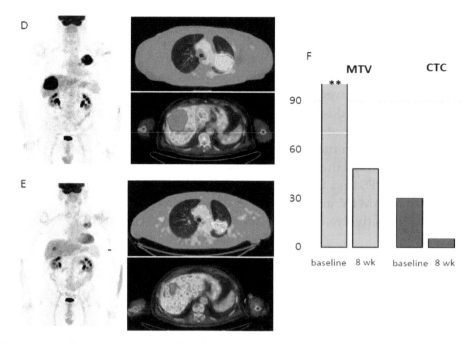

Figure 3. Two cases of progression (**A–C**) and response (**D–F**) to ICI according to metabolic parameters and CTC evaluation. (**A**) Maximum intensity projection (MIP) with two axial slices of liver and celiac node metastases at baseline. (**B**) Increase of tumor burden and appearance of further metastatic sites within the liver and in the abdominal nodes at the first restaging. (**C**) Bar graph representation of MTV (blue bars) between the baseline (49.4 mL) and the first restaging (97.2 mL). Likewise, CTC count (red bars) increased from 30 to 60. (**C**) MIP with two large lesions within the lung and liver at baseline. (**D**) 18F-fluorodeoxyglucose positron emission tomography/computed tomography (18F-FDG PET/CT) at 8 weeks, which demonstrated a decrease of overall tumor burden. (**F**) Bar graph representation of MTV (blue bars) at baseline (256.5 mL) and at 8 weeks (48 mL). Likewise CTC count (red bars) decreased from 30 to 5, * MTV= 97.2 mL; ** MTV= 256.5 mL.

Table 2. Uni- and multivariate Cox proportional hazard regression analyses for the prediction of PFS and OS.

Parameters	PFS			OS		
	Hazard Ratio	**95% IC**	***p*-Value**	**Hazard Ratio**	**95% IC**	***p*-Value**
Age (median)	1.233	0.564–2.694	ns	1.009	0.423–2.910	ns
Gender	0.346	0.156–0.768	0.009	0.329	0.119–0.905	0.031
Smoking history	1.407	0.480–4.129	ns	3.518	1.050–11.790	0.041
Histology	0.828	0.345–1.990	ns	0.907	0.291–2.822	ns
PD-L1 status	0.736	0.255–2.128	ns	0.659	0.147–2.957	ns
CTC baseline (median)	1.089	0.472–2.512	ns	1.869	0.607–5.759	ns
CTC at 8 weeks (median)	0.135	0.040–0.458	0.001	0.260	0.77–0.871	0.029
SUVmax baseline (median)	1.049	0.483–2.276	ns	0.996	0.383–2.654	ns
SUVmean baseline (median)	0.701	0.320–1.534	ns	0.839	0.312–2.257	ns
TLG baseline (median)	0.998	0.459–2.171	ns	1.016	0.389–1.534	ns
MTV baseline (median)	1.601	0.739–3.468	ns	2.473	0.934–6.551	ns
ΔSUVmax (median)	2.409	0.954–6.085	ns	0.179	0.039–0.825	0.027
ΔSUVmean (median)	1.498	0.611–3.671	ns	0.375	0.100–1.402	ns
ΔTLG (median)	0.310	0.122–787	0.014	0.751	0.241–2.346	ns
ΔMTV (median)	0.312	0.123–792	0.014	0.481	0.151–1.532	ns
Multivariate Cox proportional hazards regression analysis						
CTC at 8 weeks (median)	0.115	0.030–0.434	0.001 *	0.178	0.045–0.707	0.014 *
ΔMTV (median)	0.357	0.130–0.984	0.046 *			
ΔSUVmax (median)				0.144	0.028–0.736	0.02 *

* $p < 0.05$.

Figure 4A,B shows two cases with metabolic response by 18F-FDG PET/CT and CTC assessment before and after 8 weeks of ICI.

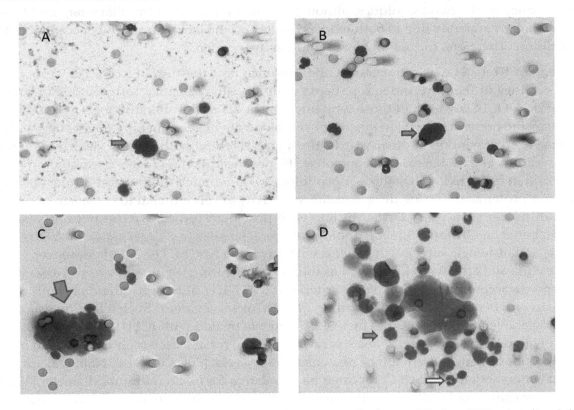

Figure 4.   Comparison of positive (**A–C**) and negative findings (**D**) for CTC visualized by May–Grünwald–Giemsa (MGG) staining at 40× magnification. (**A**) Naked nucleus (without cytoplasm), intensely stained (hypercromatic), with irregular shape and scalloped borders, suspect for carcinoma. The absence of a clearly visible cytoplasm did not permit the evaluation of the nuclear/cytoplasmic ratio. (**B**) The same as the previous image; herein, we can compare the size of the naked nucleus (arrow) with the size of neighboring leukocytes (around 3–4 times bigger). (**C**) A cluster of cells with a high nucleus/cytoplasm ratio, hypercromasia, and irregular shape of nuclei. Additionally, cells were bigger than leukocytes. (**D**) Some of the cells in this sample were degenerated. We did not take into account these cells. The remaining population (for example, the cell indicated by the blue arrow) had a nuclear size somewhat similar to that of leukocytes (yellow arrow). Where cytoplasm was present, it was granular. Thus, all of these cells were probably leukocytes. * CTC = circulating tumor cells; MGG = May–Grünwald–Giemsa.

3. Discussion

Several studies have investigated the prevalence and the prognostic role of CTC in different cancer types, including NSCLC, but only a limited number have analyzed their relationship to 18F-FDG PET/CT parameters [13,16–18]. On the other side, only a few studies have assessed the role of CTC in patients with advanced NSCLC treated with checkpoint inhibitors [19,20]. If we exclude our preliminary data [21], to the best of our knowledge, this research is the first to report a significant association between the CTC count and the tumor 18F-FDG uptake in a similar patient cohort treated with immunotherapy.

In our analysis, CTC were detected in 46% of the patients before the initiation of ICI and in 42% at the first assessment. Our detection rate was superior compared to Tamminga' study [20], that being 32% before ICI and 27% after 4 weeks, where CTC identification was performed by epithelial marker-dependent (CellSearch) technology. Moreover, our finding is consistent with previous studies in lung cancer patients, which demonstrated an overall sensitivity higher for cell size rather than marked-based approaches, although not in an ICI setting [22–26]. Nevertheless, in the abovementioned study from the Italian group [19], using another system based on cell size (i.e., Screencells Cyto), the prevalence of CTC was almost double that of our study (91% vs. 46%) in a larger population ($n = 89$). This discrepancy by the two techniques, although based on the same filter diameter, might suggest a high inter-reader variability due to both readers' skills and the lack of uniformly accepted criteria for CTC definition. Therefore, further and larger studies are needed.

Similar to Krebs et al., in our study, the presence and the number of CTC were influenced by previous lines of therapy. Indeed, patients with a positive history for previous therapy had a mean number of CTC lower than those who underwent ICI as first-line therapy ($p = 0.004$) [7]. As a consequence, the presence of CTC in the peripheral blood after chemotherapy might suggest the grade of response to treatment or, in other words, the aggressiveness of the tumor determining how fast cancer can return after a macroscopic response. Hence, residual CTC after chemotherapy could be characterized in order to identify those morphological or genetic modification-inducing expression of genes and proteins conferring drug-resistance, such as the endothelial to mesenchymal transition observed in cancer stem cells [27,28]. In line with previous studies, we did not find a significant association between CTC and clinicopathological characteristics (e.g., age, gender, tobacco exposure, tumor size, and histologic subtype) in patients with advanced NSCLC [14,29,30]. Moreover, CTC count both at baseline and after 8 weeks, as well as their change during treatment, was not associated with tumor response according to morphologic criteria (RECIST 1.1), although a trend of significance with higher mean number of CTC for the PD group ($p = 0.076$) was evident. Such a finding was consistent with the two abovementioned studies in NSCLC patients treated with ICI [19,20]. Of note, CTC were associated with durable response, defined as no progression for at least 6 months measured by RECIST 1.1, more pronounced than early tumor response at 4–6 weeks [20]. Likewise, Nair et al., prior to any therapeutic intervention for NSCLC, reported no correlation for CTC and tumor diameter [13]. On the other hand, considering EORTC criteria, we showed a significant association between patients with increased CTC and poor metabolic response by 18F-FDG PET/CT at first assessment after 8 weeks of treatment. Similarly, Punnoose and colleagues [15] demonstrated higher levels of CTC in patients classified as non-responders by metabolic criteria, although this was performed in a cohort treated with erlotinib and pertuzumab. Hence, our results confirm on one hand the prevailing cytostatic effect of ICI compared to cytocidal and, on the other, the precocious metabolic changes detected by 18F-FDG that occur earlier than morphologic changes.

We also investigated the relationship between CTC and metabolic 18F-FDG positron emission tomography (PET)-based indexes. Interestingly, we detected a significant association between higher densities of CTC after 8 weeks and metabolic tumor burden, expressed by MTV and TLG (both $p = 0.009$). A significant difference was also found between the number of CTC at 8 weeks and the percentage changes of metabolic volume (i.e., ΔMTV and ΔTLG). These findings suggest, as already stated previously, that the CTC count in the peripheral blood can reflect the entity of the tumor burden and provide valuable information on the metabolic activity, which may serve as a marker of tumor aggressiveness in advanced NSCLC. Hence, as CTC count is a marker of poor response, if our results were confirmed in a larger cohort, CTC along with metabolic indexes would be useful for monitoring disease, allowing for early cessation of treatment with checkpoint inhibitors, and switching to an alternative therapeutic regimen. Because our paper is the first in the era of checkpoint inhibitors investigating CTC and 18F-FDG PET parameters, comparison with other reports is not well applicable. Previously, some studies demonstrated a significant correlation between CTC and SUV value in patients with chemotherapy-naïve lung cancer [12–14,31]. On the contrary, Nygaard et al. did not find any association between metabolic parameters and cell-free (cf) DNA, another tumor-derived biomarker [32].

The presence of CTC is related with survival and is predictive of disease progression and death in NSCLC during chemotherapy and targeted therapies [15,23,29,33–37]. In the present study, CTC count after 8 weeks was significantly associated with PFS and OS, whereas MTV at first restaging was prognostic only for PFS, and showed a trend for OS ($p = 0.072$), in our opinion due to limited sample size. In addition, CTC and MTV were also prognostic factors when considered in conjunction. In this regard, we identified a group characterized by poor PFS presenting with high CTC and high MTV at 8 weeks. Our findings are consistent with the only two abovementioned studies, which explored the prognostic role of CTC in patients receiving ICI [19,20]. Interestingly, Tamminga et al. showed that CTC and cell-free DNA (cfDNA), although at baseline, separately and in conjunction, were significantly associated with OS in NSCLC patients receiving nivolumab [20]. Moreover, CTC count after 8 weeks was predictive for both PFS and OS, along with ΔMTV and ΔSUVmax for PFS and OS, respectively, suggesting that large and highly metabolic tumors could have the potential of shedding a high number of CTC in the bloodstream, increasing the possibility to metastasize at distant sites.

These findings may be particularly interesting for patients in whom no tumor tissue is available for other predictive analysis. On the same line, Fiorelli et al. identified SUVmax as an independent predictor for CTC presence after surgery in NSCLC patients [31].

Nevertheless, our study had some shortcomings. First, a limited sample size, and second, we did not evaluate PD-L1 expression on CTC. Recently, Ilié et al. demonstrated that patients who had PD-L1-negative CTC 6 months after the start of checkpoint inhibitors benefitted from immunotherapy, highlighting CTC as a heterogeneous population worthy of further investigation [33]. Third, we did not investigate the genetic features of CTC, which could open a new frontier in the understanding of therapy resistance. Finally, we did not collect other circulating markers, such as cfDNA, known as potential biomarkers in cancer patients.

4. Materials and Methods

4.1. Patients and Study Design

The current study was conducted following the approval of the local institutional review board and in accordance with the Declaration of Helsinki and Good Clinical Practice guidelines (Prot. Nr. CE Humanitas ex D.M. 8/2/2013 335/17). Written informed consent was obtained in all cases. The trial was registered at www.clinicaltrials.gov (NCT03563482). Between April 2017 and March 2019, 35 patients (23 males, 12 females) affected by metastatic or relapsed NSCLC were referred to our hospital, Humanitas Clinical and Research Center, for treatment with ICI, and were prospectively enrolled. ICI therapy was administered intravenously at a dose of 3 mg/kg every 2 weeks for nivolumab or at a fixed dose of 200 mg every 3 weeks for pembrolizumab.

All patients performed whole-body contrast-enhanced CT, 18F-FDG PET/CT scan, and peripheral blood sample for CTC isolation at baseline and at the first restaging after approximately 8 weeks (after three cycles for pembrolizumab and atezolizumab, and after four cycles for nivolumab). The patients' epidemiologic and clinical characteristics are reported in Table 3.

Table 3. Patients' characteristics at baseline.

Characteristics	N (%)
Patients	35
Median age (range)	77 (51–86)
Gender	
Male	23 (65.7)
Female	12 (34.3)
Smoking status	
Never	5 (14.3)
Former	19 (54.3)
Smoker	11 (31.4)
ECOG PS	
0	18 (51.4)
≥1	17 (48.6)

Table 3. *Cont.*

Characteristics	N (%)
Therapy line	
0	9 (25.7)
1	14 (40)
≥2	12 (34.3)
Metastatic sites	
1–2	16 (45.7)
>2	19 (54.3)
Histology	
Adeno	24 (68.6)
Squamous	7 (20)
Poorly differentiated	34 (8.6)
Sarcomatoid	1 (2.8)
Tumor PD-L1 status	
Negative	7 (20)
Positive	14 (40)
Not evaluable *	14 (40)

* Programmed cell death ligand 1 (PD-L1) could not be evaluated in 14 patients as biopsied material was of insufficient quality or quantity.

4.2. CTC Isolation and Enumeration

For CTC detection, 10 mL of blood was collected in EDTA (ethylenediaminetetraacetic acid) tubes and processed within 2 h on the Isolation by Size of Tumor/Trophoblastic Cells (ISET) platform (Rarecells, Paris, France). Peripheral blood was filtered through the ISET polycarbonate membrane containing 10 filter-spots with calibrated 8 μm diameter cylindrical pores, each spot representing the filtration of 1 mL of blood. The membrane was cut into two parts containing four and six spots per part. Four spots were stained using a freshly made May–Grünwald–Giemsa (MGG) solution according to the technique described by Hofman and colleagues [29] for 5 min with undiluted May–Grünwald, and subsequently for 5 min with 50% diluted May–Grünwald and 40 min in 10% diluted Giemsa, followed by rinsing with water. Membranes were then air-dried and mounted with limonene mounting medium (Sigma-Aldrich, St. Louis, MO, USA) and kept in the dark at room temperature. Stained spots were examined under a light microscopy (Olympus BX51, Olympus Corporation, Shinjuku, Tokyo, Japan) at 10× and subsequently digitized at 40× magnification. All images were analyzed by two cytopathologists blinded to the study data. CTC were recognized on the basis of four cytopathological features: (a) nuclear hyperchromatism, (b) increased nuclear volume, (c) irregular nuclear borders, and (d) increased nucleus-to-cytoplasm ratio. Cells were defined as CTC when all four abovementioned criteria were fulfilled, as previously described by Hofman and colleagues [29]. A dedicated pathologist analyzed and counted CTC present in the membranes (four spots per patient). A panel of features obtainable after magnification is illustrated in Figure 3.

4.3. 18F-FDG PET/CT and Image Analysis

Patients fasted at least 6 h before intravenous administration of 250–500 MBq of fluorodeoxyglucose (FDG) in a quiet room. Images were acquired 60 min after tracer injection using two scanners accredited by EANM Research Ltd. (EARL) program [38]: (a) Siemens Biograph LSO (lutetium oxyorthosilicate) 6 scanner (Siemens Erlangen, Munich, Germany), with an integrated 6-slice CT; and (b) GE Discovery PET/CT 690 (General Electric Healthcare, Waukesha, WI, USA), with an integrated 64-slice CT. Attenuation-correction images were obtained with a low-dose CT (120 kV, 30 mA). Unenhanced low-dose CT was performed at 140 kV and 40 mA for attenuation correction of emission data and anatomic localization of the PET dataset. PET sinograms were reconstructed by means of an ordered-subset expectation maximization iterative reconstruction algorithm (three iterations; eight subsets). Images were displayed on a GE ADW4.6 workstation (GE Healthcare, Waukesha,

WI, USA) and interpreted by two experienced nuclear medicine physicians. From 18F-FDG PET/CT images, the following parameters were measured: SUVmax, SUVmean, MTV, and TLG; MTV was assessed using a PETVCAR (GE Healthcare, Waukesha, WI, USA) workstation and was computed using an SUVmax threshold of 41%; TLG was computed as MTV × SUVmean. Percentage reduction between baseline and restaging was calculated using the formula: [(8 weeks SUVmax − pretreatment SUVmax)/pretreatment SUVmax] × 100 for SUVmax; similarly for the other metabolic parameters.

4.4. Tumor Response Assessment

Early tumor response, after approximately 8 weeks of treatment, was measured using the revised RECIST 1.1 criteria [39]. Four categories were identified: complete response (CR), disappearance of all target lesions; PR, reduction of at least 30% in the sum of diameters of target lesions; PD, increase of at least 20% in the sum of diameters of target lesions or appearance of new lesions; SD, neither CR, nor PR or PD.

Metabolic response was evaluated according to EORTC criteria with the following categories: complete metabolic response (CMR), complete resolution of 18F-FDG uptake within all lesions; PMR, reduction of at least 25% in the sum of SUVmax; PMD, increase of at least 25% in the sum of SUVmax or appearance of new 18F-FDG avid lesions that are typical of cancer and not related to inflammation or infection; SMD, neither CMR, nor PMR or PMD [40].

4.5. Statistical Analysis

Descriptive statistics for clinical, imaging, and pathologic variables were determined using the median (range) or media with SD as appropriate.

Associations of CTC with clinical and metabolic characteristics were studied by means of t-tests and Mann–Whitney U tests for continuous variables and χ^2 tests or Fisher's exact test for categorical variables.

Clinical outcomes were evaluated in terms of PFS, defined as the interval from the date of initiation of ICI to the date of either disease progression or death, and OS calculated as the duration between the date of initiation of immunotherapy and the date of death. For the univariate and multivariate analyses of survival, Cox's proportional hazard model was employed as well as the log-rank test with Kaplan–Meier analysis. All statistical analyses were carried out using the Statistical Package for Social Sciences, version 23.0, for Windows (SPSS, Chicago, IL, USA), and p-values < 0.05 were considered as being statistically significant.

5. Conclusions

In our study, analyzing for the first-time concomitant CTC and metabolic parameters in NSCLC patients receiving ICI, we observed that CTC number was modulated by previous therapeutic interventions. Moreover, the presence of elevated CTC count was an additional prognostic and predictor factor along with metabolic tumor burden. Further large-scaled studies confirming the clinical utility of CTC in combination with metabolic PET-based parameters in this setting are now warranted.

Author Contributions: Conceptualization, E.L., L.T. and A.C.; methodology, A.C., E.L., S.M., F.G.C., S.R., D.F. and L.T.; software, E.L., A.C.; formal analysis, A.C., S.M., F.G.C., D.F.; investigation, E.L., A.C.; resources, E.L., L.T.; data curation, E.L.; writing—original draft preparation, A.C.; writing—review and editing, A.C., E.L., S.M., F.G.C., S.R., D.F. and L.T.; supervision, E.L.; project administration, E.L.; funding acquisition, E.L. All authors have read and agreed to the published version of the manuscript.

Acknowledgments: The Italian Association for Research on Cancer (AIRC—Associazione Italiana per la Ricerca sul Cancro) is acknowledged for the support on this research. ISET machine is available thanks to a grant from LILT (Lega Italiana per la Lotta contro i Tumori). The authors are particularly grateful to the Immunology Research Lab (D. Qehajaj, F. Grizzi) and to the Thoracic Surgery of Humanitas (G. Veronesi, E. Dieci, P. Novellis) for the support on research.

References

1. Chen, D.S.; Mellman, I. Oncology meets immunology: The cancer immunity cycle. *Immunity* **2013**, *39*, 1–10. [CrossRef] [PubMed]

2. Tanaka, F.; Yoneda, K.; Kondo, N.; Hashimoto, M.; Takuwa, T.; Matsumoto, S.; Okumura, Y.; Rahman, S.; Tsubota, N.; Tsujimura, T.; et al. Circulating tumor cell as a diagnostic marker in primary lung cancer. *Clin. Cancer Res.* **2009**, *15*, 6980–6986. [CrossRef] [PubMed]

3. Krebs, M.G.; Metcalf, R.L.; Carter, L.; Brady, G.; Blackhall, F.H.; Dive, C. Molecular analysis of circulating tumour cells-biology and biomarkers. *Nat. Rev. Clin. Oncol.* **2014**, *11*, 129–144. [CrossRef] [PubMed]

4. Hayes, D.F.; Cristofanilli, M.; Budd, G.T.; Ellis, M.J.; Stopeck, A.; Miller, M.C.; Matera, J.; Allard, W.J.; Doyle, G.V.; Terstappen, L.W. Circulating tumor cells at each follow-up time point during therapy of metastatic breast cancer patients predict progression-free and overall survival. *Clin. Cancer Res.* **2006**, *12*, 4218–4224. [CrossRef] [PubMed]

5. Cohen, S.J.; Punt, C.J.; Iannotti, N.; Saidman, B.H.; Sabbath, K.D.; Gabrail, N.Y.; Picus, J.; Morse, M.; Mitchell, E.; Miller, M.C.; et al. Relationship of circulating tumor cells to tumor response, progression-free survival, and overall survival in patients with metastatic colorectal cancer. *J. Clin. Oncol.* **2008**, *26*, 3213–3221. [CrossRef]

6. de Bono, J.S.; Scher, H.I.; Montgomery, R.B.; Parker, C.; Miller, M.C.; Tissing, H.; Doyle, G.V.; Terstappen, L.W.; Pienta, K.J.; Raghavan, D. Circulating tumor cells predict survival benefit from treatment in metastatic castration-resistant prostate cancer. *Clin. Cancer Res.* **2008**, *14*, 6302–6309. [CrossRef]

7. Frick, M.A.; Feigenberg, S.J.; Jean-Baptiste, S.R.; Aguarin, L.A.; Mendes, A.; Chinniah, C.; Swhisher-McClure, S.; Berman, A.; Levin, W.; Cengel, K.; et al. Circulating tumor cells are associated with recurrent disease in patients with early stage non-small cell lung cancer. *Clin. J. Cancer Res.* **2020**. [CrossRef]

8. Hofman, V.; Ilie, M.; Long, E.; Guibert, N.; Selva, E.; Washetine, K.; Mograbi, B.; Mouroux, J.; Vénissac, N.; Reverso-Meinietti, J.; et al. Detection of circulating tumour cells from lung cancer patients in the era of targeted therapy: Promises, drawbacks and pitfalls. *Curr. Mol. Med.* **2014**, *14*, 440–456. [CrossRef]

9. Paesmans, M.; Berghmans, T.; Dusart, M.; Garcia, C.; Hossein-Foucher, C.; Lafitte, J.J.; Mascaux, C.; Meert, A.P.; Roelandts, M.; Scherpereel, A.; et al. Primary tumor standardized uptake value measured on fluorodeoxyglucose positron emission tomography is of prognostic value for survival in non-small cell lung cancer: Update of a systematic review and meta-analysis by the European Lung Cancer Working Party for the International Association for the Study of Lung Cancer Staging Project. *J. Thorac. Oncol.* **2010**, *5*, 612–619.

10. Sharma, A.; Mohan, A.; Bhalla, A.S.; Vishnubhatla, S.; Pandey, A.K.; Bal, C.S.; Kumar, R. Role of various semiquantitative parameters of 18F-FDG PET/CT studies for interim treatment response evaluation in non-small-cell lung cancer. *Nucl. Med. Commun.* **2017**, *38*, 858–867. [CrossRef]

11. Huang, W.; Fan, M.; Liu, B.; Fu, Z.; Zhou, T.; Zhang, Z.; Gong, H.; Li, B. Value of metabolic tumor volume on repeated 18F-FDG PET/CT for early prediction of survival in locally advanced non-small cell lung cancer treated with concurrent chemoradiotherapy. *J. Nucl. Med.* **2014**, *55*, 1584–1590. [CrossRef] [PubMed]

12. Morbelli, S.; Alama, A.; Ferrarazzo, G.; Coco, S.; Genova, C.; Rijavec, E.; Bongioanni, F.; Biello, F.; Dal Bello, M.G.; Barletta, G.; et al. Circulating Tumor DNA Reflects Tumor Metabolism Rather Than Tumor Burden in Chemotherapy-Naive Patients with Advanced Non-Small Cell Lung Cancer: 18F-FDG PET/CT Study. *J. Nucl. Med.* **2017**, *58*, 1764–1769. [CrossRef] [PubMed]

13. Nair, V.S.; Keu, K.V.; Luttgen, M.S.; Kolatkar, A.; Vasanawala, M.; Kuschner, W.; Iagaru, A.H.; Hoh, C.; Shrager, J.B.; Loo, B.W., Jr.; et al. An observational study of circulating tumor cells and 18F-FDG PET uptake in patients with treatment-naive non-small cell lung cancer. *PLoS ONE* **2013**, *8*, e67733. [CrossRef] [PubMed]

14. Bayarri-Lara, C.I.; de Miguel Pérez, D.; Cueto Ladrón de Guevara, A.; Rodriguez Fernández, A.; Puche, J.L.; Sánchez-Palencia Ramos, A.; Ruiz Zafra, J.; Giraldo Ospina, C.F.; Delgado-Rodríguez, M.; Expósito Ruiz, M.; et al. Association of circulating tumour cells with early relapse and 18F-fluorodeoxyglucose positron emission tomography uptake in resected non-small-cell lung cancers. *Eur. J. Cardiothorac. Surg.* **2017**, *52*, 55–62. [CrossRef]

15. Punnoose, E.A.; Atwal, S.; Liu, W.; Raja, R.; Fine, B.M.; Hughes, B.G.; Hicks, R.J.; Hampton, G.M.; Amler, L.C.; Pirzkall, A.; et al. Evaluation of circulating tumor cells and circulating tumor DNA in non-small cell lung cancer: Association with clinical endpoints in a phase II clinical trial of pertuzumab and erlotinib. *Clin. Cancer Res.* **2012** *18*, 2391–2401. [CrossRef]

16. Cristofanilli, M.; Budd, G.T.; Ellis, M.J.; Stopeck, A.; Matera, J.; Miller, M.C.; Reuben, J.M.; Doyle, G.V.; Allard, W.J.; Terstappen, L.W.; et al. Circulating tumor cells, disease progression, and survival in metastatic breast cancer. *N. Engl. J. Med.* **2004**, *351*, 781–791. [CrossRef]

17. Huang, X.; Gao, P.; Song, Y.; Sun, J.; Chen, X.; Zhao, J.; Xu, H.; Wang, Z. Meta-analysis of the prognostic value of circulating tumor cells detected with the CellSearch System in colorectal cancer. *BMC Cancer* **2015**, *15*, 202. [CrossRef]

18. Scher, H.I.; Heller, G.; Molina, A.; Attard, G.; Danila, D.C.; Jia, X.; Peng, W.; Sandhu, S.K.; Olmos, D.; Riisnaes, R.; et al. Circulating tumor cell biomarker panel as an individual-level surrogate for survival in metastatic castration-resistant prostate cancer. *J. Clin. Oncol.* **2015**, *33*, 1348–1355. [CrossRef]

19. Alama, A.; Coco, S.; Genova, C.; Rossi, G.; Fontana, V.; Tagliamento, M.; Giovanna Dal Bello, M.; Rosa, A.; Boccardo, S.; Rijavec, E.; et al. Prognostic Relevance of Circulating Tumor Cells and Circulating Cell-Free DNA Association in Metastatic Non-Small Cell Lung Cancer Treated with Nivolumab. *J. Clin. Med.* **2019**, *8*, 1011. [CrossRef]

20. Tamminga, M.; de Wit, S.; Hiltermann, T.J.N.; Timens, W.; Schuuring, E.; Terstappen, L.W.M.M.; Groen, H.J.M. Circulating tumor cells in advanced non-small cell lung cancer patients are associated with worse tumor response to checkpoint inhibitors. *J. Immunother. Cancer.* **2019**, *7*, 173. [CrossRef]

21. Monterisi, S.; Castello, A.; Toschi, L.; Federico, D.; Rossi, S.; Veronesi, G.; Lopci, E. preliminary data on circulating tumor cells in metastatic NSCLC patients candidate to immunotherapy. *Am. J. Nucl. Med. Mol. Imaging* **2019**, *9*, 282–295. [PubMed]

22. Hofman, V.; Ilie, M.I.; Long, E.; Selva, E.; Bonnetaud, C.; Molina, T.; Vénissac, N.; Mouroux, J.; Vielh, P.; Hofman, P. Detection of circulating tumor cells as a prognostic factor in patients undergoing radical surgery for non-small-cell lung carcinoma: Comparison of the efficacy of the CellSearch Assay™ and the isolation by size of epithelial tumor cell method. *Int. J. Cancer* **2011**, *129*, 1651–1660. [CrossRef] [PubMed]

23. Krebs, M.G.; Hou, J.M.; Sloane, R.; Lancashire, L.; Priest, L.; Nonaka, D.; Ward, T.H.; Backen, A.; Clack, G.; Hughes, A. Analysis of circulating tumor cells in patients with non-small cell lung cancer using epithelial marker-dependent and -independent approaches. *J. Thorac. Oncol.* **2012**, *7*, 306–315. [CrossRef]

24. Pailler, E.; Adam, J.; Barthélémy, A.; Oulhen, M.; Auger, N.; Valent, A.; Ward, T.H.; Backen, A.; Clack, G.; Hughes, A.; et al. Detection of circulating tumor cells harboring a unique ALK rearrangement in ALK-positive non-small-cell lung cancer. *J. Clin. Oncol.* **2013**, *31*, 2273–2281. [CrossRef]

25. Farace, F.; Massard, C.; Vimond, N.; Drusch, F.; Jacques, N.; Billiot, F.; Laplanche, A.; Chauchereau, A.; Lacroix, L.; Planchard, D.; et al. A direct comparison of CellSearch and ISET for circulating tumour-cell detection in patients with metastatic carcinomas. *Br. J. Cancer* **2011**, *105*, 847–853. [CrossRef] [PubMed]

26. Illie, M.; Szafer-Glusman, E.; Hofman, V.; Long-Mira, E.; Suttmann, R.; Darbonne, W.; Butori, C.; Lalvée, S.; Fayada, J.; Selva, E.; et al. Expression of MET in circulating tumor cells correlates with expression in tumor from advanced-stage lung cancer patients. *Oncotarget* **2017**, *8*, 26112–26121. [CrossRef] [PubMed]

27. Shibue, T.; Weinberg, R.A. EMT, CSCs, and drug resistance: The mechanistic link and clinical implications. *Nat. Rev. Clin. Oncol.* **2017**, *14*, 611–629. [CrossRef]

28. Lecharpentier, A.; Vielh, P.; Perez-Moreno, P.; Planchard, D.; Soria, J.C.; Farace, F. Detection of circulating tumour cells with a hybrid (epithelial/mesenchymal) phenotype in patients with metastatic non-small cell lung cancer. *Br. J. Cancer* **2011**, *105*, 1338–1341. [CrossRef]

29. Hofman, V.; Bonnetaud, C.; Ilie, M.I.; Vielh, P.; Vignaud, J.M.; Fléjou, J.F.; Lantuejoul, S.; Piaton, E.; Mourad, N.; Butori, C.; et al. Preoperative circulating tumor cell detection using the isolation by size of epithelial tumor cell method for patients with lung cancer is a new prognostic biomarker. *Clin. Cancer Res.* **2011**, *17*, 827–835. [CrossRef]

30. Zhang, Z.; Xiao, Y.; Zhao, J.; Chen, M.; Xu, Y.; Zhong, W.; Xing, J.; Wang, M. Relationship between circulating tumour cell count and prognosis following chemotherapy in patients with advanced non-small-cell lung cancer. *Respirology* **2016**, *21*, 519–525. [CrossRef]

31. Fiorelli, A.; Accardo, M.; Carelli, E.; Angioletti, D.; Santini, M.; Di Domenico, M. Circulating tumor cells in diagnosing lung cancer: Clinical and mophological analysis. *Ann. Thorac. Surg.* **2015**, *99*, 1899–1905. [CrossRef] [PubMed]

32. Nygaard, A.D.; Holdgaard, P.C.; Spindler, K.L.; Pallisgaard, N.; Jakobsen, A. The correlation between cell-free DNA and tumour burden was estimated by PET/CT in patients with advanced NSCLC. *Br. J. Cancer* **2014**, *110*, 363–368. [CrossRef] [PubMed]

33.   Ilié, M.; Szafer-Glusman, E.; Hofman, V.; Chamorey, E.; Lalvée, S.; Selva, E.; Leroy, S.; Marquette, C.H.; Kowanetz, M.; Hedge, P.; et al. Detection of PD-L1 in circulating tumor cells and white blood cells from patients with advanced non-small-cell lung cancer. *Ann. Oncol.* **2018**, *29*, 193–199. [CrossRef] [PubMed]

34.   de Wit, S.; van Dalum, G.; Lenferink, A.T.M.; Tibbe, A.G.J.; Hiltermann, T.J.N.; Groen, H.J.M.; van Rijn, C.J.; Terstappen, L.W. The detection of EpCAM+ and EpCAM− circulating tumor cells. *Sci. Rep.* **2015**, *5*, 12270. [CrossRef] [PubMed]

35.   Muinelo-Romay, L.; Vieito, M.; Abalo, A.; Nocelo, M.A.; Barón, F.; Anido, U.; Brozos, E.; Vázquez, F.; Aguín, S.; Abal, M. Evaluation of circulating tumor cells and related events as prognostic factors and surrogate biomarkers in advanced NSCLC patients receiving first-line systemic treatment. *Cancers* **2014**, *6*, 153–165. [CrossRef] [PubMed]

36.   Juan, O.; Vidal, J.; Gisbert, R.; Muñoz, J.; Maciá, S.; Gómez-Codina, J. Prognostic significance of circulating tumor cells in advanced non-small cell lung cancer patients treated with docetaxel and gemcitabine. *Clin. Transl. Oncol.* **2014**, *16*, 637–643. [CrossRef]

37.   Krebs, M.G.; Sloane, R.; Priest, L.; Lancashire, L.; Hou, J.-M.J.M.; Greystoke, A.; Ward, T.H.; Ferraldeschi, R.; Hughes, A.; Clack, G.; et al. Evaluation and prognostic significance of circulating tumor cells in patients with non-small-cell lung cancer. *J. Clin. Oncol.* **2011**, *29*, 1556–1563. [CrossRef]

38.   Boellaard, R.; Delgado-Bolton, R.; Oyen, W.J.; Giammarile, F.; Tatsch, K.; Eschner, W.; Verzijlbergen, F.J.; Barrington, S.F.; Pike, L.C.; Weber, W.A.; et al. FDG PET/CT: EANM procedure guidelines for tumour imaging: Version 2.0. *Eur. J. Nucl. Med. Mol. Imaging* **2015**, *42*, 328–354. [CrossRef]

39.   Eisenhauer, E.; Therasse, P.; Bogaerts, J.; Schwartz, L.H.; Sargent, D.; Ford, R.; Dancey, J.; Arbuck, S.; Gwyther, S.; Mooney, M.; et al. New response evaluation criteria in solid tumours: Revised RECIST guideline (version 1.1). *Eur. J. Cancer* **2009**, *45*, 228–247. [CrossRef]

40.   Young, H.; Baum, R.; Cremerius, U.; Herholz, K.; Hoekstra, O.; Lammertsma, A.A.; Pruim, J.; Price, P. Measurement of clinical and subclinical tumour response using [18F]-fluorodeoxyglucose and positron emission tomography: Review and 1999 EORTC recommendations. European Organization for Research and Treatment of Cancer (EORTC) PET Study Group. *Eur. J. Cancer.* **1999**, *35*, 1773–1782. [CrossRef]

5

Multiparametric MRI for Prostate Cancer Detection: New Insights into the Combined Use of a Radiomic Approach with Advanced Acquisition Protocol

Serena Monti [1], Valentina Brancato [1,*], Giuseppe Di Costanzo [2], Luca Basso [1], Marta Puglia [2], Alfonso Ragozzino [2], Marco Salvatore [1] and Carlo Cavaliere [1]

[1] IRCCS SDN, 80143 Naples, Italy; smonti@sdn-napoli.it (S.M.); lbasso@sdn-napoli.it (L.B.); direzionescientifica@sdn-napoli.it (M.S.); ccavaliere@sdn-napoli.it (C.C.)

[2] Ospedale S. Maria delle Grazie, 80078 Pozzuoli, Italy; giupe7700@yahoo.it (G.D.C.); martapuglia@alice.it (M.P.); alfonsoragozzino@gmail.com (A.R.)

*   Correspondence: vbrancato@sdn-napoli.it

Abstract: Prostate cancer (PCa) is a disease affecting an increasing number of men worldwide. Several efforts have been made to identify imaging biomarkers to non-invasively detect and characterize PCa, with substantial improvements thanks to multiparametric Magnetic Resonance Imaging (mpMRI). In recent years, diffusion kurtosis imaging (DKI) was proposed to be directly related to tissue physiological and pathological characteristic, while the radiomic approach was proven to be a key method to study cancer imaging phenotypes. Our aim was to compare a standard radiomic model for PCa detection, built using T2-weighted (T2W) and Apparent Diffusion Coefficient (ADC), with an advanced one, including DKI and quantitative Dynamic Contrast Enhanced (DCE), while also evaluating differences in prediction performance when using 2D or 3D lesion segmentation. The obtained results in terms of diagnostic accuracy were high for all of the performed comparisons, reaching values up to 0.99 for the area under a receiver operating characteristic curve (AUC), and 0.98 for both sensitivity and specificity. In comparison, the radiomic model based on standard features led to prediction performances higher than those of the advanced model, while greater accuracy was achieved by the model extracted from 3D segmentation. These results provide new insights into active topics of discussion, such as choosing the most convenient acquisition protocol and the most appropriate postprocessing pipeline to accurately detect and characterize PCa.

Keywords: prostate cancer; PI-RADS; radiomics; magnetic resonance imaging; diffusion kurtosis imaging; dynamic contrast-enhanced magnetic resonance imaging

1. Introduction

Prostate cancer (PCa) is the second most common malignant neoplasm among men [1]. The early detection and grading of PCa are crucial for patient management and long-term survival evaluation.

The prostate cancer screening paradigm commonly consists of a serum prostate-specific antigen (PSA) test, a digital rectal examination, a transrectal ultrasound, and prostatic biopsies, but each of these methods has its disadvantages, spanning from low accuracy, i.e., when PSA is used alone, to invasiveness, i.e., in transrectal examinations or biopsies.

Recently, the use of a multiparametric Magnetic Resonance Imaging (mpMRI) approach, combining anatomic T1 or T2-weighted (T2W) images with functional MRI methods as Diffusion Weighted Imaging (DWI) and Dynamic Contrast Enhanced (DCE) imaging, provided substantial improvements in non-invasive prostate cancer detection and characterization [2–4]. In fact, the imaging approach, besides its non-invasiveness, can give "in vivo" information on the entire tumor volume, thereby reducing inaccuracies due to sampling errors in histopathological analyses.

The Prostate Imaging-Reporting and Data System (PI-RADS) was developed in 2013, and then updated in 2015 (PI-RADS v2) [5], in order to standardize the use of mpMRI in PCa imaging. This technology provides a scale indicating how likely an mpMRI finding from T2W, DWI, and DCE is related to a clinically significant cancer. The PI-RADS score ranges from one, which indicates a very low probability of malignancy, to five, which indicates a very high probability that a lesion is malignant. Since its introduction, the PI-RADS classification has played a very important role in PCa diagnosis [6], proving to be a useful tool for the detection of prostatic lesions and their characterization in terms of aggressiveness. However, due to its definition, PI-RADS scoring can be affected by subjectivity and inter-/intra-operator variability [7], which are factors that may compromise PCa assessment. Moreover, it is not unusual to find benign and malignant lesions with similar imaging findings, making it challenging to detect the nature of prostatic lesions [8]. It should also be considered that lesions classified as having a PI-RADS score of three are usually lesions termed as "intermediate" or "equivocal on the presence of clinically significant cancer" [9]. The abovementioned limitations of PI-RADS, together with an ever-growing volume of medical images for each patient and the development of increasingly powerful image acquisition and processing techniques, have led to an increasing interest in new quantitative approaches to analyze mpMRI images [10].

In particular, non-Gaussian diffusion models were proposed to better describe diffusion signal behaviors, which are directly related to tissue physiological and pathological characteristics, and to overcome the possible limitation of standard DWI. One of the most used models in the field of prostate cancer is diffusion kurtosis imaging (DKI), although this technique requires more advanced MRI sequences, longer acquisition time, and specific postprocessing tools compared with standard DWI. DKI parameters, namely, the diffusion coefficient D and the deviation from normal distribution coefficient K, proved to be very useful for PCa detection and characterization [11–14].

On the other hand, a radiomic approach proved to be a key method to study cancer imaging phenotypes, reflecting underlying clinical and pathological information, as well as gene expression patterns [15–18]. Radiomics, in fact, refers to the extraction of a large number of quantitative features from medical images [19], thereby revealing heterogeneous tumor metabolism and anatomy [20,21]. This high-throughput extraction is preparatory to a process of data mining [17] for studies of associations with or predictions of different clinical outcomes [22], thereby giving important prognostic information about disease. The potential of radiomics to extensively characterize intratumoral heterogeneity has shown promise regarding the prediction of treatment responses and outcomes, differentiating benign and malignant tumors, and assessing genetic relationships in many cancer types [23,24].

Several radiomic studies were performed to discriminate PCa from noncancerous tissues, to differentiate between cancers with different Gleason scores, and also to compare radiomic diagnostic capabilities with those of PI-RADS scores [8,25–28]. All of these studies computed radiomic features from standard mpMRI acquisition, including T2W, Apparent Diffusion Coefficient (ADC) computed from a classical Gaussian diffusion model, and eventually DCE images. Feature extraction starting from 2D regions of interest (ROIs) was performed in some of these studies, while 3D volumes of interest (VOI) was utilized in others. Only few works, to the best of our knowledge, applied radiomic approach to DKI imaging; Wang et al. [29] investigated whether radiomic features extracted from T2W, ADC, D, K, and the quantitative perfusion parameter K^{trans} could help to improve the diagnostic performance of structured PI-RADS v2 in clinically relevant PCa. In the study by Hectors et al. [30], radiomics features extracted from T2W, ADC, and DKI maps were correlated with Gleason score, gene expression signatures and cancer-related gene expression levels. Toivonen et al. [31] developed and evaluated a classification system for Gleason score predictions using radiomics features from T2W, DWI, and DKI. However, none of these fully investigated the added value of combining the complex radiomic processing approach with the advanced DKI mathematical model for PCa detection.

The aim of our study was to fully investigate this issue. We obtained mpMRI radiomic signatures to discriminate between 4–5 PI-RADS PCa and healthy tissue (HT) in a standard model, computed using T2W and ADC alone, and using more advanced technology, which included using DKI and quantitative DCE pharmacokinetic parameters [32]. Besides comparing the accuracies obtained by these two radiomic signatures, we also evaluated the differences found in prediction performances when using 2D ROIs or 3D VOIs.

2. Results

First and second order radiomic features (described in detail in the Materials and Methods section) were extracted from T2W, ADC, DKI, and quantitative DCE pharmacokinetic parameters (volume transfer constant from the plasma compartment to the extravascular extracellular space, K^{trans}; rate constant for transfer between the extravascular extracellular space and the blood compartment, K_{ep}; volume of extravascular extracellular space per unit volume of tissue, v_e; the initial area under the enhancement curve, iAUC).

The initial sets of features were composed of 120 features for two of the three analyzed classification tasks, i.e., PI-RADS 4–5 vs. HT on 3D VOI in the advanced model (adv3D), which was computed using first order features from T2W, ADC, D, K, and quantitative DCE pharmacokinetic parameters, and PI-RADS 4–5 vs. HT on 2D ROI in the advanced model (adv2D). The third feature set was composed of 44 features for the classification task PI-RADS 4–5 vs. HT on 3D VOI in the standard model (std3D), which was computed using first and second order features from T2W and ADC.

Considering that, for a single patient, more than one segmentation can be obtained, i.e., both lesion and HT can be obtained from the same prostate and more lesions or more healthy regions in the same subject, a total of 118 3D VOIs were segmented (69 PCa and 49 HT); correspondingly, 118 2D ROIs were extracted.

For each classification task, a reduced feature set was computed according to a stepwise forward feature selection scheme. Each feature set, as reported in Table 1, was composed of the 25 top-ranked features in the gain equation.

Table 1. Reduced feature set for each classification task. For each feature, the image from which it was extracted is indicated. For std3D, whether it is a first or second order feature and the feature name are also indicated. Abbreviations: T2W = T2-weighted; ADC = Apparent Diffusion Coefficient; D = diffusion coefficient of Diffusion Kurtosis Imaging (DKI) model; K = deviation from normal distribution coefficient; iAUC = initial area under the enhancement curve; v_e = volume of extravascular extracellular space per unit volume of tissue; K_{ep} = ; K^{trans} = ; Max = maximum; Mad = mean absolute deviation; Min = minimum; Rms = root mean square; Std = standard deviation; GLCM = Gray Level Co-occurrence Matrix.

adv3D	adv2D	std3D
D—Mean	ADC—Rms	ADC—Mean
D—Energy	T2W—Energy	ADC—Energy
iAUC—Median	K^{trans}—Median	ADC—GLCM Auto Correlation
v_e—Min	T2—Std	ADC—Max
T2W—Max	K—Mad	ADC—Min
K—Mad	K—Std	T2W—Max
ADC—Max	D—Max	T2W—Std
ADC—Min	T2W—Max	T2W—Mean
T2W—Std	ADC—Energy	ADC—Rms
K—Std	D—Mean	ADC—Median
ADC—Energy	ADC—Max	T2W—Variance
K—Variance	D—Energy	T2W—Energy

Table 1. *Cont.*

adv3D	adv2D	std3D
T2W—Variance	T2W—Variance	T2W—Rms
T2W—Rms	K—Variance	ADC—GLCM Sum Average
D—Max	D—Rms	T2W—Median
D—Min	D—Median	T2W—Mad
T2—Mad	ADC—Mean	T2W—GLCM Correlation
K_{ep}—Median	T2W—Mean	ADC—Skewness
T2W—Energy	K—Rms	T2W—GLCM Homogeneity
T2W—Mean	ADC—Median	T2W—Uniformity
D—Rms	T2W—Mad	T2—Entropy
K^{trans}—Min	K^{trans}—Mean	T2—GLCM Dissimilarity
K^{trans}—Mean	T2W—Median	T2—Min
D—Median	iAUC—Median	ADC—Uniformity
ADC—Mean	T2W—Rms	ADC—GLCM Correlation

For each reduced feature set, multivariable logistic regression models of order from 1 to 10 were obtained and their prediction performances for the different classification tasks are reported in Figures 1 and 2, where the comparisons between adv3D/adv2D and adv3D/std3D are shown, respectively.

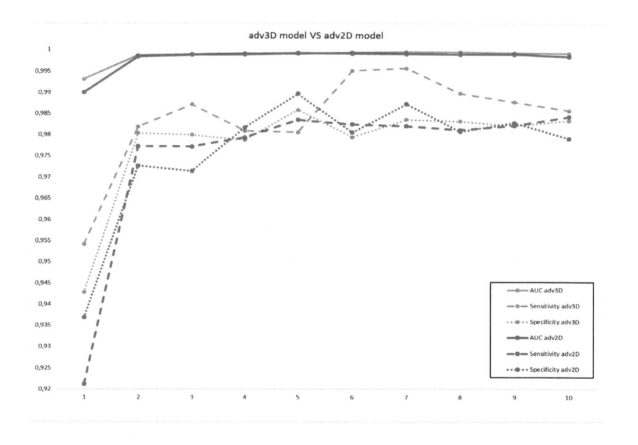

Figure 1. Area under the receiver operating characteristics curve (AUC) (full line), sensitivity (dashed line), and specificity (dotted line) of the multivariable models for adv3D (in blue) and adv2D (in red), for model orders from 1 to 10.

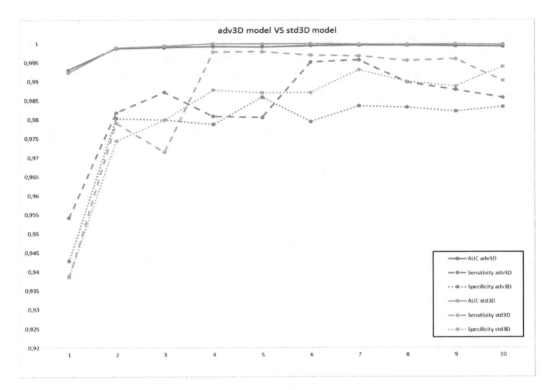

Figure 2. Area under the receiver operating characteristics curve (AUC) (full line), sensitivity (dashed line), and specificity (dotted line) of the multivariable models for adv3D (in blue) and std3D (in yellow), for model orders from 1 to 10.

By inspecting the curves in Figures 1 and 2, very similar and good results were obtained by the three classification models. In more detail, from the comparison between the adv3D and adv2D comparable results in terms of AUC, the sensitivity was higher for adv3D, except for model order 5; this was in contrast with specificity, which was higher on average for adv2D. On the other hand, the comparison between adv3D and std3D highlighted higher results for std3D, except for low order models.

For adv3D, the best model was order 7 based on the T2W mean, Max, Mad, Rms, ADC energy, Min, and K variance. Order 5 was chosen for adv2D based on T2W Mad, ADC mean, median, energy, and K^{trans} median. Finally, order 4 was selected for std3D based on T2W mean and Min, ADC energy, and Min.

3. Discussion

In this work, the added value of combining the radiomic processing approach with the advanced DKI mathematical model for PCa detection was investigated. The main aim was to compare a standard radiomic model built using T2W and ADC with an advanced one which included DKI and quantitative DCE pharmacokinetic parameters in terms of PCa diagnostic accuracy. In addition, we evaluated the differences found in prediction performances when using 2D ROIs or 3D VOIs.

The obtained results of AUC, sensitivity, and specificity were extremely high for all the classification tasks tested (PI-RADS 4–5 vs. HT on adv3D, PI-RADS 4–5 vs. HT on adv2D, and PI-RADS 4–5 vs. HT on std3D), reaching values up to 0.99 for AUC and 0.98 for both sensitivity and specificity. These performances were comparable to those obtained by Chen et al. [27] in their logistic regression model, which was built by incorporating T2W sequences and ADC maps to classify PCa vs. non-PCa tissues. However, in their work, Chen et al. included also shape features, which were deliberately not considered in our models in order to avoid possible biases in feature values introduced by the delineation of HT VOI/ROI which did not follow anatomical boundaries, as in the case of tumor lesions.

Looking at the variables included in the best predictive model chosen for each classification task, the recurrence of ADC energy as a common feature was observed. Interestingly, this index of tumor heterogeneity was previously found to be a promising quantitative imaging biomarker for characterizing cancer imaging phenotypes, since it was associated with tumor gene expression, tumor metabolism, tumor stage, patient prognosis, and treatment response in several studies on different cancer types [33].

To the best of our knowledge, only a few previous works [29–31] performed radiomic studies on prostate cancer, including DKI model parameters, to detect clinically relevant PCa and to evaluate PCa aggressiveness. Even though a direct comparison is not directly applicable, considering the different populations and imaging approaches, some parallels can be carefully drawn with the work by Wang et al. [29], which partially shared our aim and also considered the Toft perfusion model. Those authors found that the best ranked features for PCa detection were extracted from D and K, while pharmacokinetic features were not highly ranked in their classification model. Similarly, in our adv3D model, the majority of the best ranked features (see Table 1) were extracted from DKI and ADC (which was not included in the models by Wang et al. [29]), while few features were derived from the Toft parameters.

In this study, looking in particular at the comparison between standard and advanced models, radiomic approaches based on a standard feature set (T2w and ADC) led to a predictive model with higher AUC, sensitivity, and specificity values than those of the predictive model based on the advanced feature set. It should be noted that the DKI and DCE features, even though they contributed to the features set after the first reduction step, survived only to a minor extent in the final selected models and minimally contributed K variance in the adv3D model and K^{trans} median in the adv2D model. These results suggest that the inclusion of radiomic features derived from DCE and DKI models does not provide a clear added value for PCa detection. On one hand, this would justify the choice to exclude DCE from dominant sequences for PI-RADSv2 score assessment, which is still a topic of discussion [34–36]; on the other hand, this would be food for thought regarding the complex debate of the financial benefits of including time- and computational-demanding DKI acquisition in prostate mpMRI acquisition protocol [14]. Regarding the comparison of the 3D and 2D advanced models, high diagnostic performances were shown by both advanced models, although the sensitivity was slightly lower and the specificity higher for the model built using 2D ROI, even though the resulting AUCs were similar and above 0.99, thereby suggesting great accuracy for the quantitative parameters extracted from VOI. This confirmed the hypothesis that tridimensional regions of interest allow for a more complete description of the lesion [37] and increased the number of points included in the statistical feature computation, thereby leading to results that were, in principle, more reliable and less vulnerable to sampling errors [38].

Our study presents several limitations. First of all, even if the lesions selected as PI-RADS 4–5 were confirmed during biopsy, uncertainty in histological radiological correlations may still remain when determining HT VOIs performed on the basis of radiological images. Such uncertainties could be ruled out using MR-guided biopsy techniques, which could adopt the advantages of new technologies, such as 3D printing, and could be used to develop personalized mold from diagnostic images to obtain histopathological slices exactly corresponding to the acquired slice in mpMRI, as an example [39]. In addition, due to the small sample size (< 100 cases), we could not evaluate the prediction accuracy for a nonbinary classification task (i.e., the additional inclusion of PI-RADS 3 lesions), neither could we test the reproducibility of the proposed method in a separate validation group of patients.

4. Materials and Methods

4.1. Patient Cohort

The study was approved by the Institutional Review Board (9/19). All mpMRI data acquired from March 2017 to August 2018 from a single center were retrospectively checked. A total of 65 patients were selected according to the following inclusion criteria: PI-RADS 4–5 at mpMRI, PSA > 4 ng/mL, age older than 18 years at the time of the study, and available results of biopsy. Exclusion criteria included inadequate MR images and unbiopsied lesions.

4.2. MR Imaging

mpMRI examinations were performed on a 3T Biograph mMR (Siemens Healthcare, Erlangen, Germany) with a body surface coil. The imaging protocols included a T2W (Repetition Time [TR] = 4010 ms, Echo Time [TE] = 112 ms, in plane field of view [FOV] = 200×200 mm^2, number of slices = 26, resolution = 0.6×0.6 mm2, slice thickness = 3 mm), DWI (TR = 7000 ms, TE = 86 ms, in plane FOV = 260×220 mm^2, number of slices = 26, resolution = 2×2 mm^2, slice thickness = 3 mm, b values = 0, 250, 500 (4 averages), 1000, 1500 (6 averages), 2000, 2500 (8 averages) s/mm^2), 6 gradient echo Volumetric Interpolated Breath-hold Examination (VIBE) sequences at variable flip angles (FAs) for T1 mapping (TR = 5.58 ms, TE = 1.83 ms, FAs = ($2°, 5°, 8°, 12°, 15°, 20°$), in plane FOV = $243 \times 260 \times 80$ mm^3, slice gap 20%, resolution = $1.4 \times 1.4 \times 3.0$ mm^3), and a dynamic scan with 60 consecutives phases with a VIBE sequence (TR = 5.58 ms, TE = 1.83 ms, FA = 20°, FOV = $243 \times 260 \times 80$ mm^3, resolution = $1.4 \times 1.4 \times 3.0$ mm^3, temporal resolution = 9 s/phase). Intravenous contrast injections started at the end of the first phase of dynamic scan at a dose of 0.1 mmol/kg of body weight and at the highest rate compatible with the patient's age and compliance (up to 5 mL/s)

4.3. PI-RADS

The PI-RADS assignment was performed by two radiologists experienced in urogenital imaging. They inspected, in consensus, T2W, DWI, ADC maps, and DCE images in order to identify prostatic lesions in accordance to PI-RADS v2 guidelines [40]. Of the PI-RADS 4 and PI-RADS 5 lesions, 100% were confirmed to be cancer on biopsy.

4.4. ADC and DKI Maps Calculation

ADC maps were computed using the in-line software of the Biograph scanner, selecting b-values from 0 to 1500. DKI maps, i.e., D and K, were computed using a voxel-wise fitting procedure implemented in Matlab (The MathWorks Inc., Natick, MA, USA).

4.5. Pharmacokinetic Map Calculation

Pharmacokinetic maps were obtained with the commercial software Tissue 4D (Siemens Healthcare, Erlangen, Germany). After an automated step of motion correction of the VIBE sequences at variable FAs with the dynamic VIBE sequence, the Toft model [41] was chosen for pharmacokinetic parameter calculations. The arterial input function (AIF) used for the analysis was set to "intermediate", on the basis of population-based AIFs built in Tissue 4D. Finally, 3D maps of K^{trans}, K_{ep}, v_e, and iAUC were obtained [23].

4.6. Image Preprocessing

Before feature extraction, some preprocessing steps were performed for each subject, i.e., the image acquired at b = 0 was non-rigidly coregistered to the T2W image in order to correct for spatial distortion typical of DWI acquisition. The registration was performed using the Elastix software (v. 4.9.0 [42]), and the resulting transform was used to warp the volumes acquired at the other b-values and the corresponding ADC, D, and K maps. In addition, K^{trans}, K_{ep}, v_e, and iAUC maps were resampled to match the resolution of the T2W image.

4.7. VOI/ROI Segmentation

3D VOI segmentations were manually obtained. Two experienced radiologists were asked to consensually draw the 3D VOI in the biopsied lesions with PI-RADS 4–5 and in HT on T2W images, while also looking at the b = 1000 coregistered volume. During the segmentation procedure, the radiologists were blinded to both the histological results and all clinical information relative to the retrospective prostate MR images. The segmentation was done using in-house developed software for region labeling. The 2D ROIs were automatically obtained in Matlab from 3D VOIs, with the 2D section with the longest major axis chosen for each.

4.8. Feature Extraction

The first order features were extracted from T2W, ADC, D, K, K^{trans}, K_{ep}, v_e, and iAUC for the 3D VOIs and 2D ROIs. First, each image was normalized, limiting its dynamics within the segmentation to $\mu \pm 3\sigma$ [43], then 13 first order features were extracted from the intensity histogram computed on 256 bins, namely, energy, entropy, kurtosis, maximum (Max), mean, mean absolute deviation (Mad), median, minimum (Min), root mean square (Rms), skewness, standard deviation (Std), uniformity, and variance.

In addition, second order features were also computed for the T2W and ADC images. Gray Level Co-occurrence Matrix (GLCM) [44], which was computed by 3D analysis of the tumor region with 26-voxel connectivity, was chosen, simultaneously taking into account the neighboring properties of the voxels in all 3D directions [45] after image quantization on 32 grey levels. The obtained features included energy, contrast, entropy, homogeneity, correlation, sum average, variance, dissimilarity, and auto correlation.

4.9. Multivariable Analysis

Three classification tasks were analyzed: PI-RADS 4–5 vs. HT on 3D VOI in the adv3D, which was computed using first order features from T2W, ADC, D, K, K^{trans}, K_{ep}, v_e, and iAUC, PI-RADS 4–5 vs. HT on 2D ROI in the adv2D, and PI-RADS 4–5 vs. HT on 3D VOI in the std3D, which was computed using the first and second order features from T2W and ADC.

The multivariable predictive models were obtained following the method described by Vallières et al. [45], using an imbalance-adjusted bootstrap resampling (IABR) on 1000 samples at each step.

First, from the large initial set of features, a reduced feature set of 25 features was computed through a stepwise forward feature selection scheme for each classification task. The first feature was chosen as the one that maximized Spearman's rank correlation regarding the outcome. Then, the features were added one at a time to maximize a linear combination of Spearman's rank correlation (between the feature and the outcome) and the Maximal Information Coefficient (between the feature and the features that were yet to be included in the reduced set) [46].

Then, from the reduced feature set, logistic regression models of order i from 1 to 10 that would best predict the outcome under investigation were obtained using another stepwise forward feature selection. This procedure involved adding features that maximized the 0.632 + bootstrap area under the receiver operating characteristic curve (AUC) [47] to the ith model one by one.

Finally, for each classification task, the prediction model was obtained by choosing the order that maximized the AUC and computing the final model logistic regression coefficients for the aforementioned combination of features using IABR.

5. Conclusions

In this work, we proposed a radiomic approach to differentiate between PI-RADS 4–5 lesions and HT using different prediction models. The proposed comparisons, including one between models constructed from standard mpMR acquisition protocol (including ADC and T2W) and advanced acquisition protocol (with the addition of DCE and DKI) and another between models derived from features extracted from 3D VOIs or 2D ROIs, provided interesting insights into these sensitive discussion topics amongst the scientific community. This work paved the way toward further studies of these topics, potentially evaluating nonbinary outcomes, tumor aggressiveness, and reproducibility of the computed features in wider cohorts of patients. More extensive work could enable the scientific community to more confidentially suggest guidelines regarding the choice of the most confident, but not redundant, acquisition protocol, and of the most appropriate postprocessing pipeline to accurately detect and characterize PCa.

Author Contributions: S.M. and C.C. conceived the study; C.C., L.B., A.R., G.D.C., and M.P. enrolled the patients and acquired data; S.M., V.B., and L.B. performed the data analysis; S.M. and V.B. wrote the original draft; C.C., M.S., and A.R. reviewed and edited the manuscript. All authors read and agreed to the published version of the manuscript.

References

1. Bray, F.; Ferlay, J.; Soerjomataram, I.; Siegel, R.L.; Torre, L.A.; Jemal, A. Global cancer statistics 2018: GLOBOCAN estimates of incidence and mortality worldwide for 36 cancers in 185 countries. *CA Cancer J. Clin.* **2018**, *68*, 394–424. [CrossRef] [PubMed]

2. Hegde, J.V.; Mulkern, R.V.; Panych, L.P.; Fennessy, F.M.; Fedorov, A.; Maier, S.E.; Tempany, C.M.C. Multiparametric MRI of prostate cancer: An update on state-of-the-art techniques and their performance in detecting and localizing prostate cancer. *J. Magn. Reson. Imaging* **2013**, *37*, 1035–1054. [CrossRef] [PubMed]

3. De Rooij, M.; Hamoen, E.H.J.; Fütterer, J.J.; Barentsz, J.O.; Rovers, M.M. Accuracy of multiparametric MRI for prostate cancer detection: A meta-analysis. *Am. J. Roentgenol.* **2014**, *202*, 343–351. [CrossRef] [PubMed]

4. Fütterer, J.J.; Briganti, A.; De Visschere, P.; Emberton, M.; Giannarini, G.; Kirkham, A.; Taneja, S.S.; Thoeny, H.; Villeirs, G.; Villers, A. Can clinically significant prostate cancer be detected with multiparametric magnetic resonance imaging? A systematic review of the literature. *Eur. Urol.* **2015**, *68*, 1045–1053. [CrossRef]

5. Weinreb, J.C.; Barentsz, J.O.; Choyke, P.L.; Cornud, F.; Haider, M.A.; Macura, K.J.; Margolis, D.; Schnall, M.D.; Shtern, F.; Tempany, C.M.; et al. PI-RADS prostate imaging—Reporting and data system: 2015, version 2. *Eur. Urol.* **2016**, *69*, 16–40. [CrossRef]

6. Zhao, C.; Gao, G.; Fang, D.; Li, F.; Yang, X.; Wang, H.; He, Q.; Wang, X. The efficiency of multiparametric magnetic resonance imaging (mpMRI) using PI-RADS Version 2 in the diagnosis of clinically significant prostate cancer. *Clin. Imaging* **2016**, *40*, 885–888. [CrossRef]

7. Chung, A.G.; Shafiee, M.J.; Kumar, D.; Khalvati, F.; Haider, M.A.; Wong, A. Discovery radiomics for multi-parametric MRI prostate cancer detection. *arXiv* **2015**, arXiv:1509.00111.

8. Xu, M.; Fang, M.; Zou, J.; Yang, S.; Yu, D.; Zhong, L.; Hu, C.; Zang, Y.; Dong, D.; Tian, J.; et al. Using biparametric MRI radiomics signature to differentiate between benign and malignant prostate lesions. *Eur. J. Radiol.* **2019**, *114*, 38–44. [CrossRef]

9. Schoots, I.G. MRI in early prostate cancer detection: How to manage indeterminate or equivocal PI-RADS 3 lesions? *Transl. Androl. Urol.* **2018**, *7*, 70–82. [CrossRef]

10. Sun, Y.; Reynolds, H.M.; Parameswaran, B.; Wraith, D.; Finnegan, M.E.; Williams, S.; Haworth, A. Multiparametric MRI and radiomics in prostate cancer: A review. *Australas. Phys. Eng. Sci. Med.* **2019**, *42*, 3–25. [CrossRef]

11. Rosenkrantz, A.B.; Sigmund, E.E.; Johnson, G.; Babb, J.S.; Mussi, T.C.; Melamed, J.; Taneja, S.S.; Lee, V.S.; Jensen, J.H. Prostate cancer: Feasibility and preliminary experience of a diffusional kurtosis model for detection and assessment of aggressiveness of peripheral zone cancer. *Radiology* **2012**, *264*, 126–135. [CrossRef] [PubMed]

12. Suo, S.; Chen, X.; Wu, L.; Zhang, X.; Yao, Q.; Fan, Y.; Wang, H.; Xu, J. Non-Gaussian water diffusion kurtosis imaging of prostate cancer. *Magn. Reson. Imaging* **2014**, *32*, 421–427. [CrossRef] [PubMed]

13. Tamura, C.; Shinmoto, H.; Soga, S.; Okamura, T.; Sato, H.; Okuaki, T.; Pang, Y.; Kosuda, S.; Kaji, T. Diffusion kurtosis imaging study of prostate cancer: Preliminary findings. *J. Magn. Reson. Imaging* **2014**, *40*, 723–729. [CrossRef] [PubMed]

14. Brancato, V.; Cavaliere, C.; Salvatore, M.; Monti, S. Non-Gaussian models of diffusion weighted imaging for detection and characterization of prostate cancer: A systematic review and meta-analysis. *Sci. Rep.* **2019**, *9*, 16837. [CrossRef] [PubMed]

15. Kumar, V.; Gu, Y.; Basu, S.; Berglund, A.; Eschrich, S.A.; Schabath, M.B.; Forster, K.; Aerts, H.J.W.L.; Dekker, A.; Fenstermacher, D.; et al. Radiomics: The process and the challenges. *Magn. Reson. Imaging* **2012**, *30*, 1234–1248. [CrossRef]

16. Lambin, P.; Rios-Velazquez, E.; Leijenaar, R.; Carvalho, S.; Van Stiphout, R.G.P.M.; Granton, P.; Zegers, C.M.L.; Gillies, R.; Boellard, R.; Dekker, A.; et al. Radiomics: Extracting more information from medical images using advanced feature analysis. *Eur. J. Cancer* **2012**, *48*, 441–446. [CrossRef]

17. Gillies, R.J.; Kinahan, P.E.; Hricak, H. Radiomics: Images are more than pictures, they are data. *Radiology* **2016**, *278*, 563–577. [CrossRef]

18. Aerts, H.J.W.L.; Velazquez, E.R.; Leijenaar, R.T.H.; Parmar, C.; Grossmann, P.; Cavalho, S.; Bussink, J.; Monshouwer, R.; Haibe-Kains, B.; Rietveld, D.; et al. Decoding tumour phenotype by noninvasive imaging using a quantitative radiomics approach. *Nat. Commun.* **2014**, *5*, 4006. [CrossRef]

19. Incoronato, M.; Aiello, M.; Infante, T.; Cavaliere, C.; Grimaldi, A.M.; Mirabelli, P.; Monti, S.; Salvatore, M. Radiogenomic analysis of oncological data: A technical survey. *Int. J. Mol. Sci.* **2017**, *18*, 805. [CrossRef]

20. Diehn, M.; Nardini, C.; Wang, D.S.; McGovern, S.; Jayaraman, M.; Liang, Y.; Aldape, K.; Cha, S.; Kuo, M.D. Identification of noninvasive imaging surrogates for brain tumor gene-expression modules. *Proc. Natl. Acad. Sci. USA* **2008**, *105*, 5213–5218. [CrossRef]

21. Segal, E.; Sirlin, C.B.; Ooi, C.; Adler, A.S.; Gollub, J.; Chen, X.; Chan, B.K.; Matcuk, G.R.; Barry, C.T.; Chang, H.Y.; et al. Decoding global gene expression programs in liver cancer by noninvasive imaging. *Nat. Biotechnol.* **2007**, *25*, 675–680. [CrossRef] [PubMed]

22. Li, H.; Zhu, Y.; Burnside, E.S.; Huang, E.; Drukker, K.; Hoadley, K.A.; Fan, C.; Conzen, S.D.; Zuley, M.; Net, J.M.; et al. Quantitative MRI radiomics in the prediction of molecular classifications of breast cancer subtypes in the TCGA/TCIA data set. *npj Breast Cancer* **2016**, *2*, 16012. [CrossRef] [PubMed]

23. Monti, S.; Aiello, M.; Incoronato, M.; Grimaldi, A.M.; Moscarino, M.; Mirabelli, P.; Ferbo, U.; Cavaliere, C.; Salvatore, M. DCE-MRI pharmacokinetic-based phenotyping of invasive ductal carcinoma: A radiomic study for prediction of histological outcomes. *Contrast Media Mol. Imaging* **2018**, *2018*, 5076269. [CrossRef] [PubMed]

24. Yip, S.S.F.; Aerts, H.J.W.L. Applications and limitations of radiomics. *Phys. Med. Biol.* **2016**, *61*, R150–R166. [CrossRef] [PubMed]

25. Chaddad, A.; Kucharczyk, M.J.; Niazi, T. Multimodal radiomic features for the predicting gleason score of prostate cancer. *Cancers* **2018**, *10*, 249. [CrossRef] [PubMed]

26. Chaddad, A.; Niazi, T.; Probst, S.; Bladou, F.; Anidjar, M.; Bahoric, B. Predicting Gleason score of prostate cancer patients using radiomic analysis. *Front. Oncol.* **2018**, *8*, 630. [CrossRef]

27. Chen, T.; Li, M.; Gu, Y.; Zhang, Y.; Yang, S.; Wei, C.; Wu, J.; Li, X.; Zhao, W.; Shen, J. Prostate cancer differentiation and aggressiveness: Assessment with a radiomic-based model vs. PI-RADS v2. *J. Magn. Reson. Imaging* **2019**, *49*, 875–884. [CrossRef]

28. Hermie, I.; Van Besien, J.; De Visschere, P.; Lumen, N.; Decaestecker, K. Which clinical and radiological characteristics can predict clinically significant prostate cancer in PI-RADS 3 lesions? A retrospective study in a high-volume academic center. *Eur. J. Radiol.* **2019**, *114*, 92–98. [CrossRef]

29. Wang, J.; Wu, C.J.; Bao, M.L.; Zhang, J.; Wang, X.N.; Zhang, Y.D. Machine learning-based analysis of MR radiomics can help to improve the diagnostic performance of PI-RADS v2 in clinically relevant prostate cancer. *Eur. Radiol.* **2017**, *27*, 4082–4090. [CrossRef]

30. Hectors, S.J.; Cherny, M.; Yadav, K.K.; Beksaç, A.T.; Thulasidass, H.; Lewis, S.; Davicioni, E.; Wang, P.; Tewari, A.K.; Taouli, B. Radiomics features measured with multiparametric magnetic resonance imaging predict prostate cancer aggressiveness. *J. Urol.* **2019**, *202*, 498–505. [CrossRef]

31. Toivonen, J.; Perez, I.M.; Movahedi, P.; Merisaari, H.; Pesola, M.; Taimen, P.; Boström, P.J.; Pohjankukka, J.; Kiviniemi, A.; Pahikkala, T.; et al. Radiomics and machine learning of multisequence multiparametric prostate MRI: Towards improved non-invasive prostate cancer characterization. *PLoS ONE* **2019**, *14*, e0217702. [CrossRef] [PubMed]

32. Franiel, T.; Hamm, B.; Hricak, H. Dynamic contrast-enhanced magnetic resonance imaging and pharmacokinetic models in prostate cancer. *Eur. Radiol.* **2011**, *21*, 616–626. [CrossRef] [PubMed]

33. Dercle, L.; Ammari, S.; Bateson, M.; Durand, P.B.; Haspinger, E.; Massard, C.; Jaudet, C.; Varga, A.; Deutsch, E.; Soria, J.C.; et al. Limits of radiomic-based entropy as a surrogate of tumor heterogeneity: ROI-area, acquisition protocol and tissue site exert substantial influence. *Sci. Rep.* **2017**, *7*, 7952. [CrossRef] [PubMed]

34. Greer, M.D.; Brown, A.M.; Shih, J.H.; Summers, R.M.; Marko, J.; Law, Y.M.; Sankineni, S.; George, A.K.; Merino, M.J.; Pinto, P.A.; et al. Accuracy and agreement of PIRADSv2 for prostate cancer mpMRI: A multireader study. *J. Magn. Reson. Imaging* **2017**, *45*, 579–585. [CrossRef] [PubMed]

35. Greer, M.D.; Shih, J.H.; Lay, N.; Barrett, T.; Kayat Bittencourt, L.; Borofsky, S.; Kabakus, I.M.; Law, Y.M.; Marko, J.; Shebel, H.; et al. Validation of the dominant sequence paradigm and role of dynamic contrast-enhanced imaging in PI-RADS version 2. *Radiology* **2017**, *285*, 859–869. [CrossRef] [PubMed]

36. Taghipour, M.; Ziaei, A.; Alessandrino, F.; Hassanzadeh, E.; Harisinghani, M.; Vangel, M.; Tempany, C.M.; Fennessy, F.M. Investigating the role of DCE-MRI, over T2 and DWI, in accurate PI-RADS v2 assessment of clinically significant peripheral zone prostate lesions as defined at radical prostatectomy. *Abdom. Radiol.* **2019**, *44*, 1520–1527. [CrossRef]

37. Parmar, C.; Velazquez, E.R.; Leijenaar, R.; Jermoumi, M.; Carvalho, S.; Mak, R.H.; Mitra, S.; Shankar, B.U.; Kikinis, R.; Haibe-Kains, B.; et al. Robust radiomics feature quantification using semiautomatic volumetric segmentation. *PLoS ONE* **2014**, *9*, e102107. [CrossRef]

38. O'Connor, J.P.B.; Rose, C.J.; Waterton, J.C.; Carano, R.A.D.; Parker, G.J.M.; Jackson, A. Imaging intratumor heterogeneity: Role in therapy response, resistance, and clinical outcome. *Clin. Cancer Res.* **2015**, *21*, 249–257. [CrossRef]

39. Baldi, D.; Aiello, M.; Duggento, A.; Salvatore, M.; Cavaliere, C. MR imaging-histology correlation by tailored 3d-printed slicer in oncological assessment. *Contrast Media Mol. Imaging* **2019**, *2019*, 1071453. [CrossRef]

40. Vargas, H.A.; Hötker, A.M.; Goldman, D.A.; Moskowitz, C.S.; Gondo, T.; Matsumoto, K.; Ehdaie, B.; Woo, S.; Fine, S.W.; Reuter, V.E.; et al. Updated prostate imaging reporting and data system (PIRADS v2) recommendations for the detection of clinically significant prostate cancer using multiparametric MRI: Critical evaluation using whole-mount pathology as standard of reference. *Eur. Radiol.* **2016**, *26*, 1606–1612. [CrossRef]

41. Tofts, P.S.; Parker, G.J.M. DCE-MRI: Acquisition and analysis techniques. In *Clinical Perfusion MRI: Techniques and Applications*; Cambridge University Press: Cambridge, UK, 2013; pp. 58–74.

42. Klein, S.; Staring, M.; Murphy, K.; Viergever, M.A.; Pluim, J.P.W. Elastix: A toolbox for intensity-based medical image registration. *IEEE Trans. Med. Imaging* **2010**. [CrossRef]

43. Collewet, G.; Strzelecki, M.; Mariette, F. Influence of MRI acquisition protocols and image intensity normalization methods on texture classification. *Magn. Reson. Imaging* **2004**, *22*, 81–91. [CrossRef] [PubMed]

44. Haralick, R.M.; Dinstein, I.; Shanmugam, K. Textural features for image classification. *IEEE Trans. Syst. Man Cybern.* **1973**, *3*, 610–621. [CrossRef]

45. Vallières, M.; Freeman, C.R.; Skamene, S.R.; El Naqa, I. A radiomics model from joint FDG-PET and MRI texture features for the prediction of lung metastases in soft-tissue sarcomas of the extremities. *Phys. Med. Biol.* **2015**, *60*, 5471–5496. [CrossRef] [PubMed]

46. Reshef, D.N.; Reshef, Y.A.; Finucane, H.K.; Grossman, S.R.; McVean, G.; Turnbaugh, P.J.; Lander, E.S.; Mitzenmacher, M.; Sabeti, P.C. Detecting novel associations in large data sets. *Science* **2011**, *334*, 1518–1524. [CrossRef] [PubMed]

47. Sahiner, B.; Chan, H.P.; Hadjiiski, L. Classifier performance prediction for computer-aided diagnosis using a limited dataset. *Med. Phys.* **2008**, *35*, 1559–1570. [CrossRef]

6

Subtypes of Ovarian Cancer and Ovarian Cancer Screening

Masafumi Koshiyama [1,2,*], **Noriomi Matsumura** [1] **and Ikuo Konishi** [1,3]

1   Department of Gynecology and Obstetrics, Kyoto University, Graduate School of Medicine, Sakyo-ku, Kyoto 606-8507, Japan; noriomi@kuhp.kyoto-u.ac.jp (N.M.); konishi@kuhp.kyoto-u.ac.jp (I.K.)
2   Department of Women's Health, Graduate School of Human Nursing, The University of Shiga Prefecture, 2500 Hassakacho, Hikone, Shiga 522-8533, Japan
3   Department of Obstetrics and Gynecology, National Hospital Organization Kyoto Medical Center, Fushimi-ku, Kyoto 612-8555, Japan
*   Correspondence: koshiyamam@nifty.com

Academic Editor: Edward J. Pavlik

Abstract: Ovarian cancer is the foremost cause of gynecological cancer death in the developed world, as it is usually diagnosed at an advanced stage. In this paper we discuss current issues, the efficacy and problems associated with ovarian cancer screening, and compare the characteristics of ovarian cancer subtypes. There are two types of ovarian cancer: Type I carcinomas, which are slow-growing, indolent neoplasms thought to arise from a precursor lesion, which are relatively common in Asia; and Type II carcinomas, which are clinically aggressive neoplasms that can develop de novo from serous tubal intraepithelial carcinomas (STIC) and/or ovarian surface epithelium and are common in Europe and the USA. One of the most famous studies on the subject reported that annual screening using CA125/transvaginal sonography (TVS) did not reduce the ovarian cancer mortality rate in the USA. In contrast, a recent study in the UK showed an overall average mortality reduction of 20% in the screening group. Another two studies further reported that the screening was associated with decreased stage at detection. Theoretically, annual screening using CA125/TVS could easily detect precursor lesions and could be more effective in Asia than in Europe and the USA. The detection of Type II ovarian carcinoma at an early stage remains an unresolved issue. The resolving power of CA125 or TVS screening alone is unlikely to be successful at resolving STICs. Biomarkers for the early detection of Type II carcinomas such as STICs need to be developed.

Keywords: subtypes; two types of ovarian cancer; ovarian cancer screening; CA125; transvaginal sonography

1. Introduction

Ovarian cancer is the foremost cause of gynecological cancer death and is overall one of the most frequent causes of fatal malignancy in women [1]. The symptoms are often nonspecific, hampering early detection, so the majority of patients present with advanced-stage disease.

Screening is defined as the application of a test or a combination of tests to an asymptomatic at-risk population to detect a disease at an earlier and more curable stage. In 2011, an examination of a screening program for prostate, lung, colorectal, and ovarian cancer (PLCO) in the USA revealed that annual screening using CA125/transvaginal sonography (TVS) did not markedly reduce the ovarian cancer mortality rate [2,3]. While this finding suggests that it is not possible to detect ovarian cancer at an earlier curable stage, it is possible to question the validity of these data.

Recently, the characteristics of several subtypes of ovarian cancer have been elucidated by the findings from histopathological, molecular, and genetic studies. Ovarian cancer can be roughly divided into two broad categories: Type I, in which precursor lesions in the ovaries have clearly been described; and Type II, in which such lesions have not been clearly described and tumors may develop de novo from the tubal and/or ovarian surface epithelium [4]. Understanding these characteristics is important in the effort to reduce ovarian cancer mortality.

This study first describes the characteristics of the subtypes of ovarian cancer and the results of several large-scale studies of ovarian cancer screening. We discuss current issues, the efficacy and problems associated with ovarian cancer screening, and make comparisons of the characteristics of ovarian cancer subtypes.

2. Ovarian Carcinoma Types

2.1. Type I Carcinoma

Type I carcinomas are generally slow-growing indolent neoplasms, and their precursor lesions in the ovaries have been clearly described [4].

2.1.1. Endometrioid Carcinoma and Clear Cell Carcinoma

Clear cell and endometrioid carcinomas are believed to arise from endometriosis of the ovary. Among malignant transformation cases of endometriotic cyst, serial transvaginal ultrasonography (USG) examinations revealed an increase in the cyst size [5]. Increased risks of ovarian carcinoma arising from endometriosis were associated with infertility, early menarche, and late menopause [6]. Pathologically, the co-existence of ovarian carcinoma and endometriosis is frequently observed, and in such cases endometriosis is called "atypical endometriosis", a putative precursor lesion including atypia of the cell nucleus [7].

Carcinogenesis of endometrioid and clear cell carcinomas arising from endometriotic cysts is significantly influenced by the microenvironment in the precursors [8]. The content of an endometriotic cyst (including free iron in old blood) is thought to be associated with cancer development through the induction of persistent oxidative stress [9]. The epithelial cells in the cyst are exposed to oxidative stress and hypoxia. Thus, they are subject to increased cellular and DNA damage, have less efficient DNA repair, and are easily transformed [10,11].

Somatic mutations in the ARID1A tumor-suppressor gene have been frequently identified in clear cell carcinoma. BAF250a encoded by ARID1A is a member of the SWItch/sucrose nonfermentable (SWI/SNF) complex. We recently reported that clear cell carcinomas exhibiting the loss of one or multiple SWI/SNF complex subunits demonstrated aggressive behaviors and poor prognosis [12].

2.1.2. Mucinous Carcinoma

A subset of mucinous carcinomas is thought to develop in association with ovarian benign teratomas; however, the majority of mucinous carcinomas do not show any teratomatous components [13,14]. Other theories of an ontogeny include origin from mucinous metaplasia of surface epithelial inclusions, endometriosis, and Brenner tumors [5,14]; however, these observations are relatively uncommon, except for Müllerian endocervical mucinous or mixed borderline tumors [15,16].

Morphological transitions from cystadenoma to a mucinous borderline tumor (MBT) to intraepithelial carcinoma and invasive carcinoma have occasionally been observed [17]. An increasing frequency of KRAS mutations at codons 12 and 13 has been reported in cystadenomas, MBTs, and mucinous carcinomas [18–21]. These findings support the hypothesis of the "mucinous adenoma–carcinoma sequence" [17,22] and the view that mucinous carcinomas may develop in a step-wise fashion from mucinous cystadenomas and MBTs.

2.1.3. Low-Grade Serous Carcinoma

Low-grade serous carcinomas are very rare tumors. They are genetically stable and are characterized by their low number of genetic mutations; therefore, they develop slowly from the precursors and behave in an indolent fashion. They are also thought to grow in a step-wise fashion from benign serous cystadenoma to serous borderline tumors (SBTs), and then to low-grade serous carcinoma.

p53 mutations are uncommon in low-grade serous carcinoma [23]. These carcinomas have a DNA content and level of copy number alterations that closely resembles that of SBTs [24,25].

One theory of the origin of these tumors is that they are derived from ovarian epithelial inclusions that have undergone Müllerian metaplasia [26]. The exposure of the mesothelial cells to the ovarian stromal microenvironment may result in transformation to Müllerian epithelium.

Another theory is that serous tumors may be derived from a secondary Müllerian system, arising from the embryological remnants of the proximal Müllerian ducts located within the ovarian hilm [27,28]. However, a new theory suggests that low-grade serous carcinoma may be derived from the fallopian tube. The premise is that shed tubal epithelial cells can implant on the ovarian surface epithelium, followed by the formation of inclusion cysts and transforming serous carcinoma [29,30].

2.2. Type II Carcinoma

Type II carcinomas are clinically aggressive neoplasms and may develop de novo from the tubal and/or ovarian surface epithelium.

High-Grade Serous Carcinoma

High-grade serous carcinomas account for 68% of ovarian cancer and have the worst prognosis, as they are high-grade clinically aggressive neoplasms that are usually diagnosed at an advanced stage. They show TP53 gene mutations in nearly 80% of cases [31–34] and have a high Ki67 proliferation index (50%–75%). Chromosomal rearrangements are common and associated with gene instability. Mutations in the BRCA 1 and 2 genes are associated with 90% of hereditary high-grade serous carcinoma cases [35].

Recently, analyses of gene expression microarray data from The Cancer Genome Atlas (TCGA) project have revealed that high-grade serous carcinoma can be classified into one of four gene expression subtypes: mesenchymal, immunoreactive, proliferative, and differentiated [36,37]. Our group reported that the progression-free and overall survival were best in the immunoreactive group, whereas the overall survival was worst in the mesenchymal transition group ($p < 0.001$ for each) [38]. Expression of vascular endothelial growth factor (VEGF) inhibits tumor immunity through the accumulation of myeloid-derived suppressor cells, and contributes to poor prognosis [39].

These tumors may develop de novo from the tubal and/or ovarian surface epithelium. In 2001, Piek et al. [40] found new transformations from hyperplastic to dysplastic lesions on tubal segments removed from women who had either BRCA mutations or a strong family history of ovarian carcinoma and underwent a risk-reducing bilateral salpingo-oophorectomy (BSO). These dysplastic lesions within the tubal epithelium are termed "serous tubal intraepithelial carcinomas" (STIC) and microscopic disease.

A very early abnormality termed "secretory cell outgrowths" (SCOUTs) was recently reported in tubal epithelia [41]. The TP53 signatures were the next earliest entities, and have an immunohistochemical definition of "p53-positive with a low proliferative index (Ki67 < 10%)". Developing later were "serous tubal intraepithelial lesions" (STILs) [42], also known as "transitional intraepithelial lesions of the tube" (TILTs) by some authors. These have proliferative p53 signatures, tubal dysplasia, and even tubal epithelial atypia [40,43]. Lastly, these turned into STICs; thus, STICs appear to be associated with the development of serous carcinoma.

It was recently reported that the junction of the fallopian tube epithelium with the mesothelium of the tubal serosa might be a potential site for carcinogenesis [44]. Carcinomas arising from this junctional zone can easily invade the extensive lymphovascular system under the tubal epithelium and rapidly spread throughout the abdominal cavity.

In contrast, ovarian hilum cells have shown increased transformation potential after the inactivation of tumor suppressor genes transformation-related protein 53 (Trp53) and retinoblastoma 1 (Rb1) in mice [45]. These stem cells may also be the origin of high-grade serous carcinoma.

3. Large-Scale Studies of Ovarian Cancer Screening

Ovarian cancer screening was once thought to be ineffective, but has recently been reported to result in a better prognosis than without screening [46].

3.1. A Screening Program for Prostate, Lung, Colorectal, and Ovarian Cancer

One large-scale study of ovarian cancer screening examined a screening program for prostate, lung, colorectal, and ovarian cancer (PLCO) in the USA, performed using a randomized controlled trial (RCT) [2,3]. The annual screening in this study was performed by transvaginal sonography and CA125 level measurements.

The PLCO screening arm involved 78,216 women receiving either annual screening ($n = 39,105$) or the usual care ($n = 39,111$). Ovarian cancer was diagnosed in 212 patients (0.54%) in the screening group and 176 patients (0.45%) in the standard care group. The stage distribution in the screening group was as follows: 32 (15%) cases of Stage I disease, 15 (7%) cases of Stage II disease, 120 (57%) cases of Stage III disease, and 43 (20%) cases of Stage IV disease, indicating that 77% of patients had cancer at Stage III or higher. The distribution of cancer histologies included 116 (80%) cases of serous carcinomas, five (3%) cases of mucinous carcinomas, 19 (13%) cases of endometrioid carcinomas, and six (4%) cases of clear cell carcinomas, indicating that most cases involved serous cancers.

The authors concluded that annual screening did not reduce the ovarian cancer mortality rate compared with standard care. Based on this report, ovarian cancer screening is not considered to be effective.

3.2. Re-Analysis of the PLCO Screening Data

We obtained the authors' datasets and performed a new analysis. We divided the patients who were diagnosed with ovarian cancer into two groups. One group included 101 patients whose ovarian cancers were detected through annual screening (CA125 and/or TVS) or within one year after screening. The other group included 344 patients in the screening group whose ovarian cancers were found at more than one year after screening due to the patient experiencing symptoms, as well as patients in the no screening and control groups. We previously reported these results [47]. The prognosis was significantly better in the patients in the former group than in those in the latter group (median survival: 6.1 vs. 3.3 years, $p = 0.0017$). Additionally, the first group contained significantly fewer Stage IV cases than the second group (13% vs. 29%, respectively, $p = 0.005$).

We identified two weaknesses in the PLCO screening: the group undergoing annual screening included many women who never received screening, and many patients with ovarian cancer in the screening group were diagnosed incidentally more than one year after screening, and as such could not be related to the direct effect of screening.

3.3. The United Kingdom Collaborative Trial of Ovarian Cancer Screening

The United Kingdom Collaborative Trial of Ovarian Cancer Screening (UKCTOCS) is an RCT of 202,638 women (control: 101,359; multimodal screening (MMS): 50,640; TVS alone: 50,639) [48–50]. The MMS protocol included annual CA125 screening interpreted using a patented "Risk of Ovarian Cancer" algorithm (ROCA) with TVS as a second-line test [51,52]. Ovarian cancer was diagnosed in 38 (0.08%) patients in the MMS group and 32 (0.06%) patients in the TVS group. The distribution of the cancer histologies was similar to that of the PLCO group. The distribution of the cancer stages in the MMS group was as follows: 17 (45%) patients with Stage I disease, 2 (5%) patients with Stage II disease, 19 (50%) patients with Stage III disease, and 0 (0%) patients with Stage IV disease, which was similar to that of the TVS group. Recently, a UK team reported on the final mortality, citing an overall average mortality reduction of 20%, and a reduction of 8% in years 0–7 and 28% in years 7–14 in the MMS group, compared with the no screening group [46]. They suggested that this late effect of screening was predictable given the unavoidable time interval from randomization to diagnosis and finally death. Therefore, their interpretation was that MMS screening was more effective after seven years of screening.

Very recently, Pavik pointed out two problems raised by the work of the UKCTOCS [53]. The UKCTOCS results from the analysis using the Cox proportional hazards model and the Royston–Parmar flexible parametric model indicated only small differences between the MMS and TVS modalities that were not statistically significant (estimated mortality reduction for years 7–14: 23% MMS vs. 21% TVS with the Royston–Parmar flexible parametric model). Another problem was that an expected lack of CA125 expression (20%) produces CA125-negative ovarian carcinomas that cannot be expected to be detected in the MMS group.

3.4. The Kentucky Screening Study

In the Kentucky Screening Study, single-arm annual TVS screenings of 37,293 women was performed [54,55]. The stage distribution of the 47 invasive ovarian cancers was as follows: 22 (47%) Stage I lesions, 11 (23%) Stage II lesions, 14 (30%) Stage III lesions, and 0 (0%) Stage IV lesions, with a 70% rate of Early-Stage (I/II) disease. The distribution of cancer histologies included 38% with serous carcinomas, 2% with mucinous carcinomas, 26% with endometrioid carcinomas, 4% with clear cell carcinomas, and 30% with others. The survival rate at five years of the patients with ovarian cancer in the annual screening group was better than that of the patients with ovarian cancer who did not undergo screening (74.8% ± 6.6% vs. 53.7% ± 2.3%, $p < 0.001$). Histologically, compared with the PLCO data, the rate of serous carcinomas was relatively low and the rate of endometrioid carcinomas was relatively high.

The authors concluded that annual TVS screening was associated with a decreased stage at detection, as well as a decrease in the case-specific ovarian cancer mortality. However, this study was not an RCT.

3.5. The Japanese Study

In Japan, the results of the Shizuoka Cohort Study of Ovarian Cancer Screening have been reported [56]. This study was an RCT of 82,487 low-risk postmenopausal women (intervention group: 41,688, control group: 40,799) who were screened using annual TVS and CA125 levels. The total number of cases of ovarian cancer in the screening group was 27 (0.06%). The stage distribution in the intervention group was as follows: 17 (63%) cases of Stage I disease, 1 (4%) case of Stage II disease, 7 (26%) cases of Stage III disease, and 2 (7%) cases of Stage IV disease. The distribution of the cancer histologies included 8 (30%) cases of serous carcinomas, 4 (15%) cases of mucinous carcinomas, 5 (19%) cases of endometrioid carcinomas, 9 (33%) cases of clear cell carcinomas, and 1 (4%) case of "other". Histologically, most of these cases involved cancers other than serous carcinoma. The proportion of Stage I/II ovarian cancers was higher in the screening group (67%) than in the control group (44%). The rate of complete surgical excision was higher in the screening group (21; 78%) than in the control group (15; 47%) ($p = 0.018$). However, the mortality rates are unknown, which again is problematic.

4. Differing Histological Subtypes of Ovarian Carcinoma among Races

In Europe, the USA, and Asia, there are significant differences in the rates of histological subtypes of ovarian carcinoma [57–62]. As we reported previously, the rate of aggressive ovarian cancer such as high-grade serous cancer (Type II) is significantly higher in Europe and the USA than in Asia ($p < 0.001$) [47]. For example, the rates of Type I vs. Type II are, 24% vs. 48% in Europe (including the UK); 24% vs. 66% in Denmark; and 30% vs. 45% in the USA. Conversely, Type I carcinomas—indolent carcinomas arising from precursors—are relatively common in Asia. For example, the rates of Type I vs. Type II are 53% vs. 33% in Japan; 58% vs. 24% in Hong Kong; and 66% vs. 34% in

Korea. These results theoretically imply that ovarian cancer screening using CA125/TVS would be more effective in Asia than in Europe and the USA, as the precursors or ovarian cancer can be detected at an earlier stage, thereby reducing the mortality.

5. Conclusions

We presented characteristics of subtypes of ovarian cancer, summarized in Table 1. Type I carcinomas are generally slow-growing indolent neoplasms, and their precursor lesions in the ovaries have clearly been described and are easily detected. Conversely, Type II carcinomas are clinically aggressive neoplasms and may develop de novo from the tubal and/or ovarian surface epithelium. The efficacy of ovarian cancer screening depends on the subtypes of ovarian cancer. Type I ovarian carcinomas are relatively common in Asia, while Type II ovarian carcinomas are relatively common in Europe and the USA. Therefore, annual ovarian cancer screening may improve the prognoses in Asia to a substantially greater degree than in Europe and the USA, as precursors or early-stage Type I ovarian carcinomas can be detected using CA125/TVS in those regions. Furthermore, it is possible to improve the prognosis or induce down-staging of Type II ovarian carcinomas, even in Europe and the USA. The detection of Type II ovarian carcinoma at an early stage remains an unresolved issue. We have likely failed to notice the presence of STICs using CA125/TVS screening alone, as neither method showed positive findings in women with STICs. Biomarkers for the early detection of Type II carcinomas such as STICs are therefore urgently needed [53].

Table 1. Characteristics of two types of ovarian carcinoma.

	Type I	Type II
Behavior	Indolent	Aggressive
Genetic instability	Not very unstable	Very unstable
TP 53 mutation	Low	High
BRCA1/BRCA2 mutation	Low	High
Ki 67 proliferative index	10%–15%	50%–75%
Histological subtype	Endometrioid Clear cell Mucinous Low grade serous	High grade serous
Precursor	Benign cyst	s/o Tubal dysplasia (de novo starting)
Discover a precursor	Easy	Difficult
Incidence	Asia > Europe, USA	Europe, USA > Asia

Acknowledgments: We would like to thank Christine D. Berg and PLCO Project Team who graciously sent the PLCO data to us. We also thank John Rensselaer van Nagell Jr. and Edward John Pavlik for offering the data of the Kentucky Screening Study.

Author Contributions: Masafumi Koshiyama wrote the paper. Noriomi Matsumura and Ikuo Konishi contributed to the design and preparation of the paper.

References

1.   Ozor, R.F.; Rubin, S.C.; Thomas, G.M.; Robboy, S.J. Epithelial ovarian cancer. In *Principles and Practice of Gynecologic Oncology*; Hoskin, W.J., Perez, C.A., Young, R.C., Eds.; Lippincott Williams & Wilkins: Philadelphia, PA, USA, 2000; pp. 981–1057.

2.   Buys, S.S.; Partridge, E.; Greene, M.H.; Prorok, P.C.; Reding, D.; Riley, T.L.; Hartge, P.; Fagerstrom, R.M.; Ragard, L.R.; Chia, D.; et al. Ovarian cancer screening in the Prostate, Lung, Colorectal and Ovarian (PLCO) Cancer Screening Trial: Findings from the initial screen of a randomized trial. *Am. J. Obstet. Gynecol.* **2005**, *193*, 1630–1639. [CrossRef] [PubMed]

3. Buys, S.S.; Patridge, E.; Black, A.; Johnson, C.C.; Lamerato, L.; Isaacs, C.; Reding, D.; Greenlee, R.T.; Yokochi, L.A.; Kessel, B.; et al. Effect of screening on ovarian cancer mortality: The Prostate, Lung, Colorectal and ovarian (PLCO) cancer screening randomized controlled trial. *JAMA* **2011**, *305*, 2295–2303. [CrossRef] [PubMed]

4. Koshiyama, M.; Matsumura, N.; Konishi, I. Recent concepts of ovarian carcinogenesis: Type I and Type II. *Biomed. Res. Int.* **2014**, *2014*, 934261. [CrossRef] [PubMed]

5. Horiuchi, A.; Itoh, K.; Shimizu, M.; Nakai, I.; Yamazaki, T.; Kimura, K.; Suzuki, A.; Shiozawa, I.; Ueda, N.; Konishi, I. Toward understanding the natural history of ovarian carcinoma development: A clinicopathological approach. *Gynecol. Oncol.* **2003**, *88*, 309–317. [CrossRef]

6. Van Gorp, T.; Amant, F.; Neven, P.V. Endometriosis and the development of malignant tumors of the pelvis. A review of literature. *Best Pract. Res. Clin. Obstet. Gynecol.* **2004**, *18*, 349–371. [CrossRef] [PubMed]

7. Mandai, M.; Yamaguchi, K.; Matsumura, N.; Konishi, I. Ovarian cancer in endometriosis:molecular biology, pathology, and clinical management. *Int. J. Clin. Oncol.* **2009**, *14*, 383–391. [CrossRef] [PubMed]

8. Mandai, M.; Matsumura, N.; Baba, T.; Yamaguchi, K.; Hamanishi, J.; Konishi, I. Ovarian clear cell carcinoma as a stress-responsive cancer: Influence of the microenvirinment on the carcinogenesis and cancer phenotype. *Cancer Lett.* **2011**, *310*, 129–133. [CrossRef] [PubMed]

9. Yamaguchi, K.; Mandai, M.; Toyokuni, S.; Hamanishi, J.; Higuchi, T.; Takakura, K.; Fujii, S. Contents of endometriotic cysts, especially the high concentration of free iron, are a possible cause of carcinogenesis in the cysts through the iron-induced persistent oxidative stress. *Clin. Cancer Res.* **2008**, *4*, 32–40. [CrossRef] [PubMed]

10. Coquelle, A.; Toledo, F.; Stern, S.; Bieth, A.; Debatisse, M. A new role for hypoxia in tumor progression: Induction of fragile site triggering genomic rearrangements and formation of complex DMs and HSRs. *Mol. Cell* **1998**, *2*, 259–265. [CrossRef]

11. Meng, A.X.; Jalali, F.; Cuddihy, A.; Chan, N.; Bindra, R.S.; Glazer, P.M.; Bristow, R.G. Hypoxia down-regulates DNA double strand break repair gene expression in prostate cancer cells. *Radiother. Oncol.* **2005**, *76*, 168–176. [CrossRef] [PubMed]

12. Abou-Taleb, H.; Yamaguchi, K.; Matsumura, N.; Murakami, R.; Nakai, H.; Higasa, K.; Amano, Y.; Abiko, K.; Yoshioka, Y.; Hamanishi, J.; et al. Comprehensive assessment of the expression of the SWI/SNF complex defines two distinct prognosis subtypes of ovarian clear cell carcinoma. *Oncotarget* **2016**, *7*, 54758–54770. [PubMed]

13. Czriker, M.; Dockerty, M. Mucinous cystadenomas and mucinous cystadenocarcinomas of the ovary; a clinical and pathological study of 355 cases. *Cancer* **1954**, *7*, 302–310. [CrossRef]

14. Woodruff, J.D.; Bie, L.S.; Sherman, R.J. Mucinous tumors of the ovary. *Obstet. Gynecol.* **1960**, *16*, 699–712. [PubMed]

15. Rutgers, J.; Scully, R.E. Ovarian mullerian mucinous papillary cystadenomas of borderline malignancy. A clinicopathologic analysis. *Cancer* **1988**, *61*, 340–348. [CrossRef]

16. Lim, D.; Oliva, E. Precursors and pathogenesis of ovarian carcinoma. *Pathology* **2013**, *45*, 229–242. [CrossRef] [PubMed]

17. Mandai, M.; Konishi, I.; Kuroda, H.; Komatsu, T.; Yamamoto, S.; Nanbu, K.; Matsushita, K.; Fumumoto, M.; Yamabe, H.; Mori, T. Heterogeneous distribution of K-RAS-mutated epithelia in mucinous ovarian tumors with special reference to histopathology. *Hum. Pathol.* **1998**, *29*, 34–40. [CrossRef]

18. Enomoto, T.; Weghorst, C.M.; Inoue, M.; Tanizawa, O.; Rice, J.M. K-RAS activation occurs frequently in mucinous adenocarcinomas and rarely in other common epithelial tumors of the human ovary. *Am. J. Pathol.* **1991**, *139*, 777–785. [PubMed]

19. Ichikawa, Y.; Nishida, M.; Suzuki, H.; Yoshida, S.; Tsunoda, H.; Kudo, T.; Uchida, K.; Miwa, M. Mutation of KRAS protooncogene is associated with histological subtypes in human mucinous ovarian tumors. *Cancer Res.* **1994**, *54*, 33–35. [PubMed]

20. Caduff, R.F.; Svoboda-Newman, S.M.; Ferguson, A.W.; Johnston, C.M.; Frank, T.S. Comparison of mutations of Ki-RAS and p53 immmunoreactivity in borderline and malignant epithelial ovarian tumors. *Am. J. Surg. Pathol.* **1999**, *23*, 323–328. [CrossRef] [PubMed]

21. Gemignani, M.L.; Schlaerth, A.C.; Bogomolniy, F.; Barakat, R.R.; Lin, O.; Soslow, R.; Venkatraman, E.; Royd, J. Role of *KRAS* and *BRAF* gene mutations in mucinous ovarian carcinoma. *Gynecol. Oncol.* **2003**, *90*, 378–381. [CrossRef]

22. Mok, S.C.; Bell, D.A.; Knapp, R.C.; Fishbaugh, P.M.; Welch, W.R.; Muto, M.G.; Berkowitz, R.S.; Tsao, S.W. Mutation of K-RAS protooncogene in human ovarian epithelial tumors of borderline malignancy. *Cancer Res.* **1993**, *53*, 1489–1492. [PubMed]

23. Singer, G.; Stohr, R.; Cope, L.; Dehari, R.; Hartmann, A.; Cao, D.F.; Wang, T.L.; Kurman, R.J.; Shih, I.M. Patterns of p53 mutations separate ovarian serous borderline tumors and low- and high-grade carcinomas and provide support for a new model of ovarian carcinogenesis: A mutational analysis with immunohistochemical correlation. *Am. J. Surg. Pathol.* **2005**, *29*, 218–224. [CrossRef] [PubMed]

24. Pradham, M.; Davidson, B.; Trope, C.G.; Danielsen, H.E.; Abeler, V.M.; Risberq, B. Gross genomic alteration differ between serous borderline tumors and serous adenocarcinomas-an image cytometric DNA ploidy analysis of 307 cases with histogenetic implications. *Virchows Arch.* **2009**, *454*, 677–683. [CrossRef] [PubMed]

25. Kuo, K.T.; Guan, B.; Feng, Y.; Mao, T.L.; Jinawath, N.; Wang, Y.; Kurman, R.J.; Shih, I.M.; Wang, T.L. Analysis of DNA copy number alterations in ovarian serous tumors identifies new molecular genetic changes in low-grade and high-grade carcinomas. *Cancer Res.* **2009**, *69*, 4036–4042. [CrossRef] [PubMed]

26. Feeley, K.M.; Wells, M. Precursor lesions of ovarian epithelial malignancy. *Histopathology* **2001**, *38*, 87–95. [CrossRef] [PubMed]

27. Lauchlan, S.C. The secondary Mullerian system. *Obstet. Gynecol. Surv.* **1972**, *27*, 133–146. [CrossRef] [PubMed]

28. Dubeau, L. The cell of origin of ovarian epithelial tumours. *Lancet Oncol.* **2008**, *9*, 1191–1197. [CrossRef]

29. Kurman, R.J.; Vang, R.; Junge, J.; Hannibai, C.G.; Kjaer, S.K.; Shih, I.M. Papillary tubal hyperplasia: The putative precursor of ovarian atypical proliferative (borderline) serous tumors, noninvasive implants, and endosalpingiosis. *Am. J. Surg. Pathol.* **2011**, *35*, 1605–1614. [CrossRef] [PubMed]

30. Li, J.; Abushahin, N.; Pang, S.; Xiang, L.; Chambers, S.K.; Fadare, O.; Kong, B.; Zheng, W. Tubal origin of "ovarian" low-grade serous carcinoma. *Mod. Pathol.* **2011**, *24*, 1488–1499. [CrossRef] [PubMed]

31. Koshiyama, M.; Konishi, I.; Mandai, M.; Komatsu, T.; Yamamoto, S.; Nanbu, K.; Mori, T. Immunohistochemical analysis of p53 protein and 72kDa heat shock protein (HSP72) expression in ovarian carcinomas: Correlation with clinicopathology and sex steroid receptor status. *Virchows Arch.* **1995**, *425*, 603–609. [CrossRef] [PubMed]

32. Santin, A.D.; Zhan, F.; Bellone, S.; Palmieri, M.; Cane, S.; Bignotti, E.; Anfossi, S.; Gokden, M.; Dunn, D.; Romann, J.J.; et al. Gene expression profiles in primary ovarian serous papillary tumors and normal ovarian epithelium: Identification of candidate molecular markers for ovarian cancer diagnosis and therapy. *Int. J. Cancer* **2004**, *112*, 14–25. [CrossRef] [PubMed]

33. Salani, R.; Kurman, R.J.; Giuntoli, R., II; Gardner, G.; Bristow, R.; Wang, T.L.; Shih, I.M. Assessment of TP53 mutation using purified tissue samples of ovarian serous carcinomas reveals a higher mutation rate than previously reportedand does not correlate with drug resistance. *Int. J. Gynecol. Cancer* **2008**, *18*, 487–491. [CrossRef] [PubMed]

34. Cho, K.R.; Shih, I.M. Ovarian cancer. *Ann. Rev. Pathol.* **2009**, *4*, 287–313. [CrossRef] [PubMed]

35. Christie, M.; Oehler, M.K. Molecular pathology of epithelial ovarian cancer. *J. Br. Menopause Soc.* **2006**, *12*, 57–63. [CrossRef] [PubMed]

36. Cancer Genome Atlas Research Network. Integrated genomic analyses of ovarian carcinoma. *Nature* **2011**, *474*, 609–615.

37. Verhaak, R.G.; Tamayo, P.; Yang, J.Y.; Hubbard, D.; Zhang, H.; Creighton, C.J.; Fereday, S.; Lawrence, M.; Carter, S.L.; Mermel, C.H.; et al. Cancer Genome Atlas Research Network: Prognostically relevant gene signatures of high-grade serous ovarian carcinoma. *J. Clin. Investig.* **2013**, *123*, 517–525. [PubMed]

38. Murakami, R.; Matsumura, N.; Mandai, M.; Yoshihara, K.; Tanabe, H.; Nakai, H.; Yamanoi, K.; Abiko, K.; Yoshioka, Y.; Hamanishi, J.; et al. Establishment of a novel histopathological classification of high-grade serous ovarian carcinoma correlated with prognostically distinct gene expression subtypes. *Am. J. Pathol.* **2016**, *186*, 1103–1113. [CrossRef] [PubMed]

39. Horikawa, N.; Abiko, K.; Matsumura, N.; Hamanishi, J.; Baba, T.; Yamaguchi, K.; Yoshioka, Y.; Koshiyama, M.; Konishi, I. Expression of vascular endothelial growth factor in ovarian cancer inhibits tumor immunity through the accumulation of myeloid-derived suppressor cells. *Clin. Cancer Res.* **2017**, *23*, 587–599. [CrossRef] [PubMed]

40. Piek, J.M.; van Diest, P.J.; Zweemer, R.P.; Janse, J.W.; Poort-Keesom, R.J.; Menko, F.H.; Gille, J.J.; Jonqsma, A.P.; Pals, G.; Kenemans, P.; et al. Dysplastic changes in prophylactically removed fallopian tubes of women predisposed to developing ovarian cancer. *J. Pathol.* **2001**, *195*, 451–456. [CrossRef] [PubMed]

41. Chen, E.Y.; Mehra, K.; Mehrad, M.; Ning, G.; Miron, A.; Mutter, G.L.; Monte, N.; Quade, B.J.; McKeon, F.D.; Yassin, Y.; et al. Secretory cell outgrowth, PAX2 and serous carcinogenesis in the fallopian tube. *J. Pathol.* **2010**, *222*, 110–116. [CrossRef] [PubMed]

42. Gross, A.L.; Kurman, R.J.; Vang, R.; Shih, I.M.; Visvanathan, K. Precursor lesions of high-grade serous ovarian carcinoma: Morphological and molecular characteristics. *J. Oncol.* **2010**, *2010*, 126295. [CrossRef] [PubMed]

43. Carcangiu, M.L.; Radice, P.; Manoukian, S.; Spatti, G.; Gobbo, M.; Penstti, V.; Crucianelli, R.; Pasini, B. Atypical epithelial proliferation in Fallopian tubes in prophylactic salpingo-oophorectomy specimens from *BRCA*1 and *BRCA*2 germline mutation carriers. *Int. J. Gynecol. Pathol.* **2004**, *23*, 35–40. [CrossRef] [PubMed]

44. Seidman, J.D.; Yemelyanova, A.; Zaino, R.J.; Kurman, R.J. The fallopian tube-peritoneal junction: A potential site of carcinogenesis. *Int. J. Gynecol. Pathol.* **2011**, *30*, 4–11. [CrossRef] [PubMed]

45. Flesken-Nikitin, A.; Hwang, C.I.; Cheng, C.Y.; Michurina, T.V.; Enikolopov, G.; Nikitin, A.Y. Ovarian surface epithelium at the junction area contains a cancer-prone stem cell niche. *Nature* **2013**, *495*, 241–245. [CrossRef] [PubMed]

46. Jacobs, I.J.; Menon, U.; Ryan, A.; Gentry-maharai, A.; Burnell, M.; Kalsi, J.K.; Amso, N.N.; Apostolidou, S.; Benjamin, E.; Cruickshank, D.; et al. Ovarian cancer screening and mortality in the UK collaborative trial of ovarian cancer screening (UKCTOCS): A randomized controlled trial. *Lancet* **2016**, *387*, 945–956. [CrossRef]

47. Koshiyama, M.; Matsumura, M.; Konishi, I. Clinical efficacy of ovarian cancer screening. *J. Cancer* **2016**, *25*, 1311–1316. [CrossRef] [PubMed]

48. Menon, U.; Gentry-Maharaj, A.; Hallett, R.; Ryan, A.; Burnell, M.; Sharma, A.; Lewis, S.; Davies, S.; Philpott, S.; Lopes, A.; et al. Sensitivity and specificity of multimodal and ultrasound screening for ovarian cancer, and stage distribution of detected cancers: Results of the prevalence screen of the UK Collaborative Trial of Ovarian Cancer Screening (UKCTOCS). *Lancet Oncol.* **2009**, *10*, 327–340. [CrossRef]

49. Sharma, A.; Gentr-Maharaj, A.; Burnell, M.; Fourkala, E.O.; Campbell, S.; Amso, N.; Seif, M.W.; Ryan, A.; Parmar, M.; Jacobs, I.; et al. Assessing the malignant potential of ovarian inclusion cysts in postmenomausal women within the UK Collaborative Trial of Ovarian Cancer Screening (UKCTOCS): A prospective cohort study. *Gynecol. Oncol.* **2012**, *119*, 207–219.

50. Sharma, A.; Apostolidou, S.; Burnell, M.; Fourkala, E.O.; Campbell, S.; Amso, N.; Seif, M.W.; Ryan, A.; Parmar, M.; Jacobs, I.; et al. Risk of epithelial ovarian cancer in asymptomatic women with ultrasound-detected ovarian masses: A prospective cohort study within the UK collaborative trial of ovarian cancer screening (UKCTOCS). *Ultrasound Obstet. Gynecol.* **2012**, *40*, 338–344. [CrossRef] [PubMed]

51. Skates, S.J.; Xu, F.J.; Yu, Y.H.; Sjövall, K.; Einhorn, N.; Chang, Y.C.; Bast, R.C., Jr.; Knapp, R.C. Toward an optimal algorithm for ovarian cancer screening with longitudinal tumormarkers. *Cancer* **1995**, *76*, 2004–2010. [CrossRef]

52. Skates, S.J. Ovarian cancer screening: Develop of the risk of ovarian cancer algorithm (ROCA) and ROCA screening trials. *Int. J. Gynecol. Cancer* **2012**, *22*, S24–S26. [CrossRef] [PubMed]

53. Pavlik, E.D. Ovarian cancer screening effectiveness: A realization from the UK collaborative trial of ovarian cancer screening. *Womens Health* **2016**, *12*, 475–479. [CrossRef] [PubMed]

54. van Nagell, J.R., Jr.; DePriest, P.D.; Ueland, F.R.; DeSimone, C.P.; Cooper, A.L.; McDonald, J.M.; Pavlik, E.J.; Kryscio, R.J. Ovarian cancer screening with annual tranvaginal sonography: Findings of 25,000 women screened. *Cancer* **2007**, *109*, 1887–1896. [CrossRef] [PubMed]

55. van Nagell, J.R., Jr.; Miller, R.W.; DeSimone, C.P.; Ueland, F.R.; Podzielinski, I.; Goodrich, S.T.; Elder, J.W.; Huang, B.; Kryscio, R.J.; Pavlik, E.J. Long-term survival of women with epithelial ovarian cancer detected by ultrasonographic screening. *Obstet. Gynecol.* **2011**, *118*, 1212–1221. [CrossRef] [PubMed]

56. Kobayashi, H.; Yamada, Y.; Sato, T.; Sakata, M.; Kawaguchi, R.; Kanayama, S.; Shigetomi, H.; Haruta, S.; Tsuji, Y.; Ueda, S.; et al. A randomized study of screening for ovarian cancer: A multicenter study in Japan. *Int. J. Gynecol. Cancer* **2008**, *18*, 414–420. [CrossRef] [PubMed]

57. Sperling, C.; Noer, M.C.; Christensen, I.J.; Nielsen, M.L.; Lidegaard, Ø.; Høgdall, C. Comorbidity is an independent prognosis factor for the survival of ovarian cancer: A Danish register-based cohort study from a clinical database. *Gynecol. Oncol.* **2013**, *129*, 97–102. [CrossRef] [PubMed]

58. Gram, I.T.; Lukanova, A.; Brill, I.; Lund, E.; Overvad, K.; Tjønneland, A.; Clavel-Chabbert-Buffet, N.; Bamia, C.; Trichopoulou, A.; Zylis, D.; et al. Cigarette smoking and risk of histological subtypes of epithelial ovarian cancer in the EPIC cohort study. *Int. J. Cancer* **2012**, *130*, 2204–2210. [CrossRef] [PubMed]

59. Goodman, M.; Howe, H.L. Descriptive epidemiology of ovarian cancer in the United State, 1992–1997. *Cancer* **2003**, *97*, 2615–2630. [CrossRef] [PubMed]

60. Japan Society of Obstetrics and Gynecology. Statistics of gynecologic tumors in Japan. *Acta Obstet. Gynaecol. Jpn.* **2012**, *64*, 1029–1141.

61. Wong, K.H.; Mang, O.W.; Au, K.H.; Law, S.C. Incidence, mortality, and survival trends of ovarian cancer in Hong Kong, 1997 to 2006: A population-based study. *Hong Kong Med. J.* **2012**, *18*, 466–474. [PubMed]

62. Chung, H.H.; Hwang, S.Y.; Jung, K.W.; Won, Y.J.; Shin, H.R.; Kim, J.W.; Lee, H.P. Gynecologic Oncology Committee of Korean Society of Obstetrics and Gynecology. Ovarian cancer incidence and survival in Korea: 1993–2002. *Int. J. Gynecol. Cancer* **2007**, *17*, 595–600. [CrossRef] [PubMed]

7

The Role of 18F-FDG PET/CT in Staging and Prognostication of Mantle Cell Lymphoma: An Italian Multicentric Study

Domenico Albano [1], Riccardo Laudicella [2], Paola Ferro [3], Michela Allocca [4], Elisabetta Abenavoli [4], Ambra Buschiazzo [5], Alessia Castellino [6], Agostino Chiaravalloti [7,8], Annarosa Cuccaro [9], Lea Cuppari [10], Rexhep Durmo [1], Laura Evangelista [11], Viviana Frantellizzi [12], Sofya Kovalchuk [13], Flavia Linguanti [4], Giulia Santo [14], Matteo Bauckneht [15,*] and Salvatore Annunziata [16] on behalf of Young Italian Association of Nuclear Medicine (AIMN) Working Group

[1] Nuclear Medicine, University of Brescia, Spedali Civili Brescia, 25123 Brescia, Italy; doalba87@libero.it (D.A.); rexhep.durmo@gmail.com (R.D.)
[2] Nuclear Medicine Unit, Department of Biomedical and Dental Sciences and Morpho-Functional Imaging, University of Messina, 98125 Messina, Italy; riclaudi@hotmail.it
[3] Nuclear Medicine Department, IRCCS San Raffaele Hospital, 20132 Milan, Italy; paola.paolina01@gmail.com
[4] Nuclear Medicine Unit, Department of Experimental and Clinical Biomedical Sciences, University of Florence, 50134 Florence, Italy; michimedn2@gmail.com (M.A.); elisabettabenavoli@gmail.com (E.A.); flavialinguanti@hotmail.it (F.L.)
[5] Nuclear Medicine Department, S. Croce e Carle Hospital Cuneo, 12100 Cuneo, Italy; ambra.buschiazzo@gmail.com
[6] Hematology Division, S. Croce e Carle Hospital Cuneo, 12100 Cuneo, Italy; castellino.al@ospedale.cuneo.it
[7] Department of Biomedicine and Prevention, University Tor Vergata, 00133 Rome, Italy; agostino.chiaravalloti@gmail.com
[8] IRCCS Neuromed, 86077 Pozzilli, Italy
[9] Istituto di Ematologia, Fondazione Policlinico Universitario A. Gemelli IRCCS, Università Cattolica del Sacro Cuore, 00168 Rome, Italy; annarosa.cuccaro@gmail.com
[10] Nuclear Medicine and Molecular Imaging Unit, Veneto Institute of Oncology IOV-IRCCS, 35128 Padua, Italy; lea.cuppari@aulss2.veneto.it
[11] Nuclear Medicine Unit, Department of Medicine – DIMED, University of Padua, 35121 Padua, Italy; laura.evangelista@unipd.it
[12] Department of Molecular Medicine, Sapienza University of Rome, 00185 Rome, Italy; viviana.frantellizzi@uniroma1.it
[13] Hematology Unit, Department of Experimental and Clinical Biomedical Sciences, University of Florence, 50134 Florence, Italy; sofya.kovalchuk@unifi.it
[14] Nuclear Medicine Unit, Department of Interdisciplinary Medicine, University of Bari Aldo Moro, 70124 Bari, Italy; giuliasanto92@gmail.com
[15] Nuclear Medicine, IRCCS Policlinico San Martino, 16132 Genova, Italy
[16] Institute of Nuclear Medicine, Fondazione Policlinico Universitario A. Gemelli IRCCS, Università Cattolica del Sacro Cuore, 00168 Rome, Italy; salvatoreannunziata@live.it
* Correspondence: matteo.bauckneht@hsanmartino.it or matteo.bauckneht@gmail.com

Abstract: Mantle cell lymphoma (MCL) is an aggressive lymphoma subtype with poor prognosis in which 18F-FDG-PET/CT role in treatment response evaluation and prediction of outcome is still unclear. The aim of this multicentric study was to investigate the role of 18F-FDG-PET/CT in staging MCL and the prognostic role of Deauville criteria (DC) in terms of progression-free survival (PFS) and overall survival (OS). We retrospectively enrolled 229 patients who underwent baseline and end-of-treatment (eot) 18F-FDG-PET/CT after first-line therapy. EotPET/CT scans were visually interpreted according to DC. The sensitivity, specificity, positive predictive value, negative predictive value and accuracy of PET/CT for evaluation of bone marrow (BM) were 27%, 100%, 100%, 48% and

57%, respectively. The sensitivity, specificity, positive predictive value, negative predictive value and accuracy of PET/CT for evaluation of the gastrointestinal (GI) tract were 60%, 99%, 93%, 90% and 91%, respectively. At a median follow-up of 40 months, relapse occurred in 104 cases and death in 49. EotPET/CT results using DC significantly correlated with PFS, not with OS. Instead, considering OS, only MIPI score was significantly correlated. In conclusion, we demonstrated that MCL is an FDG-avid lymphoma and 18F-FDG-PET/CT is a useful tool for staging purpose, showing good specificity for BM and GI evaluation, but suboptimal sensitivity. EotPET/CT result was the only independent significant prognostic factor that correlated with PFS.

Keywords: mantle cell lymphoma; 18F-FDG PET/CT; prognosis; Deauville criteria

---

1. Introduction

Mantle cell lymphoma (MCL) accounts for 3% to 6% of all non-Hodgkin lymphoma and it is an aggressive lymphoma subtype with a high recurrence and mortality rate [1]. In the era of personalized and precision medicine, strong prognostic tools are needed in all lymphoma subtypes, such as MCL, to accurately predict possible further relapse of disease or death and to improve their treatment management. For this end-point, both clinical and imaging parameters are nowadays available, such as clinical scores and fluorine-18-fluorodeoxyglucose positron emission tomography/computed tomography (18F-FDG-PET/CT) derived parameters. MCL International Prognostic Index (MIPI) is the first prognostic index suited for MCL patients and may serve as an important tool to facilitate risk-adapted treatment decisions in patients with advanced stage MCL [2]. At the same time, FDG-PET/CT at the end of first-line therapy is recognized as a powerful prognostic tool in many lymphoma subtypes. The Deauville score criteria (DC) and subsequent Lugano criteria were proposed in this setting and nowadays they are commonly accepted as a tool to evaluate response to treatment and prognosis in both interim and end-of-therapy setting in some lymphoma subtypes as in Hodgkin lymphoma (HL) and large B-cell lymphoma (DLBCL) [3,4]. For other less common lymphoma subtypes such as MCL, there is no clear scientific evidence of the role of these criteria in treatment evaluation and prognostication, although theoretically they can be considered valid. A recent editorial by Bailly et al. [5] underlined the lack of scientific evidences of a proven role of these criteria in MCL. Moreover, 18F-FDG-PET/CT at baseline has been recently evaluated to complete the staging of disease at diagnosis, with possible implication of different prognostic risk in the follow-up. The aim of this study was to evaluate the role of 18F-FDG-PET/CT in patients with MCL as follows: assessing its power in staging MCL; evaluating DC as a predictive tool in response to therapy and as a prognostic tool in terms of progression-free survival (PFS) and overall survival (OS); testing the combination of clinical and imaging parameters in order to identify different risk classes able to predict the outcomes.

2. Results

2.1. Tumor Characteristics

Among 229 patients with histological proven MCL, there was a prevalence of male ($n = 172$) compared to female ($n = 57$); the average age was 65.1 years (range: 29–88). Patients were staged according to the Ann Arbor system as follows: stage I ($n = 4$), stage II ($n = 9$), stage III ($n = 32$) and stage IV ($n = 184$). B-symptoms, bulky disease and splenomegaly were described in 65, 40 and 101 patients, respectively. LDH level resulted high in 93 cases, β2-microglobulin in 65 and MIPI score was greater than 6 in 130 patients. Proliferative index Ki-67 was available in 183 patients, being low in 65 (36%) and high in 118 (64%) subjects. Baseline features of the patients are summarized in Table 1.

Table 1. Baseline features of our population.

Variables		Patients n (%)	Average (Range)
Age (years)			65.1 (29–88)
Sex			
	male	172 (75%)	
	female	57 (25%)	
Tumor stage at diagnosis (Ann Arbor)			
	I	4 (2%)	
	II	9 (4%)	
	III	32 (14%)	
	IV	184 (80%)	
Blastoid variant		26 (11%)	
B symptoms		65 (28%)	
LDH			
	≤245 U/L	121 (57%)	
	>245 U/L	93 (43%)	
β2-microglobulin			
	≤2.8 mg/L	108 (62%)	
	>2.8 mg/L	65 (38%)	
MIPI score			
	low-intermediate (≤6)	99 (43%)	
	high-intermediate (>6)	130 (57%)	
Bulky disease		40 (17%)	
Splenomegaly		101 (44%)	
Ki-67 score			
	≤15%	65 (36%)	
	>15%	118 (64%)	

LDH: lactate dehydrogenase; MIPI: mantle cell lymphoma international prognostic index.

2.2. 18F-FDG PET/CT Evaluation for Initial Staging

All patients had abnormal 18F-FDG PET/CT showing the presence of at least one lesion with increased FDG uptake consistent with MCL. 18F-FDG PET/CT scans detected nodal disease in 216 (94%) patients. Splenic involvement was detected by PET/CT in 100 (44%) patients.

Considering bone marrow (BM) biopsy as reference, BM disease was reported in 136 (59%) patients, while 18F-FDG PET/CT showed a focal uptake, compatible with BM involvement, in 37 (16%) subjects. Sensitivity (SE), specificity (SP), positive predictive value (PPV), negative predictive value (NPV) and accuracy (AC) of 18F-FDG-PET/CT in evaluating BM were 27% (20–35%), 100% (96–100%), 100%, 48% (46–51%) and 57% (50–63%); negative likelihood ratio was 0.73. No false positive findings for BM involvement were registered at PET/CT; however, 99 false negative findings were registered (Table 2). Agreement between the two techniques was low (Cohen's k = 0.23).

Table 2. Agreement between 18F-FDG PET/CT and BM biopsy and GI endoscopy findings.

PET/CT Findings	BM Biopsy		GI Endoscopy	
	Positive	Negative	Positive	Negative
Positive	37 (16%)	0 (0%)	28 (12%)	2 (1%)
Negative	99 (43%)	93 (41%)	19 (8%)	180 (79%)
Total	136 (59%)	93 (41%)	47 (21%)	182 (79%)

BM: bone marrow; GI: gastrointestinal.

18F-FDG PET/CT resulted positive for gastrointestinal (GI) tract involvement in 30 (13%) cases: among them, in 13 showing gastric uptake, 1 in gastro-duodenal junction uptake, 2 in the duodenum, 12 in the colon, 1 in sigma and 1 in the cecum. Considering GI endoscopy as standard of reference, 47 patients had a GI involvement of MCL. SE, SP, PPV, NPV and AC of 18F-FDG-PET/CT were 60% (44–74%), 99% (96–100%), 93% (78–98%), 90% (87–93%), 91% (86–94%) respectively; positive and negative likelihood ratios were 54.21 and 0.41, respectively (Table 2). Agreement between the two techniques was quite good (Cohen's k = 0.67).

2.3. Role of 18F-FDG PET/CT in Predicting Survival

Application of Deauville Criteria

According to DC, 186 (81%) patients were categorized as eotPET negative (score 1–3) (Figure 1) and 43 (19%) as a positive scan (score 4–5) (Figure 2). At a median follow-up of 40 months, relapse and/or progression of lymphoma was found in 104 patients with a mean time of 31.2 months (range: 3–145) from the diagnosis, and death was found in 49 cases with a mean time of 33.9 months (range 3–145). Considering patients with relapse/progression of disease, a negative eotPET/CT scans applying DC were registered in 74 cases, whilst a positive scan in 30 (in particular, Deauville score 4 in thirteen cases and Deauville score 5 in seventeen). Instead, among patients who died during the course of the disease, eotPET/CT applying DC was positive in 20 (in particular, score 4 in seven cases and score 5 in thirteen) and negative in 27 (in particular, score 1 in 17 subjects, score 2 in nine and score 3 in one). Patients with eot positive PET/CT underwent subsequent second-line chemotherapy regimen according to institutional protocol.

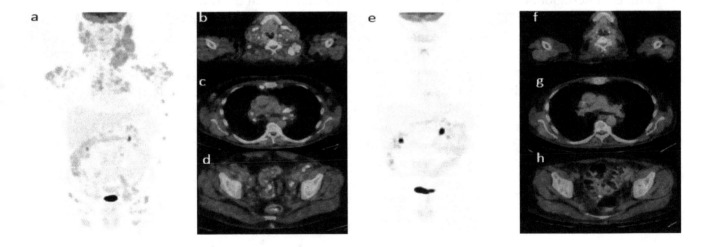

Figure 1. Emblematic example of complete metabolic response. A representative case of a 56-year-old male with stage III MCL. (**a**) Baseline maximum intensity projection (MIP), showing diffuse hypermetabolic disease in (**b**) laterocervical, (**c**) mediastinal and (**d**) iliac nodes. (**e**) PET/CT after chemotherapy showing a complete metabolic response (Deauville score 1) with no 18F-FDG uptake (**f–h**) with the disappearance of previous lesions.

The median PFS and OS were 28 months (range 3–145 months) and 34 months (range 3–145 months) respectively; with estimated 2-year PFS and OS rates of 73% and 84%, and 3-year PFS and OS rates of 56% and 75%, respectively.

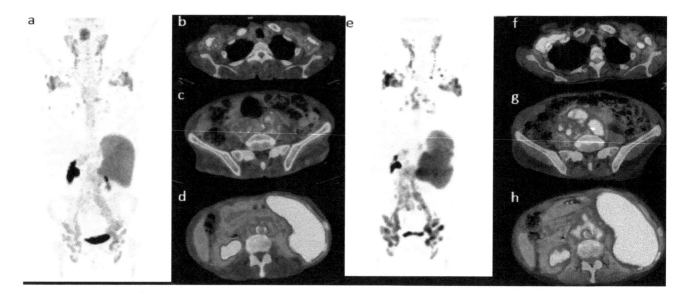

Figure 2. Emblematic example of progressive disease. A representative case of a 65-year-old male with stage III MCL. (**a**) Baseline maximum intensity projection (MIP, showing diffuse hypermetabolic disease in (**b**) laterocervical, axillary, (**c**) iliac and (**d**) inguinal nodes and in spleen. (**e**) PET/CT after chemotherapy showing a metabolic progression of disease (Deauville score 5) with the appearance of new lesions (**f–h**).

At univariate analysis, DC and MIPI score were the only parameters significantly related to PFS (Figure 3); other clinical/pathological features (sex, age, splenomegaly, bulky disease, stage, blastoid variant, β2-microglobulin and LDH level) were not associated with the outcome. PFS was significantly shorter in patients with eotPET/CT DC positive compared to negative (12 vs. 32 months, $p < 0.001$). At multivariate analysis, only metabolic feature (Deauville score) was confirmed to be an independent prognostic factor for PFS ($p < 0.001$). Combining DC (≤ 3 and >3) and MIPI score (≤ 6 and >6), PFS was significantly longer in eotPET negative patients independently from MIPI score ($p < 0.001$) (Figure 4). Median PFS was 82 months in patients with low-intermediate MIPI score (≤ 6) and a negative eotPET/CT (DC ≤ 3); 62 months in patients with high MIPI score (>6) and a negative eotPET/CT; 25 months in patients with low-intermediate MIPI score and a positive eotPET/CT (DC 4 or 5), and 12 months in patients with high MIPI score and a positive eotPET/CT.

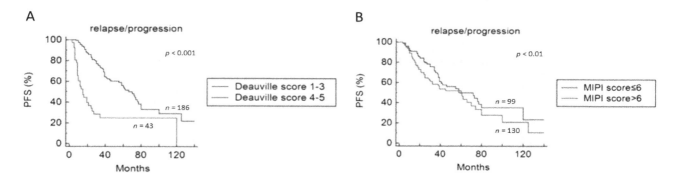

Figure 3. Progression-free survival (PFS) curves according to end-of-treatment PET/CT results using (**A**) Deauville criteria and (**B**) MIPI score.

Instead, considering OS, only MIPI score resulted as significantly correlated (Figure 5), both at univariate and multivariate analysis ($p = 0.017$) (Table 3). EotPET/CT according to DC did not predict OS (31 vs. 37.5 months, $p = 0.814$) (Figure 5).

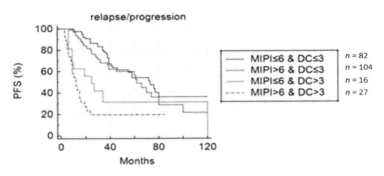

Figure 4. Progression-free survival curve combining MIPI score and Deauville score groups.

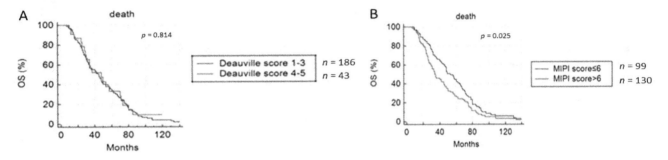

Figure 5. Overall survival (OS) curves according to end-of-treatment PET/CT results using (**A**) Deauville criteria and (**B**) MIPI score.

Table 3. Univariate and multivariate analyses for PFS and OS.

Variables	Univariate Analysis		Multivariate Analysis	
	p-Value	HR (95% CI)	*p*-Value	HR (95% CI)
	PFS			
Sex	0.451	0.845 (0.548–1.306)		
Age	0.153	1.530 (0.838–3.097)		
MIPI score	0.009	0.713 (0.482–1.056)	0.174	1.219 (0.915–1.623)
LDH level	0.163	0.742 (0.488–1.128)		
B2 microglobulin	0.458	0.831 (0.511–1.353)		
Ki-67 score	0.066	0.653 (0.415–1.028)		
Bulky disease	0.153	1.722 (0.992–2.987)		
Splenomegaly	0.087	0.703 (0.472–01049)		
Stage acc Ann Arbor	0.855	0.957 (0.589–1.531)		
Blastoid variant	0.185	0.598 (0.282–1.270)		
Deauville score	<0.001	0.137 (0.073–0.259)	<0.001	4.059 (2.573–6.403)
Treatment regimen	0.655	0.857 (0.519–1.243)		
	OS			
Sex	0.211	1.759 (0.577–6.033)		
Age	0.375	1.270 (0.722–2.369)		
MIPI score	0.025	0.711 (0.527–0.959)	0.017	1.204 (1.032–1.403)
LDH level	0.709	0.942 (0.690–1.287)		
B2 microglobulin	0.524	1.128 (0.778–1.635)		
Ki67 score	0.195	1.250 (0.891–1.754)		
Bulky disease	0.390	0.828 (0.539–1.272)		
Splenomegaly	0.287	0.846 (0.622–1.150)		
Stage acc Ann Arbor	0.393	0.859 (0.606–1.217)		
Blastoid variant	0.075	0.618 (0.363–1.051)		
Deauville score	0.814	1.055 (0.671–1.660)		
Treatment regimen	0.598	1.001 (0.571–1.460)		

PFS: progression-free survival; OS: overall survival; HR: hazard ratio; CI: confidence interval; N: number.

Treatment regimen (R-CHOP regimen vs. other chemotherapy regimen) did not influence outcome survival considering both PFS and OS.

3. Discussion

MCL is an aggressive B-cell non-Hodgkin lymphoma with a fast-growing course, high-risk of relapse and need for early treatment. Patients affected by MCL typically present with advanced-stage disease and extranodal involvement with a predilection for BM and GI tract, where routine conventional techniques such as CT have a suboptimal accuracy [6]. A correct and an early identification of initial and extranodal disease may be crucial because it could potentially affect patient's management and therapeutic choice. 18F-FDG PET/CT has shown a high accuracy in the detection of nodal involvement [7–9], but a low sensitivity in BM and GI tract, being inadequate to replace BM biopsy and GI endoscopy in disease staging [10–12]. In the present study, we demonstrated a very low sensitivity of PET/CT in the evaluation of BM involvement (27%), but with a specificity equal to 100%. No case of false-positive findings on BM at PET/CT were recorded, but there were 99 cases of false-negative PET. Thus, the need for BM biopsy seems to be mandatory in case of negative BM PET/CT. Previous studies [10–12] reported a very low pretreatment PET scan accuracy to detect BM involvement, very low with sensitivity ranging from 12% to 51%. A comparison between our paper and others is not easy due to the different population number and features evaluated. Recently, Morgan et al. [13] projected a voxel-based analysis of the iliac bones for classifying BM disease in MCL founding a good sensitivity and specificity (100% and 87.5%, respectively); this method seems to be very promising but less practical and reproducible and it has been validated only on a small sample of patients. The potential role of 18F-FDG PET/CT in evaluating lymphoma BM involvement remains a challenge; this is a non-invasive technique well studied in HL and DLBCL, but with controversial and limited evidence [14,15]. Several studies have proven that 18F-FDG PET/CT can be an accurate method for the evaluation of BM involvement in patients affected by DLBCL considering focal highly 18F-FDG-avid lesions as reference standard; on the other hand the absence of a focal uptake does not exclude the presence of BM involvement. Our results confirmed similar evidences also in MCL, suggesting to avoid a BM biopsy in case of positive PET/CT scan.

Also, for the GI tract, our results showed that 18F-FDG PET/CT revealed a good specificity but a low sensitivity (60%), being in agreement with other published papers [9,12,16]. It was already demonstrated that an increased 18F-FDG bowel uptake may be common, especially in diabetic patients [17,18], thus reducing the diagnostic accuracy of the evaluation of this district.

Another crucial topic to consider in MCL is the prognostication; nowadays, neither clinical nor imaging prognostic markers are available in MCL setting. MIPI score [2] was an attempt created to better classify patients with MCL and predict prognosis, but its validation has shown conflicting results [19,20]. Other histopathological features, such as blastoid variant and Ki-67 score, have been investigated without shared evidence [21]. Instead, the prognostic value of 18F-FDG-PET/CT in MCL remains under debate [16,22–25]. In 2009, a five-point scale system called Deauville criteria (DC) was introduced to analyze 18F-FDG PET/CT results after treatment in lymphoma [26]; this scale used the mediastinum and liver activity as the reference standard, and has been recommended for reporting both interim and end-of-treatment PET for FDG-avid lymphoma (both HL and NHL, especially DLBCL) [3,4,27]. In our paper, we tried to validate this score also in MCL, obtaining some strong results; patients with a negative end-of-treatment PET/CT (DC1-3) had significantly longer PFS than patients with a positive PET/CT (DC4,5). Similar results in small cohort of patients were reported by other authors [20,22,28]. However, this evidence was not confirmed for OS, where DC seems to not influence the outcome survival. This could be explained to the fact that eotPET/CT results were used to guide subsequent management and further treatments, as second-line chemotherapy regimen.

The treatment of MCL is a challenge and often stays unsatisfactory; complete responses to the standard chemotherapy regimens are not common. Czuczman et al. [29] in a multicenter open-label single-arm phase II study showed that the complete metabolic response at PET/CT was a predictor of outcome survival. In addition to qualitative 18F-FDG PET/CT analysis using DC, also semiquantitative PET/CT parameters have been studied as prognostic factors, like SUVmax, with controversial results. Karam et al. [30] and Bodet-Milin et al. [16], in patients affected by MCL, suggested SUVmax thresholds of 5 and 6, respectively, to stratify patients into high-risk versus low-risk groups and to predict OS and disease-free survival. On the other hand, no prognostic impact of SUVmax was demonstrated by other groups [10,12,24]. Recently in the LyMa-PET Project [23], it was demonstrated that SUVmax was the only independent prognostic factor for PFS and OS; moreover, authors suggested a scoring system combining MIPI and SUVmax (using a cutoff of 10.3) to help the outcome prediction. In our study, eotPET/CT results using DC were superior than the MIPI score in PFS, while for OS only the MIPI score resulted as an independent prognostic factor.

Instead, no clinical or histological variables, like blastoid variant and B2 microglobulin, showed significant association with outcome survival in our analysis; this is partially in contradiction with literature [1] and related probably to heterogeneity of population studied.

Also, Ki-67 score seems not to be related to PET/CT features and outcome survival despite that in other lymphoma subtypes significant correlation was demonstrated [31,32].

The present study has some limitations. First, this is a retrospective multicentric study, so heterogeneous features in our population in terms of clinical baseline parameters and treatment schemes could be found. Despite this, so far and to best of our knowledge, the present study is the first large series of MCL patients aimed to assess the diagnostic and prognostic role of 18F-FDG PET/CT. Second, although this study showed the independent prognostic value for PFS of end-of-treatment PET/CT, the role of semi-quantitative PET/CT parameters, in terms of SUVs, should be further analyzed. Third, more complex statistical analysis, like a deep learning approach, might have improved data analysis.

4. Materials and Methods

4.1. Patients

Between January 2007 and December 2018 in nine Italian Nuclear Medicine Centers, 229 patients with newly diagnosed, histologically proven MCL were retrospectively enrolled. The histopathological diagnosis was based on the World Health Organization criteria [33]. The inclusion criteria were as follows: patients with a histological confirmation of MCL; age ≥18 years; availability of BM biopsy and GI endoscopy at time of diagnosis; availability of baseline and end of treatment 18F-FDG PET/CT results in all patients; and availability of clinical/radiologic follow-up data for at least 12 months. Patients with concomitant malignancies were excluded. We further reviewed the follow medical records of these patients: epidemiological features (age at diagnosis, sex), clinical data (tumor stage, MIPI score, bulky disease, splenomegaly, B symptoms, lactate-dehydrogenase (LDH) level, β2-microglobulin level), histopathological data (Ki-67 score, blastoid variant), metabolic features by 18F-FDG PET/CT, treatment modalities and follow-up data. LDH level, β2-microglobulin and MIPI score were dichotomized using cutoff values of 245 U/L, 2.8 mg/L and 6 respectively. Tumor stage according to Ann Arbor classification was divided in early (I and II) and advanced (III and IV) disease. The bulky disease was defined when the maximum width was equal or greater than one-third of the internal transverse diameter of the thorax or at an alternative site as any mass measuring 10 cm or more by any imaging study. Proliferative activity, expressed by Ki-67 score, was available in 183 patients; average Ki-67 was 25% (range 1–95%). The Ki-67 expression level was arbitrarily dichotomized using a cut-off of 15% as suggested by other authors [24,34].

All patients were treated according to the institution's standard protocol with chemotherapy regimen related to the stage of disease, age and institutional internal protocol. Eighty-two patients were treated according to R-CHOP (Rituximab, Cyclophoshpamide, Hydroxydaunomycin, Oncovin, Prednisone) regimen, sixty-eight with R-DHAP (dexamethasone, cytarabine, cisplatin), thirty-nine with R-Bendamustina, twenty-four with BCVPP (Carmustine, Cyclophosphamide, Vinblastine, Procarbazine, and Prednisone), twelve with MBVD (Myocet+BVD). In one case, chemotherapy was followed by the involved field radiotherapy. Four patients (2%) underwent only radiotherapy due to the early stage of disease (stage I).

4.2. 18F-FDG PET/CT Imaging and Interpretation

All patients underwent baseline 18F-FDG PET/CT and a subsequent PET/CT at completion of first-line therapy (eotPET/CT). PET/CT studies were performed following EANM guidelines [35]. Baseline PET/CT was performed within 14 days before the first cycle of chemotherapy and end-of-treatment PET/CT was done at least three weeks after the completion of chemotherapy or 12 weeks after completion of radiotherapy.

18F-FDG-PET/CT was performed after at least 6 h of fasting and with glucose level lower than 150 mg/dL. An activity of 3.5–4.5 MBq/Kg of 18F-FDG was administered intravenously and scans were acquired about 60 min after injection, usually from the skull basis to the mid-thigh. Owing to the multicenter nature of the study, the exams were acquired on different PET/CT scanners: Discovery STE or 690 (GE Healthcare Technologies, Milwaukee, Wisconsin, USA), Discovery IQ (GE Healthcare Technologies), Discovery LS (GE Healthcare Technologies), Gemini TFEGXL (Philips Medical Systems, Cleveland, OH, USA) and Biograph 16 (Siemens Healthcare, Erlangen, Germany). Standard parameters used were: CT: 80 mA, 120 Kv without contrast; 2.5–4 min per bed-PET-step of 15 cm; the reconstruction was performed in a 128×128 matrix and with a 60 cm field-of-view.

Patients were instructed to void before imaging acquisition, no oral or intravenous contrast agents were administrated and no bowel preparation was used for any patient; written consent was obtained before studies. The PET images were visually analyzed and readers had knowledge of clinical history. PET/CT scans were interpreted visually by two nuclear medicine physicians (DA, SA) with experience in this field and the discordance was resolved by a consensus between the two imaging readers.

For the interpretation of images, each focal tracer uptake deviating from physiological distribution and background and uptake higher than liver activity was considered as suggestive for lymphoma.

In the evaluation of BM involvement, PET/CT findings were considered positive in the presence of isolated/multiple focal uptakes in the BM that could not be explained by benign findings on the underlying CT scan or patient's medical history (like fractures, spondylodiscitis, etc.). In the evaluation of GI involvement, PET/CT findings were considered positive in the presence of isolated/multiple intense focal uptakes in the GI tract. Accuracy of 18F-FDG PET/T results was evaluated considering further evaluations: lesions with 18F-FDG PET/CT uptakes were considered as true-positives if further analyses confirmed the malignant nature, and false-positive if further evaluations showed no malignant lesions. Lesions without 18F-FDG PET/CT uptakes were considered as true negative if further analyses confirmed the absence of neoplastic lesions and false-negative if further evaluations showed malignant ones. Eot 18F-FDG PET/CT was interpreted by visual analysis using the Deauville 5-point scale [4]. According to Deauville Criteria (DC), 18F-FDG PET was interpreted as follows: 1 = no uptake above background, 2 = uptake equal to or lower than mediastinum, 3 = uptake higher than mediastinum and lower than liver, 4 = uptake moderately increased compared to the liver and 5 = uptake markedly increased compared to the liver. Eot 18F-FDG PET/CT scans were considered negative for scores 1 to 3 and positive for scores 4 to 5.

4.3. Statistical Analysis

Our statistical analysis was carried out using MedCalc Software version 17.1 for Windows (Ostend, Belgium). Categorical variables were described as the calculation of simple and relative frequencies, while the numeric variables were described as average, minimum and maximum. We calculated SE, SP, PPV, NPV and AC based on Bayes's law, with 95% confidence intervals, considering final diagnosis as a reference.

The PFS was calculated from the date of diagnosis of MCL to the date of first relapse, progression of disease or the last follow-up date. The OS was calculated from the date of diagnosis of MCL to the date of death from any cause or the last follow-up date.

Survival curves were plotted according to the Kaplan–Meier method and differences between several groups were investigated by using a two-tailed log rank test. Cox regression was used to evaluate the hazard ratio (HR) and its confidence interval (CI). A p-value of <0.05 was considered statistically significant and the adjusted significant p-value after Bonferroni's correction was 0.038.

5. Conclusions

In conclusion, in this study, we demonstrated that MCL is an FDG-avid lymphoma and that 18F-FDG PET/CT is a useful tool for staging purpose, which should be considered in the diagnostic flow-chart of this patients in concert with other modalities.

PET/CT showed good specificity for BM and GI evaluation but suboptimal sensitivity. Moreover, eotPET post-therapy PET/CT results, evaluated according to Deauville criteria, can be considered powerful prognostic information in order to stratify the progressive patients.

Author Contributions: Study concept and design, D.A., S.A., R.L., M.B.; recruitment and collection data, D.A., S.A., M.B., R.D., A.B., A.C. (Alessia Castellino), L.C., P.F., V.F., A.C. (Agostino Chiaravalloti), F.L., E.A., M.A., G.S., A.C. (Annarosa Cuccaro), S.K.; quality control of data and algorithm, L.E., M.B., R.L.; data analysis, statistical analysis and interpretation, D.A., S.A.; manuscript preparation, D.A., S.A., R.L., M.B.; editing, review, supervision, approval final version of the manuscript, all authors.

References

1. Vose, J.M. Mantle cell lymphoma: 2017 update on diagnosis, risk-stratification, and clinical management. *Am. J. Hematol.* **2017**, *92*, 806–813. [CrossRef] [PubMed]
2. Hoster, E.; Dreyling, M.; Klapper, W.; Gisselbrecht, C.; van Hoof, A.; Kluin-Nelemans, H.C.; Pfreundschuh, M.; Reiser, M.; Metzner, B.; Einsele, H.; et al. A new prognostic index (MIPI) for patients with advanced-stage mantle cell lymphoma. *Blood* **2008**, *111*, 558–565. [CrossRef] [PubMed]
3. Barrington, S.F.; Mikhaeel, N.G.; Kostakoglu, L.; Meignan, M.; Hutchings, M.; Müeller, S.P.; Schwartz, L.H.; Zucca, E.; Fisher, R.I.; Trotman, J.; et al. Role of imaging in the staging and response assessment of lymphoma: Consensus of the International Conference on Malignant Lymphomas Imaging Working Group. *J. Clin. Oncol.* **2014**, *32*, 3048–3058. [CrossRef] [PubMed]
4. Cheson, B.D.; Fisher, R.I.; Barrington, S.F.; Cavalli, F.; Schwartz, L.H.; Zucca, E.; Lister, T.A. Recommendations for initial evaluation, staging, and response assessment of Hodgkin and non-Hodgkin lymphoma: The Lugano classification. *J. Clin. Oncol.* **2014**, *32*, 3059–3068. [CrossRef] [PubMed]
5. Bailly, C.; Carlier, T.; Touzeau, C.; Arlicot, N.; Kraeber-Bodéré, F.; Le Gouill, S.; Bodet-Milin, C. Interest of FDG-PET in the Management of Mantle Cell Lymphoma. *Front Med (Lausanne)* **2019**, *6*, 70. [CrossRef]
6. Maddocks, K. Update on Mantle cell lymphoma. *Blood* **2018**, *132*, 1647–1656. [CrossRef]
7. Gill, S.; Wolf, M.; Prince, H.M.; Januszewicz, H.; Ritchie, D.; Hicks, R.J.; Seymour, J.F. 18F Fluorodeoxyglucose positron emission tomography scanning for staging, response assessment, and disease surveillance in patients with Mantle cell lymphoma. *Clin. Lymphoma Myeloma* **2008**, *8*, 158–165. [CrossRef]
8. Alavi, A.; Shrikanthan, S.; Aydin, A.; Talanow, R.; Schuster, S. Fluorodeoxyglucose-positron-emission tomography findings in Mantle cell lymphoma. *Clin. Lymphoma Myeloma Leuk.* **2011**, *11*, 261–266. [CrossRef]
9. Albano, D.; Ferro, P.; Bosio, G.; Fallanca, F.; Re, A.; Tucci, A.; Ferreri, A.J.M.; Angelillo, P.; Gianolli, L.; Giubbini, R.; et al. Diagnostic and Clinical Impact of Staging 18F-FDG PET/CT in Mantle-Cell Lymphoma: A Two-Center Experience. *Clin. Lymphoma Myeloma Leuk.* **2019**, *19*, e457–e464. [CrossRef]
10. Brepoels, L.; Stroobants, S.; De Wever, W.; Dierickx, D.; Vandenberghe, P.; Thomas, J.; Mortelmans, L.; Verhoef, G.; De Wolf-Peeters, C. Positron emission tomography in mantle cell lymphoma. *Leuk. Lymphoma* **2008**, *49*, 1693–1701. [CrossRef]
11. Cohen, J.B.; Hall, N.C.; Ruppert, A.S.; Jones, J.A.; Porcu, P.; Baiocchi, R.; Christian, B.A.; Penza, S.; Benson, D.M.; Flynn, J.; et al. Association of pre-transplantation positron emission tomography/computed tomography and outcome in mantle cell lymphoma. *Bone Marrow Transplant.* **2013**, *48*, 1212–1217. [CrossRef] [PubMed]

12. Hosein, P.J.; Pastorini, V.H.; Paes, F.M.; Eber, D.; Chapman, J.R.; Serafini, A.N.; Alizadeh, A.A.; Lossos, I.S. Utility of positron emission tomography scans in mantle cell lymphoma. *Am. J. Hematol.* **2011**, *86*, 841–845. [CrossRef] [PubMed]

13. Morgan, R.; Perry, M.; Kwak, J.; Jensen, A.; Kamdar, M. Positron emission tomography-based analysis can accurately predict bone marrow involvement with Mantle Cell Lymphoma. *Clin. Lymphoma Myeloma Leuk.* **2018**, *18*, 731–736. [CrossRef] [PubMed]

14. Adams, H.J.A.; Kwee, T.C.; de Keizer, B.; Fijnheer, R.; de Klerk, J.M.; Littooij, A.S.; Nievelstein, R.A. Systematic review and meta-analysis on the diagnostic performance of FDG-PET/CT in detecting bone marrow involvement in newly diagnosed Hodgkin lymphoma: Is bone marrow biopsy still necessary? *Ann. Oncol.* **2014**, *25*, 921–927. [CrossRef]

15. Adams, H.J.A.; Kwee, T.C.; de Keizer, B.; Fijnheer, R.; de Klerk, J.M.; Nievelstein, R.A. FDG PET/CT for the detection of bone marrow involvement in diffuse large B cell lymphoma: Systematic review and meta-analysis. *Eur. J. Nucl. Med. Mol. Imaging* **2014**, *41*, 565–574. [CrossRef]

16. Bodet-Milin, C.; Touzeau, C.; Leux, C.; Sahin, M.; Moreau, A.; Maisonneuve, H.; Morineau, N.; Jardel, H.; Moreau, P.; Gallazini-Crépin, C.; et al. Prognostic impact of 18F-fluorodeoxyglucose positron emission tomography in untreated mantle cell lymphoma: A retrospective study from GOELAMS group. *Eur. J. Nucl. Med. Mol. Imaging* **2010**, *37*, 1633–1642. [CrossRef]

17. Gontier, E.; Fourme, E.; Wartski, M.; Blondet, C.; Bonardel, G.; Le Stanc, E.; Mantzarides, M.; Foehrenbach, H.; Pecking, A.P.; Alberini, J.L. High and typical 18F-FDG bowel uptake in patients treated with metformin. *Eur. J. Nucl. Med. Mol. Imaging* **2008**, *35*, 95–99. [CrossRef]

18. Bybel, B.; Greenberg, I.D.; Paterson, J.; Ducharme, J.; Leslie, W.D. Increased F-18 FDG intestinal uptake in diabetic patients on metformin: A matched case-control analysis. *Clin. Nucl. Med.* **2011**, *36*, 452–456. [CrossRef]

19. Shah, J.J.; Fayad, L.; Romaguera, J. Mantle Cell International Prognostic Index (MIPI) not prognostic after R-hyper-CVAD. *Blood* **2008**, *112*, 2583. [CrossRef]

20. Mato, A.R.; Svodoba, J.; Feldman, T.; Zielonka, T.; Agress, H.; Panush, D.; Miller, M.; Toth, P.; Lizotte, P.M.; Nasta, S.; et al. Post-treatment (not interim) positron emission tomography-computed tomography scan status is highly predictive of outcome in mantle cell lymphoma patients treated with R-HyperCVAD. *Cancer* **2012**, *118*, 3565–3570. [CrossRef]

21. Tiemann, M.; Schrader, C.; Klapper, W.; Dreyling, M.H.; Campo, E.; Norton, A.; Berger, F.; Kluin, P.; Ott, G.; Pileri, S.; et al. Histopathology, cell proliferation indices and clinical outcome in 304 patients with mantle cell lymphoma (MCL): A clinicopathological study from the European MCL Network. *Br. J. Haematol.* **2005**, *131*, 29–38. [CrossRef] [PubMed]

22. Lamonica, D.; Graf, D.A.; Munteanu, M.C.; Czuczman, M.S. 18F-FDG PET for Measurement of Response and Prediction of Outcome to Relapsed or Refractory Mantle Cell Lymphoma Therapy with Bendamustine-Rituximab. *J. Nucl. Med.* **2017**, *58*, 62–68. [CrossRef] [PubMed]

23. Bailly, C.; Carlier, T.; Barriolo-Rieding, A.; Casasnovas, O.; Gyan, E.; Meignan, M.; Moreau, A.; Burroni, B.; Djaileb, L.; Gressin, R.; et al. Prognostic value of FDG-PET in patients with mantle cell lymphoma: Results from the LyMa-PET Project. *Haematologica* **2019**. [CrossRef] [PubMed]

24. Albano, D.; Bosio, G.; Bianchetti, N.; Pagani, C.; Re, A.; Tucci, A.; Giubbini, R.; Bertagna, F. Prognostic role of baseline 18F-FDG PET/CT metabolic parameters in mantle cell lymphoma. *Ann. Nucl. Med.* **2019**, *33*, 449–458. [CrossRef]

25. Kedmi, M.; Avivi, I.; Ribakovsky, E.; Benyamini, N.; Davidson, T.; Goshen, E.; Tadmor, T.; Nagler, A.; Avigdor, A. Is there a role for therapy response assessment with 2-[fluorine-18] fluoro-2-deoxy-D-glucose-positron emission tomography/computed tomography in mantle cell lymphoma? *Leuk. Lymphoma* **2014**, *55*, 2484–2489. [CrossRef]

26. Meignan, M.; Gallamini, A.; Haioun, C.; Polliack, A. Report on the Second International Workshop on interim positron emission tomography in lymphoma held in Menton, France, 8–9 April 2010. *Leuk Lymphoma.* **2010**, *51*, 2171–2180. [CrossRef]

27. Fallanca, F.; Alongi, P.; Incerti, E.; Ginaolli, L.; Picchio, M.; Kayani, I.; Bomanji, J. Diagnostic accuracy of FDG PET/CT for clinical evaluation at the end of treatment of HL and NHL: A comparison of the Deauville Criteria (DC) and the International Harmonization Project Criteria (IHPC). *Eur. J. Nucl. Med. Mol. Imaging* **2016**, *43*, 1837–1840. [CrossRef]

28. Klener, P.; Fronkova, E.; Belada, D.; Forsterova, K.; Pytlik, R.; Kalinova, M.; Simkovic, M.; Salek, D.; Mocikova, H.; Prochazka, V.; et al. Alternating R-CHOP and R-cytarabine is a safe and effective regimen for transplant-ineligible patients with a newly diagnosed mantle cell lymphoma. *Hematol. Oncol.* **2018**, *36*, 110–115. [CrossRef]

29. Czuczman, M.S.; Goy, A.; Lamonica, D.; Graf, D.A.; Munteanu, M.C.; van der Jagt, R.H. Phase II study of bendamustine combined with rituximab in relapsed/refractory mantle cell lymphoma: Efficacy, tolerability, and safety findings. *Ann. Hematol.* **2015**, *94*, 2025–2032. [CrossRef]

30. Karam, M.; Ata, A.; Irish, K.; Feustel, P.J.; Mottaghy, F.M.; Stroobants, S.G.; Verhoef, G.E.; Chundru, S.; Douglas-Nikitin, V.; Wong, C.O.; et al. FDG positron emission tomography/computed tomography scan may identify mantle cell lymphoma patients with unusually favorable outcome. *Nucl. Med. Comm.* **2009**, *30*, 770–778. [CrossRef]

31. Novelli, A.; Briones, J.; Flotats, A.; Sierra, J. PET/CT Assessment of Follicular Lymphoma and High Grade B Cell Lymphoma-Good Correlation with Clinical and Histological Features at Diagnosis. *Adv. Clin. Exp. Med.* **2015**, *24*, 325–330. [CrossRef] [PubMed]

32. Meyer, H.J.; Wienke, A.; Surov, A. Correlations Between Imaging Biomarkers and Proliferation Index Ki-67 in Lymphomas: A Systematic Review and Meta-Analysis. *Clin. Lymphoma Myeloma Leuk.* **2019**, *19*, 266–272. [CrossRef] [PubMed]

33. Jaffe, E.S.; Harris, N.L.; Stein, H.; Vardinam, J.W. *Tumours of Haematopoietic and Lymphoid Tissues: World Health Organization Classification of Tumours, Pathology, and Genetics*; IARC Press: Lyon, France, 2001; Volume 3.

34. Albano, D.; Bosio, G.; Camoni, L.; Farina, M.; Re, A.; Tucci, A.; Giubbini, R.; Bertagna, F. Prognostic role of baseline ^{18}F-FDG PET/CT parameters in MALT lymphoma. *Hematol. Oncol.* **2019**, *37*, 39–46.

35. Boellaard, R.; Delgado-Bolton, R.; Oyen, W.J.; Giammarile, F.; Tatsch, K.; Eschner, W.; Verzijlbergen, F.J.; Barrington, S.F.; Pike, L.C.; Weber, W.A.; et al. FDG PET/CT: EANM procedure guidelines for tumour imaging: Version 2.0. *Eur. J. Nucl. Med. Mol. Imaging* **2015**, *42*, 328–354. [CrossRef]

8

Symptoms Relevant to Surveillance for Ovarian Cancer

Robert M. Ore [1], Lauren Baldwin [1], Dylan Woolum [1], Erika Elliott [1], Christiaan Wijers [1], Chieh-Yu Chen [1], Rachel W. Miller [1], Christopher P. DeSimone [1], Frederick R. Ueland [1], Richard J. Kryscio [2], John R. van Nagell [1] and Edward J. Pavlik [1,*]

[1] Division of Gynecologic Oncology, Department of Obstetrics and Gynecology, University of Kentucky Chandler Medical Center-Markey Cancer Center, Lexington, KY 40536-0293, USA; robert.ore@uky.edu (R.M.O.); labald1@uky.edu (L.B.); dylan.woolum@uky.edu (D.W.); erikatay28@gmail.com (E.E.); christiaan.d.wijers@vanderbilt.edu (C.W.); chieh-yu.chen@uky.edu (C.-Y.C.); raware00@email.uky.edu (R.W.M.); cpdesi00@uky.edu (C.P.D.); fuela0@email.uky.edu (F.R.U.); jrvann2@email.uky.edu (J.R.v.N.)

[2] Department of Statistics, University of Kentucky Chandler Medical Center-Markey Cancer Center, Lexington, KY 40536-0293, USA; richard.kryscio@uky.edu

* Correspondence: epaul1@uky.edu

Academic Editor: Andreas Kjaer

Abstract: To examine how frequently and confidently healthy women report symptoms during surveillance for ovarian cancer. A symptoms questionnaire was administered to 24,526 women over multiple visits accounting for 70,734 reports. A query of reported confidence was included as a confidence score (CS). Chi square, McNemars test, ANOVA and multivariate analyses were performed. 17,623 women completed the symptoms questionnaire more than one time and >9500 women completed it more than one four times for >43,000 serially completed questionnaires. Reporting ovarian cancer symptoms was ~245 higher than ovarian cancer incidence. The positive predictive value (0.073%) for identifying ovarian cancer based on symptoms alone would predict one malignancy for 1368 cases taken to surgery due to reported symptoms. Confidence on the first questionnaire (83.3%) decreased to 74% when more than five questionnaires were completed. Age-related decreases in confidence were significant ($p < 0.0001$). Women reporting at least one symptom expressed more confidence (41,984/52,379 = 80.2%) than women reporting no symptoms (11,882/18,355 = 64.7%), $p < 0.0001$. Confidence was unrelated to history of hormone replacement therapy or abnormal ultrasound findings ($p = 0.30$ and 0.89). The frequency of symptoms relevant to ovarian cancer was much higher than the occurrence of ovarian cancer. Approximately 80.1% of women expressed confidence in what they reported.

Keywords: symptoms; questionnaire; certainty/uncertainty

1. Introduction

Intake forms are commonly used in clinical care and are often presented to women undergoing well-woman exams and routine gynecologic care. Guidelines exist for British general practitioners [1] as well as for American generalists [2] for collecting and evaluating information on symptoms related to ovarian cancer (OvCA). Women who report certain symptoms are candidates for testing with Ca125, pelvic ultrasound and/or referral to a gynecologic oncologist. Symptoms indicative of ovarian cancer have been included in information collected through the Patient Reported Outcomes Measurement Information System (PROMIS [3,4]) developed by NIH in the United States and integrated with electronic medical records in the ambulatory care setting [5]. Discrepancy has been described between clinician and patient symptoms reporting with many cancer-related symptoms going unrecognized [6]. The dynamics of communication between the physician and patient can be complex and lead to this discrepancy in symptoms discovery with the doctor assuming that the patient will initiate a revealing conversation while the patient expects the doctor to inquire about possible symptoms. Differences in symptoms reporting even exist between paper and electronic reporting [7].

The present report is unique in that it examines factors influencing personal confidence inherent to symptoms reporting by focusing on a large cohort of women without cancer. This report focuses on intake information specific to symptoms of ovarian cancer for deciding the possibility of malignancy. We have employed a questionnaire containing a constellation of symptoms (both related and not related to ovarian cancer) that was reported on by Goff [8]. While data challenging the power of this symptoms index to identify early-stage ovarian cancer has been reported [9,10], symptoms information cannot be ignored, otherwise delays in diagnosis can occur [11]. We have added a self-administered evaluation of reporting confidence to the Goff symptoms questionnaire in order to assess the degree to which women are confident in their responses and have analyzed serially completed questionnaires to determine how time and repeated exposure to symptoms reporting affect confidence. Contemplation of patient-reported confidence is paralleled by the judiciary system where a great deal of emphasis is placed on witness confidence in determining the credibility of testimony [12]. Our report is noteworthy because it identifies changing patient confidence in information that they report on questionnaires which should make physicians more sensitive to the reliability of patient responses.

2. Materials and Methods

Women enrolled in the ongoing ultrasound-based University of Kentucky Ovarian Cancer Screening Program [13–15] from 1987 to July 2013 consisted of both women in the general population and those of high risk based on confirmation of a primary or secondary relative diagnosed with ovarian cancer (n = 41,529). Approval was received from the University of Kentucky Institutional Review Board (IRB number 88-0021-9F6, renewed 11 August 2016). Women were recruited by physician recommendation, media announcements, and word of mouth. Women needed to be competent and understand the terms of the informed consent presented in English, or they were excluded from screening.

Participants in this screening program are characterized as health conscious (>90% medical checkups, >85% annual mammography), well educated (>50% college, ~3% not high school graduates), married (75%) and medically insured (95%) [16].

In October of 2008, participants began completing a modified symptoms questionnaire printed in English which was originally developed by Goff et al. [8]. In total, 24,526 women completed the questionnaire and 17,623 women completed the questionnaire more than once on subsequent screens, for a total of 70,734 evaluated questionnaires. The questionnaire was in the exact form as published by Goff, [8] but was modified to include the confidence of the responder as reported [9]. This modification added the question: "How confidently did you answer these questions?" The possible responses were: "no confidence" = 0, "minimally sure" = 1, "more than minimally sure" = 2, "pretty sure" = 3, "sure" = 4 and "absolutely sure" = 5. The screening sonographer queried each participant about their understanding of each symptom and was responsible for the participant providing answers to all data fields prior to screening. Sonographers gave explanations about the symptoms on the questionnaires as a clarification process prior to screening. Effort was made to model general clinical practice by presenting clarifications as necessary at every participant encounter with the questionnaire. The setting for this study was most similar to women presenting for well-woman exams or routine gynecological checkups. Each questionnaire was completed prior to screening ultrasonography. Over the course of the study 12 different sonographers were involved, each of which received individual training related to questionnaire administration.

Study eligibility, exclusions, instrumentation, protocol, criteria for designating an abnormality, data collection and storage were as previously reported [14,17–19]. In brief, criteria for eligibility were:

(1) women aged ≥ 50 years and (2) women aged 25–49 years with a documented family history of OvCA in at least one primary or secondary relative.

Participants provided their medical history, surgical history, menstrual history/menopausal status, hormonal use, and family history of cancer. Women with a known ovarian tumor or a personal history of OvCA were excluded. Ultrasound findings were designated as abnormal if ovarian volume exceeded 20 cm^3 for pre-menopausal women or 10 cm^3 for post-menopausal women, and if cysts (with septations, solid areas, or papillary projections) as well as echogenic solid structures were observed. An abnormal screening result referred exclusively to the ultrasound result *per se* and not to biomarkers or genetic testing results. Less than 100 women were observed to have free fluid on their ultrasound exam and free fluid generally resolved on their subsequent exam(s) so that free fluid was not treated as an informative predictor.

Following an abnormal ultrasonographic result, repeat screens were scheduled at intervals ranging from six weeks to six months and the symptoms questionnaire was re-administered at each screening. In the present study, the majority of screens were administered annually. The mean interval between questionnaires was 1.15 years $\pm$ 0.01 (SEM), median = 1.03 years, min = 0.02 years/max = 4.9 years, 75th percentile = 1.13 years, 90th percentile = 1.49 years, 95th percentile = 1.95 years. Criteria for *Goff symptoms* related to ovarian cancer were a symptom presenting for >12 days per month with an onset <12 months for having pelvic or abdominal pain, being unable to eat normally, feeling full quickly, feeling abdominal bloating or increased abdominal size. Symptoms *unrelated to ovarian cancer* included on the Goff questionnaire (*non-Goff symptoms*) used in the present study were: back pain, indigestion, nausea, vomiting, weight loss, urinary urgency, frequent urination, constipation, diarrhea, menstrual irregularities, bleeding after menopause, pain during intercourse, fatigue, leg swelling, difficulty breathing.

Confidence of respondents on the symptoms questionnaire was examined in terms of age, menopausal status, body mass index (BMI), hormone replacement therapy (HRT) usage, reporting *no* vs. *any* symptoms, number of Goff symptoms reported, number of non-Goff symptoms reported, number of any symptoms reported and receipt of an abnormal ultrasound screening result. Subjects with missing information listed above were excluded.

Statistical Methods

All information was entered by the sonographer performing the ultrasound into a Medlog database (Medlog Systems, Crystal Bay, NV, USA) using encodings for symptoms, severity, frequency & duration to minimize error on an electronic template organized identically to the printed questionnaire. Random audits of the data and corrections yielded estimates of accuracy greater than 98%. Significance was determined at the $p \leq 0.05$ level in order to robustly identify differences. Proportions were compared using chi-square statistics. In longitudinal analysis, McNemars test for correlated proportions in the marginals was used.

Multivariate analysis: Two binary variables were created from the symptoms confidence scores (CS): (1) *no confidence* defined as a confidence score of 0 versus all other (higher) scores and (2) *little confidence* defined as a score of 0 or 1 versus all other (higher) scores. Each was tabulated against the assessment number. It was decided to abbreviate the assessment number as 1, 2, 3, 4, or 5 plus assessments on the basis of the sample size for each value and due to the fact that the percentage of respondents with no or little confidence did not vary much beyond the fifth time the confidence score was recorded. Similar cross tabulations were done for other potential explanatory variables including BMI (recorded as less than 25, 25–29.99, or 30 plus); presence of HRT (yes or no); number of reported Goff symptoms complying with frequency (>12 days/month) and duration (<12 months) recorded as 0, 1, or 2 plus; abnormal screen (yes or no); menopausal status (premenopausal, postmenopausal, or peri-menopausal); and the number of other symptoms (non-Goff symptoms, recorded as 0, 1–10, and ≥ 11). Age at the assessment was not recoded.

To compare the percentage of "no" or "little" confidence scores among assessments, a generalized linear mixed model was constructed based on a logit link function. Confidence was rated on a six-point Likert (ordinal) scale. The model was fitted using a generalized estimating equation (GEE) procedure to account for repeated assessments on the same subject (working correlation matrix estimated using a compound symmetry assumption). This was done for both a reduced model with only assessment number as a predictor variable and then for a full model with all variables outlined above used as predictor variables. Because the results for the assessment variable were similar for each model, we report only the results for the full model. Statistical significance was determined at the 0.05 level. The GEE models were fitted using PROC GENMOD in PC-SAS, Version 9.3 (SAS Institute, Cary, NC, USA).

3. Results

The demographic characteristics of the group studied are presented in Table 1. None of these women had a diagnosis of ovarian malignancy during the study period or during 40 months of follow-up. Only a small fraction (7.1%) experienced an abnormal ultrasound exam during the study period during which they completed symptoms questionnaires. A total of 24,526 women completed 70,734 symptoms questionnaires (Table 2). The vast majority of participants (prevalence = 88.8%) at some time reported one or more of the constellation of symptoms with only 11.2% never reporting any symptom, shown in Table 2. About a third of reported symptoms (31.9%) occurred on the first questionnaire, while 68.1% had no symptoms on the first reporting. Only 11.5% did not report any symptoms after reporting symptoms on the first report, while about twice as many (20.7%) continued to report symptoms, shown in Table 2. A majority (67.8%) reported symptoms after not having symptoms on the first reporting, accounting for a 60.2% incidence, shown in Table 2. More than 9500 women completed the symptoms questionnaires four or more times, accounting for more than 43,000 symptoms questionnaires completed four or more times (Table 3). Examination of reported confidence on the symptoms questionnaires was made with confidence considered as both a confidence score >0 and >1.

Confidence (CS > 0) was highest on the first questionnaire completed (83.3% of all respondents) and decreased to 74% when five or more questionnaires were completed (Table 4). Complete lack of confidence (CS = 0) in symptoms reporting was observed in 21.1% of all responses and increased (from 16.7% to 26%) as a function of questionnaires completed (Table 4, CS = 0 line), showing decreasing confidence despite increasing experience with the symptoms questionnaire.

Table 1. Demographic characteristics of the study group at first symptom evaluation.

Variable	All, n = 24,526 Women
Age	61.7, 61 (24–99)
Parity	2.3, 2 (1–19)
Weight (pounds)	162.4, 156 (76–420)
Height (inches)	64.3, 64 (47–78)
BMI	27.6, 26.6 (12.6–80.5)
Family history of:	
Ovarian cancer	5566 (22.7)
Breast cancer	10,935 (44.6)
Colon cancer	6595 (26.9)
Personal history of:	
Breast cancer	2278 (9.3)
Colon cancer	202 (0.8)
No history of hormone replacement therapy	21,206 (86.5)
History of hormone replacement therapy	3315 (13.5)
Nulliparous	3500 (14.3)
Premenopausal	1597 (6.5)
Perimenopausal	444 (1.8)
Post menopausal	22,840 (93.1)
Abnormal exam history	1742 (7.1)
Any symptoms	18,610 (75.9)
Goff symptoms	845 (3.4)
Other symptoms	16,433 (67.0)

Data are mean, median (range) or n (%). BMI: body mass index.

Table 2. Frequency and occurrence of symptoms.

Duration Period of Data Collection Studied 15 April 2008–25 June 2013	
Women screened	24,526 (100%)
Symptoms questionnaires administered	70,734 (100%)
Questionnaires reporting symptoms	52,467 (64.3%)
Women reporting symptoms	21,789 women (88.8%) on 52,467 questionnaires
Women never reporting symptoms	2737 (11.2%)
Women reporting symptoms on first symptoms questionnaire	6956 (31.9% of women reporting symptoms)
Women reporting symptoms with no symptoms on first symptoms questionnaire	14,833 (68.1% of women reporting symptoms)
Women reporting symptoms on first symptoms questionnaire AND subsequently no symptoms reported	2503 (38.2% of women reporting symptoms on 1st questionnaire; 11.5% of all women reporting symptoms)
Women reporting symptoms on first symptoms questionnaire AND subsequently symptoms reported	4515 (68.9% of women reporting symptoms on 1st questionnaire; 20.1% of all women reporting symptoms)
Women reporting NO symptoms on first symptoms questionnaire AND subsequently symptoms	14,771 (99.6% of women with no symptoms on 1st questionnaire; 67.8% of women reporting symptoms)

Table 3. Frequency of symptom questionnaire completion.

Number of Symptoms Questionnaires Completed	Women Completing Questionnaire (n)	Total Questionnaires Completed
1	6903	6903
2	4423	8846
3	3696	11,088
4	4530	18,120
5	4168	20,840
6	714	4284
7	84	588
8	7	56
9	1	9
Total	24,526	70,734

Table 4. Confidence as a function of the number of symptoms questionnaires completed.

Confidence	Questionnair Completed	Nunber Completed	Nunber Completed	Nunber Completed	Nunber Completed	Total Completed
Confidence Score (CS)	1st	2nd	3rd	4th	5 or more	All times
0	4103 (16.7)	4055 (23)	2992 (22.7)	2226 (23.4)	1529 (26)	14,905 (21.1)
1	714 (2.9)	443 (2.5)	391 (3)	250 (2.6)	165 (2.8)	1963 (2.8)
2	506 (2.1)	411 (2.3)	349 (2.6)	226 (2.4)	172 (2.9)	1664 (2.4)
3	4090 (16.7)	1984 (11.3)	1353 (10.3)	989 (10.4)	593 (10.1)	9009 (12.7)
4	4280 (17.5)	3477 (19.7)	2774 (21)	2127 (22.4)	1289 (21.9)	13,947 (19.7)
5	10,833 (44.2)	7252 (41.2)	5341 (40.5)	3686 (38.8)	2134 (36.3)	29,246 (41.3)
Responses	24,526 (100)	17,622 (100)	13,200 (100)	9504 (100)	5882 (100)	70,734 (100)
Women completing	1	2	3	4	≥5	Questionnaires
n	6903	4423	3696	4530	4974	24526
Comparisons 1 vs. 2,3,4 or >4	$p < 0.0001$					
2 vs 3, 4		NS $p > 0.5$				
2, 3, 4 vs. >4		$p < 0.0001$				

Response scores were: "no confidence" = 0, "minimally sure" = 1, "more than minimally sure" = 2, "pretty sure" = 3, "sure" = 4 and "absolutely sure" = 5. Analysis for difference included both 0 vs. all other scores and 0 + 1 vs. all other score in both 2×2, 2×6, 2×5 contingency tables. NS: not statistically significant.

3.1. General Factors Associated with Expressions of Confidence in Symptoms Reporting

With increased age, a statistically significant decrease in confidence in symptoms reporting was observed (Table 5), with the fall-off appearing after age 60 so that the ratio of confident to non-confident women over 75 years (2.0) was half that of women under 40 (4.0), shown in Table 5.

Table 5. Confidence as a function of age.

Age, Years	Confidence n (%)			Y/N Ratio
	Women	N = No	Y = Yes	
25–40	1073 (1.5)	214 (19.9)	859 (80.1)	4.0
41–50	2911 (4.1)	562 (19.3)	2349 (80.7)	4.2
51–60	21,668 (30.6)	4094 (18.9)	17,574 (81.8)	4.3
61–74	35,900 (50.8)	8972 (25)	26,928 (75)	3.0
≥75	9182 (13)	3026 (33)	6156 (67)	2.0
Total	70,734 (100)	16,868	53,866	

For women under age 40, 80.1% (859/1073) expressed confidence in their response and this decreased to 76.1% for all women over 40 (53,007/69,661), shown in Table 5. Confidence decreased to 75.9% (50,658/66,750) for women over 50, to 73.4% (33,084/45,082) for women over 60 and to 68.9% (11,565/16,778) for women over 70 ($p < 0.0001$). Expressed confidence for postmenopausal women was 75.7% (49,100/64,831), mirroring confidence for women over 50 years of age.

The fraction of underweight (BMI ≤ 18.5) and normal weight (BMI = 18.5–24.9) women who expressed confidence in their reporting (21,263/27,932 = 76.1%) was not significantly different from overweight (BMI = 25–29.9) and obese (BMI ≥ 30) responders (32,603/42,802 = 76.2%). The fraction of women that received an abnormal screening result and expressed confidence in their reporting only differed by 1% from the fraction of women that had a normal screening result, while for only Goff symptoms the difference was 6% and not statistically significant.

Significantly more women reporting at least one symptom expressed confidence in their responses (41,984/52,379 = 80.2%) than women who reported no symptoms (11,882/18,355 = 64.7%), $p < 0.0001$. Women that reported at least one Goff symptom relevant to ovarian cancer expressed confidence with the same frequency (1597/1931 = 82.7%) as women that did not report any Goff symptoms (9895/11,871 = 83.4%). There were more women that expressed confidence who reported at least one of the symptoms (those not relevant to ovarian cancer) (37,163/45,992 = 80.8%) than women who did not report any symptoms (16,703/24,742 = 67.5%), $p < 0.0001$. Thus, participants that were the least certain about what they reported were those women who did not report having symptoms.

3.2. Longitudinal Analysis of Confidence Stability

Efforts were directed at determining if confidence scores changed as individuals completed more symptoms evaluations. Analysis focused on 17,623 individuals who completed two or more symptoms questionnaires. Results were based on individuals initially reporting some confidence (CS > 0) and tracked on the basis of the number of symptoms questionnaires that were completed. The change between the first and last confidence score was determined for each individual as increasing, decreasing or unchanged. The fraction of women that demonstrated a decrease in confidence expanded as additional questionnaires were completed (Figure 1). Confidence remained unchanged in approximately one-third of the cases (35.1%–37.4%, Table 6). Confidence scores increased in ~20% of women that initially reported some confidence (CS > 0: 18.4%–22.6%, Table 6). Decreases in confidence occurred in just under 50% of the individuals that initially reported some confidence (CS > 0: 41.4%–46%, Table 6). There was a statistically significant difference in the response distribution between individuals completing the questionnaire two to three times vs. those taking the questionnaire five or more times ($p < 0.005$), shown in Table 6. Examining paired longitudinal differences using the McNemars test showed a significant difference ($p < 0.0001$) for completing three, four, or five or more evaluations compared to two evaluations (Table 6). Thus, longitudinal analysis indicated a trending decrease of confidence scores (Table 6) in almost half of the women completing the symptoms questionnaires.

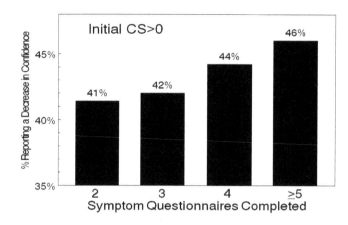

Figure 1. Confidence reported as a function of the number of symptoms questionnaires completed. Decreased confidence reported by women who originally reported confidence (CS > 0).

Table 6. Longitudinal stability as a function of the number of symptoms questionnaires completed (CS > 0).

Questionnaires Completed	Change	n	%	Comparison	Significance
2	a. Increased	827	22.6%	2 vs. 3, 4	NS
2	b. Unchanged	1318	36.0%	2 vs. ≥5	$p < 0.005$
2	c. Decreased	1518	41.4%		
2	Sub-total	3663	100.0%		
3	a. Increased	688	22.3%	3 vs. 4	NS
3	b. Unchanged	1101	35.7%	3 vs. ≥5	$p < 0.005$
3	c. Decreased	1297	42.0%		
3	Sub-total	3086	100.0%		
4	a. Increased	708	18.4%	4 vs. ≥5	NS
4	b. Unchanged	1439	37.4%		
4	c. Decreased	1702	44.2%		
4	Sub-total	3849	100.0%		
≥5	a. Increased	793	18.8%	4 vs. ≥5	NS
≥5	b. Unchanged	1478	35.1%	3 vs. ≥5	$p < 0.005$
≥5	c. Decreased	1936	46.0%	2 vs. ≥5	$p < 0.005$
≥5	Sub-total	4207	100.0%		

Significance in the table is based on chi square 3×2 contingency table analyses. $p < 0.0001$ using McNemars test for correlated proportions in the marginals of a 2×2 contingency table for initial confidence >0 where decreased paired confidence = "Yes". Comparisons were for two to five or more evaluations. Odds ratio changed from 1.18 (two vs. three evaluations) to 1.496 (two vs. five or more evaluations). $p < 0.0001$ using McNemars test for initial confidence = 0 where increased confidence = "Yes".

3.3. Multivariate Analysis

Relating the binary outcome (confidence scale) to the number of symptoms questionnaires completed was based on the frequencies reported in column 2 of Table 3 and not on arbitrarily varying the cut point to achieve significant results. The percentage of respondents expressing no confidence increased significantly from 16.7% after the first assessment ($p < 0.0001$ when each of the no confidence levels for assessments two, three, four, or five plus were compared to the first assessment). It then leveled off during assessments two, three, or four (23.0%, 22.7%, and 23.4%, respectively) which were not statistically different from each other. However, by assessment five or later, those expressing no confidence increased to 26.0% which is significant when compared to assessments two, three, or four ($p < 0.001$ in all cases). All other variables examined were significant in the multivariate model except for use of hormone replacement therapy ($p = 0.44$), and normal vs. abnormal screening exams ($p = 0.09$). Thus, although the number of women with abnormal findings is small, so it should be expected to have little effect in this study, it does not test as a confounder. Specifically, the percentage of patients expressing no confidence increased with age ($p < 0.001$). The percentage was stable through age 60 and then increased steadily from 18.8% to 32.8% by age 85; decreased for morbidly obese patients (19.9% compared to normal BMI 21.2%, ($p < 0.03$); declined with the number of other symptoms reported (symptoms unrelated to ovarian cancer) from 31.2% (score 0) to 18.5% (scores 1 through 10) to 6.4% (score 11); decreased with the number of reported Goff symptoms complying with frequency (>12 days/month) and duration (<12 months) from 21.3% at score 0 to 15.1% at score 1 to 12.1% for scores ≥ 2; and increased in postmenopausal women when compared to premenopausal women (21.3% versus 19.3%, $p < 0.0001$). Similar results were obtained for the endpoint *little confidence* (results not shown).

3.4. Symptoms Reported Relevant to Ovarian Cancer

Overall, 59.9% (42,404/70,734) of the symptoms questionnaires reported one or more of the five symptoms related to ovarian cancer, but only 3.9% (2756/70,734) met the frequency and duration criteria and did so with a significantly different distribution (Table 7. $p < 0.0001$). The overall incidence of symptoms was: abdominal bloating > pelvic pain > increased abdominal size > feeling full quickly > unable to eat normally (Table 7). In these women that were not diagnosed with an ovarian malignancy during the study period or during 40 months of follow-up, the incidence of any of the five symptoms relevant to ovarian cancer was high, but frequency and duration information significantly reduced this number. Symptom severity was significantly lower in women that did not meet the Goff-positive frequency and duration criteria ($p < 0.001$, Table 7), but did not differ with regards to reported confidence (CS = 0 vs. CS > 0). Most women (68.4%, Table 8) reported only one symptom that met the Goff criteria of frequency and duration, while 23.3% reported two and ~8% reported three or more of these symptoms (Table 8). Moreover, the incidence of symptoms was not different with respect to reported confidence (CS = 0 vs. CS > 0). Nevertheless, the 2.7% Goff-positive occurrence (Table 8: 1931/70,734) was nearly ~245 times higher than the ovarian cancer incidence for this population (11.2/100,000), [20]. Unlike one-time reports that have previously considered symptoms related to ovarian cancer, the present report is a longitudinal study of multiple reports collected over time. Consequently, a woman may be positive for the Goff ovarian cancer symptoms in the context of always meeting or sometimes meeting the frequency and duration criteria. There are also women in the present data set who, after being positive for the Goff ovarian cancer symptoms, subsequently no longer report these symptoms. Against this background, to address these considerations, we identify two groups: (A) women that at any time have reported any Goff ovarian cancer symptoms and (B) women that at any time satisfied the frequency and duration criteria for any Goff ovarian cancer symptoms. Approximately one-third of the women surveyed (7983/24,526) qualified for inclusion in Group A, while ~7% of women qualified for inclusion in Group B (1708/24,526). Our estimates mirror a recent report from the United Kingdom on ovarian cancer symptoms reported in the general population [21]. In relating these findings to the positive predictive value (PPV) which depends on prevalence (PPV = True Positives/(True Positives + False Positives)), the work presented here would yield a symptoms-estimated PPV of 0.073% or one malignancy for 1368 cases that would be taken to surgery using the sample reported on here (24,526 women filling out 70,734 questionnaires reporting 52,467 symptoms for 21,789 women) and screen-detected ovarian cancers reported previously [9]. This symptoms-estimated PPV is smaller than that reported by Rossing from a much smaller study size ($n = 1905$) [10] that would not have approached prevalence as closely as the results described here. However, despite the occurrence of symptoms being vastly higher than the incidence of ovarian cancer, ignoring symptoms is very likely to result in women being diagnosed with advanced-stage disease [11].

Table 7. Occurrence of symptoms related to ovarian cancer.

Symptom	Goff-Negative Occurrence Freq < 12 per Month and Duration > 12 Months, *n* (%)	CS = 0	Severity	CS > 0	Severity
Pelvic Pain	10,859 (25.6)	1702 (24.3)	2.1 ± 0.03	9157 (25.9)	2.1 ± 0.01
Unable to eat normally	2584 (6.1)	459 (6.6)	2.2 ± 0.06	2125 (6)	2.2 ± 0.03
Feeling full quickly	5566 (13.1)	960 (13.7)	2.2 ± 0.04	4606 (13)	2.1 ± 0.02
Abdominal bloating	14,934 (35.2)	2477 (35.4)	2.2 ± 0.02	12,457 (35.2)	2.2 ± 0.01
Increased abdominal size	8461 (20)	1396 (20)	2.3 ± 0.03	7065 (20)	2.3 ± 0.02
Total	42404 (100)	6994 (100)		35,410 (100)	
Symptom	Goff-Positive Occurrence Freq > 12 per Month and Duration < 12 Months, *n* (%)	CS = 0	Severity	CS > 0	Severity
Pelvic Pain	588 (21.3)	86 (22.6)	3.1± 0.13	502 (21.1)	3.04 ± 0.05
Unable to eat normally	244 (8.9)	36 (9.5)	3.1 ± 0.21	208 (8.8)	3.5 ± 0.09
Feeling full quickly	446 (16.2)	62 (16.3)	3.3 ± 0.15	384 (16.2)	3.2 ± 0.06
Abdominal bloating	832 (30.2)	115 (30.2)	3.5 ± 0.1	717 (30.2)	3.4 ± 0.04
Increased abdominal size	646 (23.4)	82 (21.5)	3.4 ± 0.13	564 (23.8)	3.12 ± 0.05
Total	2756 (100)	381 (100)		2375 (100)	

Severity was reported using the scale: 1 = minimal to 5 = severe (mean ± SEM). Severity Goff-negative vs. Goff-positive: $p < 0.001$.

Table 8. Occurrence of multiple symptoms.

Number of Symptoms	Goff-Positive Occurrence Freq > 12 per Month and Duration < 12 Months, *n* (%)	CS = 0	CS > 0
1	1321 (68.4)	200 (73)	1121 (67.7)
2	450 (23.3)	49 (17.9)	401 (24.2)
3	115 (6)	18 (6.6)	97 (5.9)
4	35 (1.8)	6 (2.2)	29 (1.8)
5	10 (0.5)	1 (0.4)	9 (0.5)
Total	1931 (100)	274 (100)	1657 (100)

CS = 0 vs. CS > 0: $p = 0.23$.

4. Discussion

This is the first work to examine symptoms related to ovarian cancer in a very large sample and to consider the confidence that women, all with an eventual non-surgical outcome, have in the responses they entered on a symptoms questionnaire that they completed prior to their ultrasound exam. A significant finding of the work presented here is that a large majority of women (80.1%) were confident in their reporting. Confidence was lowest (64.7%) in women who did not report any symptoms. Decreasing confidence despite increasing experience with the questionnaire was demonstrated by the finding that the fraction lacking confidence increased as a function of the number of times that the symptoms questionnaire was completed. Importantly, confidence scores in individuals followed longitudinally showed a decreasing trend in almost 50% of women. There was a significant age-related decrease in confidence, and women that did not report any symptoms were significantly less confident than women who reported at least one symptom. Importantly, confidence decreased as more symptoms were reported, including both ovarian cancer–related Goff symptoms complying with frequency (>12 days/month) and duration (<12 months), as well as other symptoms unrelated to ovarian cancer. Thus, reporting of an increased number of symptoms did not coincide with greater confidence in the results reported. Analyses of symptom severity indicated that severity was higher in women that met the Goff-positive frequency and duration criteria than in women that did not, suggesting that transient or long-standing symptoms may be of lower intensity. It is noteworthy that symptoms reporting was done prior to receiving an ultrasound exam with the result that there was no statistically significant difference in confidence between women receiving a normal vs. abnormal sonographic result.

These findings indicate that while *uncertainty in symptoms reporting* occurs to a much lesser extent than certainty, every individual's report must be carefully assessed and not unconditionally accepted. It may even be appropriate to consider serial evaluation of symptoms in order for physicians to understand the extent to which complaints continue to persist or resolve. The symptoms questionnaire utilized here includes reporting of frequency and duration in addition to the actual symptoms. Consequently, uncertainty about frequency and duration may be contributing to how an individual's response reflects confidence in what they report on the questionnaire. Memory certainly plays a role in recalling when symptoms began and how often they have occurred, and this may become more challenging as a person gets older. Thus, age-related effects on memory may be most relevant to certainty about the frequency and duration of symptoms and, with multiple co-morbidities that accumulate over time, can make it difficult to identify a "new" symptom per se or to pinpoint its onset. It is also possible that as a person gets older, they become accepting of many of the symptoms considered here occurring sporadically or episodically and as such are reluctant to declare them a symptom of anything other than age.

An impact on the healthcare delivery system arises when symptoms related to ovarian cancer are reported by women that do not have an ovarian malignancy and can result in inappropriate clinical decisions that could lead to unnecessary surgery. Some data exist supporting symptoms-based surveillance with even early cancers producing symptoms detectable by questionnaire [22]. Symptoms reporting is currently important for the identification of patients needing imaging and closer examination. Just as a lack of witness confidence in legal testimony raises questions about credibility, physicians should be sensitive to the same possibility being relevant to over-diagnosis and over-treatment if a patient may be uncertain about what they report. In addition, certainty about symptoms should not be mistaken to be related to the presence of pathology. Physicians should be made aware that confidence will decrease with age and that reporting multiple symptoms does not imply patient confidence or credibility in the report. Thus, physicians should deliberate through patient information in order to make appropriate assignments of diagnostic tests and follow-up.

The strengths of this study include the large number of patients participating, and the large number of patients completing questionnaires on more than one occasion. In addition, trained sonographers assisted participants in collecting their medical history by answering questions about the context of the questionnaires that participants were filling out. The present report focuses on the level of confidence women have in reporting symptoms as a statistical estimation and not hypothesis testing. It investigates factors that might alter this level and while this involves hypothesis testing, the large sample size assures adequate statistical power to identify some factors that do affect the reported confidence level.

The inherent weakness of a study of this nature is its subjective nature. One person's symptom may be something that someone else has become accustomed to. Subjectivity also occurred in the confidence scale; however, its gradation allowed different dichotomization points to be examined to delineate certainty from uncertainty. It is also possible that a lack of confidence associated with reporting an increased number of symptoms reflects a lack of confidence in only part of the symptoms reported on the questionnaire but not in others. This possibility was not examined in the design that was utilized because addressing this would add the burden of 63 individual confidence assessments (i.e., confidence assessments for 21 symptoms, amplified by confidence queries on severity, frequency and duration: $21 \times 3 = 63$). Understanding the context of the questionnaire certainly has an influence on confidence. The questionnaire used here included reporting of severity, frequency and duration in addition to the symptoms per se. Consequently, uncertainty about severity, frequency and duration may contribute to how an individual response reflects confidence.

Directions for future study might include an assessment of whether the levels of confidence reported here are chiefly related to completing a printed questionnaire and how they also extend to interviews with healthcare professionals. The discrepancy between clinician and patient symptoms ratings is greatest for more subjective symptoms [23]. To this end, it must be realized that clinician symptom ratings are lower than patient-reported ratings [24,25]. Consequently, care must be taken about assuming the superiority of information on symptoms gathered by clinicians and about the inferiority of patient-reported symptoms. Likewise, the results here indicate that uncertainty can exist in patient-reported symptoms.

5. Clinical Implications

Although the balance between patient confidence and uncertainty very heavily favors confidence, the level of *uncertainty in symptoms reporting* described here should be kept in mind when extracting symptoms information from patients. This principle may affect the extent to which symptoms information is relied upon or should be probed during the clinical evaluation process. The addition of psychosocial tools to evaluate the contributions of stress, anxiety and depression need to be explored to help the clinician extract the pertinent information from patient symptoms reporting so that those most at risk for malignancy can be identified.

Acknowledgments: This work will be submitted in partial fulfillment of the required thesis of Robert M. Ore for his Fellowship in Gynecologic Oncology. This work was supported by grants from the Telford Foundation, and the Department of Health and Human Services, Commonwealth of Kentucky.

Author Contributions: Robert M. Ore contributed to data summary review, abstract composition and manuscript construction; Lauren Baldwin contributed to concept development and manuscript organization; Dylan Woolum, Erika Elliott, and Christiaan Wijers contributed to data collection and review. Chieh-Yu Chen contributed to Python programming for data isolation; Rachel W. Miller, Christopher P. DeSimone, and Frederick R. Ueland contributed to manuscript preparation. Richard J. Kryscio performed statistical analysis and contributed to manuscript preparation, John R. van Nagell, contributed to manuscript preparation. Edward J. Pavlik developed the project concept, organized the data collection methodlogy, and contributed to data quality control, symptoms reporting integrity, statistical evaluation and manuscript composition. The authors are solely responsible for subject development, data collection & analysis, and composition.

References

1. National Institute for Health and Clinical Excellence. Ovarian Cancer: The Recognition and Initial Management of Ovarian Cancer. Clinical Guidelines CG122. Edited by NICE. April 2011, Volume CG122. Available online: http://www.nice.org.uk/guidance/cg122 (accessed on 22 February 2017).

2. ACOG Committee Opinion No. 280: The role of the generalist obstetrician-gynecologist in the early detection of ovarian cancer. *Obstet. Gynecol.* **2002**, *100*, 1413–1416.

3. Cella, D.; Riley, W.; Stone, A.; Rothrock, N.; Reeve, B.; Yount, S.; Amtmann, D.; Bode, R.; Buysse, D.; Choi, S.; et al. The Patient-Reported Outcomes Measurement Information System (PROMIS) developed and tested its first wave of adult self-reported health outcome item banks: 2005–2008. *J. Clin. Epidemiol.* **2010**, *63*, 1179–1194. [CrossRef] [PubMed]

4. Pilkonis, P.A.; Choi, S.W.; Reise, S.P.; Stover, A.M.; Riley, W.T.; Cella, D. Item banks for measuring emotional distress from the Patient-Reported Outcomes Measurement Information System (PROMIS): Depression, anxiety, and anger. *Assessment* **2011**, *18*, 263–283. [CrossRef] [PubMed]

5. Wagner, L.I.; Schink, J.; Bass, M.; Patel, S.; Diaz, M.V.; Rothrock, N.; Pearman, T.; Gershon, R.; Penedo, F.J.; Rosen, S.; et al. Bringing PROMIS to practice: Brief and precise symptom screening in ambulatory cancer care. *Cancer* **2015**, *121*, 927–934. [CrossRef] [PubMed]

6. Vogelzang, N.J.; Breitbart, W.; Cella, D.; Curt, G.A.; Groopman, J.E.; Horning, S.J.; Itri, L.M.; Johnson, D.H.; Scherr, S.L.; Portenoy, R.K. Patient, caregiver, and oncologist perceptions of cancer-related fatigue: Results of a tripart assessment survey. The Fatigue Coalition. *Semin. Hematol.* **1997**, *34*, 4–12. [PubMed]

7. Dupont, A.; Wheeler, J.; Herndon, I.J.E.; Coan, A.; Zafar, S.Y.; Hood, L.; Patwardhan, M.; Shaw, H.S.; Lyerly, H.K.; Abernethy, A.P. Use of tablet personal computers for sensitive patient-reported information. *J. Support. Oncol.* **2009**, *7*, 91–97. [PubMed]

8. Goff, B.A.; Mandel, L.S.; Drescher, C.W.; Urban, N.; Gough, S.; Schurman, K.M.; Patras, J.; Mahony, B.S.; Andersen, M.R. Development of an ovarian cancer symptom Index: Possibilities for earlier detection. *Cancer* **2007**, *109*, 221–227. [CrossRef] [PubMed]

9. Pavlik, E.J.; Saunders, B.A.; Doran, S.; McHugh, K.W.; Ueland, F.R.; DeSimone, C.P.; Depriest, P.D.; Ware, R.A.; Kryscio, R.J.; van Nagell, J.R., Jr. The search for meaning—Symptoms and transvaginal sonography screening for ovarian cancer. *Cancer* **2009**, *115*, 3689–3698. [CrossRef] [PubMed]

10. Rossing, M.A.; Wicklund, K.G.; Cushing-Haugen, K.L.; Weiss, N.S. Predictive value of symptoms for early detection of ovarian cancer. *J. Natl. Cancer Inst.* **2010**, *102*, 222–229. [CrossRef] [PubMed]

11. Goff, B. Symptoms associated with ovarian cancer. *Clin. Obstet. Gynecol.* **2012**, *55*, 36–42. [CrossRef] [PubMed]

12. Bornstein, B.H.; Zickafoose, D.J. "I know I know it, I know I saw it": The stability of the confidence-accuracy relationship across domains. *J. Exp. Psychol.* **1999**, *5*, 76–88. [CrossRef]

13. Higgins, R.; Nagell, J.R.; Donaldson, E.S.; Gallion, H.H.; Pavlik, E.J.; Endicott, B.; Woods, C.H. Transvaginal sonography as a screening method for ovarian cancer. *Gynecol. Oncol.* **1989**, *34*, 402–406. [CrossRef]

14. DePriest, P.D.; Gallion, H.H.; Pavilk, E.J.; Kryscio, R.K.; van Nagell, J.R. Transvaginal sonography as a screening method for the detection of early ovarian cancer. *Gynecol. Oncol.* **1997**, *65*, 408–414. [CrossRef] [PubMed]

15. Van Nagell, J.R.; Pavlik, E.J. Ovarian cancer screening. *Clin. Obstet. Gynecol.* **2012**, *55*, 43–51. [CrossRef] [PubMed]

16. Pavlik, E.J.; Johnson, T.L.; DePriest, P.D.; Andrykowski, M.A.; Kryscio, R.J.; Nagell, J.R.; van Nagell, J.R., Jr. Continuing participation supports ultrasound screening for ovarian cancer. *Ultrasound Obstet. Gynecol.* **2000**, *15*, 354–364. [CrossRef] [PubMed]

17. Ueland, F.R.; DePriest, P.; DeSimone, C.; Pavlik, E.J.; Lele, S.M.; Kryscio, R.J.; van Nagell, J.R., Jr. The accuracy of examination under anesthesia and transvaginal sonography in evaluating ovarian size. *Gynecol. Oncol.* **2005**, *99*, 400–403. [CrossRef] [PubMed]

18. Pavlik, E.J.; DePriest, P.D.; Gallion, H.H.; Ueland, F.R.; Reedy, M.B.; Kryscio, R.J.; van Nagell, J.R., Jr. Ovarian volume related to age. *Gynecol. Oncol.* **2000**, *77*, 410–412. [CrossRef] [PubMed]

19. Van Nagell, J.R.; DePriest, P.; Reedy, M.; Gallion, H.H.; Ueland, F.R.; Pavlik, E.J.; Kryscio, R.J. The efficacy of transvaginal sonographic screening in asymptomatic women at risk for ovarian cancer. *Gynecol. Oncol.* **2000**, *77*, 350–356. [CrossRef] [PubMed]

20. U.S. Cancer Statistics Working Group. United States Cancer Statistics: 1999–2013 Incidence and Mortality Web-based Report. Atlanta: U.S. Department of Health and Human Services, Centers for Disease Control and Prevention and National Cancer Institute, 2016. Available online: www.cdc.gov/uscs (accessed on 22 February 2017).

21. Lim, A.W.; Mesher, D.; Sasieni, P. Estimating the workload associated with symptoms-based ovarian cancer screening in primary care: An audit of electronic medical records. *BMC Fam. Pract.* **2014**, *15*, 1–6. [CrossRef] [PubMed]

22. Goff, B.A.; Mandel, L.; Muntz, H.G.; Melancon, C.H. Ovarian carcinoma diagnosis. *Cancer* **2000**, *89*, 2068–2075. [CrossRef]

23. Basch, E.; Iasonos, A.; McDonough, T.; Barz, A.; Culkin, A.; Kris, M.G.; Scher, H.I.; Schrag, D. Patient versus clinician symptom reporting using the National Cancer Institute Common Terminology Criteria for Adverse Events: Results of a questionnaire-based study. *Lancet Oncol.* **2006**, *7*, 903–909. [CrossRef]

24. Basch, E. The missing voice of patients in drug-safety reporting. *N. Engl. J. Med.* **2010**, *362*, 865–869. [CrossRef] [PubMed]

25. Fromme, E.K.; Eilers, K.M.; Mori, M.; Hsieh, Y.C.; Beer, T.M. How accurate is clinician reporting of chemotherapy adverse effects? A comparison with patient-reported symptoms from the Quality-of-Life Questionnaire C30. *J. Clin. Oncol.* **2004**, *22*, 3485–3490. [CrossRef] [PubMed]

9

The Impact of Normalization Approaches to Automatically Detect Radiogenomic Phenotypes Characterizing Breast Cancer Receptors Status

Rossana Castaldo, Katia Pane *, Emanuele Nicolai, Marco Salvatore and Monica Franzese

IRCCS SDN, Via E. Gianturco, 113, 80143 Naples, Italy; rcastaldo@sdn-napoli.it (R.C.);
enicolai@sdn-napoli.it (E.N.); direzionescientifica@sdn-napoli.it (M.S.); mfranzese@sdn-napoli.it (M.F.)
* Correspondence: kpane@sdn-napoli.it

Abstract: In breast cancer studies, combining quantitative radiomic with genomic signatures can help identifying and characterizing radiogenomic phenotypes, in function of molecular receptor status. Biomedical imaging processing lacks standards in radiomic feature normalization methods and neglecting feature normalization can highly bias the overall analysis. This study evaluates the effect of several normalization techniques to predict four clinical phenotypes such as estrogen receptor (ER), progesterone receptor (PR), human epidermal growth factor receptor 2 (HER2), and triple negative (TN) status, by quantitative features. The Cancer Imaging Archive (TCIA) radiomic features from 91 T1-weighted Dynamic Contrast Enhancement MRI of invasive breast cancers were investigated in association with breast invasive carcinoma miRNA expression profiling from the Cancer Genome Atlas (TCGA). Three advanced machine learning techniques (Support Vector Machine, Random Forest, and Naïve Bayesian) were investigated to distinguish between molecular prognostic indicators and achieved an area under the ROC curve (AUC) values of 86%, 93%, 91%, and 91% for the prediction of ER+ versus ER−, PR+ versus PR−, HER2+ versus HER2−, and triple-negative, respectively. In conclusion, radiomic features enable to discriminate major breast cancer molecular subtypes and may yield a potential imaging biomarker for advancing precision medicine.

Keywords: Molecular imaging; breast cancer; miRNA expression; radiogenomics; machine learning; radiomic; diagnosis; biomarker

1. Introduction

Breast cancer is the most frequently diagnosed cancer among women, and it is the second leading cause of death in women [1]. Based on the molecular receptor status, breast cancer can be classified into different subtypes with different response to therapy and prognosis. The three clinically most-useful receptors status to characterize breast cancer cells are the estrogen receptor (ER), progesterone receptor (PR), and human epidermal growth factor receptor 2 (HER2) that can impact therapy and prognosis [2].

Breast cancer is a heterogeneous disease. Indeed, HER2-positive (HER2+) breast cancers are more aggressive and show a poorer prognosis than HER2-negative (HER2−) cancers. Positive hormonal receptor status such as ER-positive (ER+) and PR-positive (PR+) tumor have lower risks of mortality than ER-negative (ER−) and/or PR-negative (PR−) disease [3–7]. Triple negative (TN) tumor (negative for all three receptors) shows a high relapsing rate, and therefore, accounts for a large portion of breast cancer deaths. Therefore, it becomes necessary to identify molecular receptor status and subsequently subtypes to select the appropriate therapy and predict the therapeutic response [8,9].

Radiomics has recently emerged as a promising tool for discovering non-invasive imaging signatures characterizing lesions such as size, shape, descriptors of the image intensity histogram and texture [10,11]. The term 'Radiomics' refers to the high-throughput extraction of quantitative features from medical images, i.e., conversion of images to mineable data, that can potentially capture tumor heterogeneity, aiding precision medicine [12]. A closely related field is 'radiogenomics', which explores the associations between imaging phenotype (radiomic data) and disease genotype (genomic patterns) [13,14]. Two public data resources such as The Cancer Genome Atlas (TCGA) and The Cancer Imaging Archive (TCIA), provide cancer genomic profiling and medical images counterpart, respectively [15,16], to promote cross-disciplinary research including radiogenomic studies [17–19].

In breast cancer, radiomic applications encompass diagnosis and better differentiation of malignant and benign entities as well as identifying ductal carcinoma in situ and invasive ductal carcinoma, for prognosis of metastatic potential, prediction of pathologic stage, lymph node involvement, molecular subtypes, and clinical outcomes [20–30].

Regarding the use of radiomic features for investigating breast cancer molecular receptor status, Agner et al. [28] extracted imaging features to differentiate TN cancers from other molecular subtypes. Yamaguchi et al. [29] investigated the relationship between heterogeneous kinetic curve pattern and molecular subtype. Blaschke et al. [31] showed that HER2-positive tumors have a greater uptake than other molecular subtypes. Li et al. [7] disclosed that the computer-aided tumor imaging phenotypes were able to differentiate between molecular prognostic biomarkers, and statistically significant associations between tumor phenotypes and receptor status were observed. Xie et al. [32] showed that whole-tumor MR multiparametric images offer a non-invasive analytical approach for breast cancer subtype classification and TN cancer cases. Guo et al. [21] demonstrated that the prediction performances by genomics alone, radiomics alone, and combined radiogenomic features showed statistically significant correlations with clinical outcomes (pathological receptors). Yoon et al. [33] used deep neural networks combining both radiomic and genomic features of invasive breast cancer, achieving high classification performance to predict pathological stage and molecular receptor status.

However, an important and often undervalued aspect in radiomic framework of analysis is features normalization relevance. In fact, data normalization methods are essential for radiomic features, due to their basic differences of scale, range, and statistical distributions. Untransformed features may have high levels of skewness, which can result in artificially low p-values in statistical analysis [34]. Moreover, neglecting feature normalization and the use of inappropriate normalization methods may lead to individual features being over or underrepresented and eventually introduce bias into developed models. Recently, normalization transformations are gaining huge interest in the era of machine learning (ML), especially in data preprocessing [35]. In the existing literature, standards to normalize quantitative radiomic features seem to be missing. None of the above-mentioned studies used a normalization method to decrease the overall bias that non-normalized features can generate in the analysis. Only Guo et al. [21] standardized the radiomic and genomic data before applying discriminative models. On the other side, several efforts have been shown to improve normalization procedures for MRI image intensity values as crucial preprocessing step. In fact, image variability and normalization steps are critical correction procedures for imaging-related batch effects before extracting quantitative radiomic features [36–40]. Although image preprocessing normalization steps are decisive to reduce technical variability across images, additional feature normalization steps are still needed and should be not overlooked.

The aim of this study is to evaluate the impact of several normalization methods to study the relationship between radiomic features and breast tumor molecular receptor ER, PR, HER2, and TN status. We integrated data from TCIA-TCGA to analyze 36 MRI radiomic features extracted from 91 biopsy proven invasive breast cancers, T1-weighted Dynamic Contrast Enhancement (DCE) Magnetic Resonance Imaging (MRI), associated with tumor molecular receptor status.

Several feature normalization approaches such as scaling, z-score, robust z-score, log-transformation, quantile, upper quartile, and whitening methods were applied to radiomic features. We compared model predictive power and the impact of radiomic feature normalization using three advanced machine learning methods (Support Vector machine (SVM), Random Forest (RF) and Naïve Bayesian (NB) methods) to differentiate among ER, PR, HER2, and TN cases.

Finally, we included TCGA breast cancer miRNAs expression profiles to explore imaging-miRNA associations.

Our data highlighted that close attention is needed to assess image-based biomarker in radiomic analysis. Thus, the aim of this study is to provide several statistical approaches to generate quantitative MRI-based signature, which may lead to more precise breast cancer prognosis and help clinicians in decision-making towards personalized medicine.

2. Materials and Methods

2.1. Dataset

All patient data used in this study were obtained from The Cancer Genome Atlas (TCGA) (available at: https://tcga-data.nci.nih.gov, accessed October 9, 2019) Breast Cancer initiative. Patients were recruited from five comprehensive cancer centers across the United States. Imaging data processing and feature extraction were conducted by [7,21,27,41]. In order to enforce imaging uniformity, breast MRI studies were acquired by 1.5-Tesla (1.5 T) magnet strength using an MRI system from GE Medical Systems (Milwaukee, Wis). The final dataset included 91 breast MRI cases.

2.1.1. Clinical Data

Table 1 shows breast cancer histological type and molecular receptors status data (ER, PR, and HER2) carried out by Immunohistochemistry (IHC) test. The results of the IHC test can be 0 (negative), 1+ (also negative), 2+ (borderline), or 3+ (positive; the HER2 protein is overexpressed). In addition, TCGA also assessed HER2 receptor protein copies in the cancer cells by Fluorescence in Situ Hybridization (FISH). The ER and PR status for our dataset samples were obtained from the TCGA data portal [21]. The HER2 status of the samples was obtained from [15]. More clinical details are reported in Table S1. Ninety-one invasive breast carcinomas with radiomic imaging profiles were available from TCIA [15,21]. All samples were primary tumors from female patients. We investigated the prediction of ER, PR, and HER2 status and triple negative (TN) of patients using radiomic features alone.

Table 1. Clinical Data.

Variables	Number
Breast Cancer Types	
Ductal carcinoma	79
Lobular carcinoma	10
Mixed	2
Molecular Receptor Status	
Estrogen Receptor (ER)	
Positive	76
Negative	15
Progesterone Receptor (PR)	
Positive	71
Negative	20
Human Epidermal Growth Factor Receptor 2 (HER2)	
Positive	12
Negative	74
Triple Negative (TN)	
Triple negative (ER–, PR–, HER2–)	12
Others	74

2.1.2. Image Data

All MRIs were acquired using a standard double-breast coil on a 1.5T GE whole-body MRI system (GE Medical Systems). In the current study, only T1-weighted, dynamic contrast-enhanced MR images were used. The imaging protocols included 1 pre-contrast image and 3 to 5 post-contrast images obtained using a T1-weighted, 3-dimensional (3D) spoiled gradient echo sequence with a gadolinium-based contrast agent (Omniscan; Nycomed-Amersham, Princeton, NJ). For further information refer to [7,21,27,41].

2.1.3. Radiomic Features

A total of 36 MRI features, computer extracted image phenotypes (CEIPs), were calculated based on the automatically derived 3D tumor segmentations [7,21]. The CEIPs were divided into the following 6 phenotype categories: size (measuring tumor dimensions), shape (quantifying the 3D geometry), morphology (combining shape and margin characteristics), enhancement texture (describing the texture of the contrast uptake in the tumor on the first postcontrast MRIs), kinetic curve assessment (describing the shape of the kinetic curve and assessing the physiologic process of the uptake and washout of the contrast agent in the tumor during the dynamic imaging series), and enhancement-variance kinetics (characterizing the time course of the spatial variance of the enhancement within the tumor) [21]. Data were extracted using version V2010 of the UChicago [27]. The complete dataset was downloaded from the TCGA Breast Phenotype Research Group Data sets (available at: https://wiki.cancerimagingarchive.net/display/DOI/TCGA + Breast + Phenotype + Research + Group + Data + sets, accessed 9 October, 2019). Information about radiomic features, including feature names, label, description, and category is listed in Table S2 and as reported by [21].

2.1.4. miRNA expression data

TCGA breast invasive carcinoma miRNA expression quantification data (raw read count, February 2018) produced on Illumina HiSeq 2000 sequencers (Illumina Ventures, San Diego, CA, USA) were downloaded using the free software R (R version 3.5.2) [42] and TCGAbiolinks R package [43].

TCGA-formatted miRNA-seq data according to the BCGSC miRNA Profiling Pipeline produces miRNA IDs with raw read counts of primary tumor (n = 1096 files for 1078 tumor cases) and normal solid tissue (n = 104 files for 104 normal cases). The miRNA raw counts (n = 1881 miRNAs), were processed as described in [44]. Then, we considered 1625 filtered and normalized miRNAs. We associated the molecular receptor ER, PR, HER2 status from [15], and filtering out NA receptor status.

Samples derived from patients with (n = 504) and without (n = 57) breast cancer were then matched with the 91 patients included in the radiomic analysis. A total of 75 samples along with the respective radiomic and genomic features were included in the radiogenomic framework.

2.2. Statistical Methods

Statistical analyses were carried out for radiomic features and genomic features alone to investigate the statistical significance of the features in detecting molecular receptor status. Associations between radiomics and genomics were also investigated in terms of correlation.

Shapiro–Wilk test was used to determine the normality of radiomic and genomic features [45].

Wilcoxon signed-rank test and Fisher's exact test were adopted to compare continuous and categorical clinical variables, respectively, between molecular receptor status (Table S1). R software (R Core Team. R: A language and environment for statistical computing. R Foundation for Statistical Computing, Vienna, Austria; http://www.R-project.org, 2019) was used to perform statistical analyses.

2.2.1. Radiomic Statistical Analysis

Seven different normalization techniques were used to normalize radiomic features. Features were standardized as the min–max normalization (i.e., scaling method), where each feature was normalized in the range from 0 to 1; z-score normalization, where each feature was normalized as $z = (x - \bar{x})/s$, where x, $\bar{x}$, and s are the feature, the mean, and the standard deviation respectively [46]; robust z-score normalization is calculated from the median absolute deviation and median absolute deviation [47]; log-transformation (base 10), a constant value $a = b - min(x)$ where b is 1 and x is the feature, was added to the data for handling negative values [48]; the upper quartile normalization divides each read count by the 75th percentile of the read counts in its sample [49]; quantile normalization, which transform the original data to remove unwanted technical variation by forcing the observed distributions to be the same and the average distribution, obtained by taking the average of each quantile across samples, is used as the reference [50,51]; lastly, whitening normalization technique from the principle component analysis (PCA), is based on a linear transformation that converts a vector of random variables with a known covariance matrix into a set of new variables whose covariance is the identity matrix, meaning that they are uncorrelated and each have variance equal to one [52].

To investigate the effect of normalization techniques on the radiomic features, Spearman's rank correlation was run between non-normalized radiomic features and normalized radiomic features for each of the seven different normalization methods. A Spearman's ρ value greater than 0.8 and significant p-value (< 0.05) between non-normalized and normalized feature (using scaling, Z-score, robust Z-score, log-transformation, upper quartile, quantile, and whitening methods) was set as threshold to identify the normalized radiomic features that were in agreement with the non-normalized radiomic features. Bland–Altman analysis was also used to investigate the agreement between the features that showed a Spearman's ρ value less than 0.08 and significant p-value. Bland–Altman procedure was used to compute 95% LoA (Limits of Agreement) [53].

For each binary problem, Wilcoxon signed-rank test was performed to investigate radiomic feature variation between two different groups (ER+ vs ER–, PR+ vs PR–, HER2+ vs HER2–, TN vs Others). Median trend or feature trend, using the following convention, was also investigated [54–56]:

- Two arrows, $\downarrow\downarrow$ (or $\uparrow\uparrow$) were used to report a significant (p-value < 0.05) decrease (or increase) of radiomic feature median in negative receptor status (ER–, PR–, HER2 +, TN);
- One arrow was used for non-significant variations: $\downarrow$ (or $\uparrow$) indicated a non-significant (p-value $>$ 0.05) decrease (or increase) of a radiomic feature median in negative receptor status (ER–, PR–, HER2+, TN).

The statistical analysis was repeated for each normalization procedure described above. Non-parametric tests such as Wilcoxon signed-rank test and Spearman's rank correlation were used since most of the radiomic features ($>90\%$) were non-normally distributed in the Shapiro–Wilk test. A p-value less than 0.05 was considered significant. Holm's correction was used for multiple hypothesis correction if necessary.

A synthetic scheme of the radiomic analysis carried out in this study is shown in Figure 1.

2.2.2. Genomic Statistical Analysis

Starting from normalized counts we evaluated differentially expressed miRNAs between tumor and normal conditions, applying the Empirical Bayes method for differential expression analysis, edgeR R package [57], combined with the Generalized Linear Model approach (GLM). Differentially Expressed miRNAs (DEmiRNAs) with a |log2 fold-change |> 1.0 (hsa-mir-135b has LogFC 0.93) and with adjusted p-values (FDR) ≤ 0.05, were defined as significant and used for downstream analysis. In addition, differentially expressed miRNAs were analyzed through the use of Ingenuity Knowledge Base, IPA (QIAGEN Inc., https://www.qiagenbioinformatics.com/products/ingenuitypathway-analysis) to assess breast cancer implications.

We investigated DEmiRNAs expression as function of the ER, PR, HER2, and TN molecular receptor status and performed the Wilcoxon signed-rank test for statistical significance.

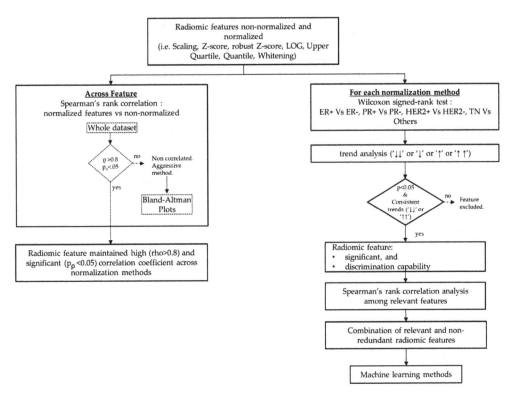

Figure 1. Radiomic analysis framework.

A p-value less than 0.05 was considered significant. Holm's correction was used for multiple hypothesis correction if necessary.

2.2.3. Radiogenomic Statistical Analysis

After identifying the statistically significant radiomic features for each receptor, Spearman's rank correlation was run between DEmiRNAs for each molecular receptor status (ER+ and ER−, PR+ and PR−, HER2+ and HER2−, TN and Others) and radiomic features. In the correlation analysis, two normalization methods were chosen for the radiomic features: upper quartile normalization method as both data types are normalized by upper quartile normalization method, and whitening-transformation method as it is the only normalization method that highlighted a significant change among radiomic features for all receptors' status.

2.3. Machine Learning Classification

The dataset was stratified random split per patient into two folders: Folder 1 (60%) was used to train and validate the classifiers; folder 2 (40%) to test the models. The reason of this split is that a classifier should be tested on an independent set of data to reduce overfitting problems and bias in the overall accuracy of the classifier [55,58].

2.3.1. Feature Selection Methods

Feature selection is a critical step to build a robust model. In fact, the number of features used in the final classifier and its cardinality should be limited by the number of subjects presenting the event to detect in order to minimize the overfitting risk in a machine learning model. Moreover, a significant small set of clinical features powerfully simplifies the clinical interpretation of the results, by pointing the attention only on the most informative and relevant features [58]. Therefore, the feature selection process was based on two main steps: relevance analysis and redundancy analysis [55]. The former was performed using the Wilcoxon signed-rank test to identify the features that changed significantly between two conditions (binary problem). The latter selected only one feature from each cluster of features mutually correlated using Spearman's rank correlation to reduce multicollinearity in the models [55].

2.3.2. Training, Validation, and Testing

Clinical outcomes have unbalanced ratio, which do not meet the assumptions of most machine learning-based models. To tackle this problem, Synthetic Minority Over-sampling Technique (SMOTE) was applied to balance the datasets [59]. It has been shown that SMOTE is a robust technique to overcome unbalanced dataset problems with a variety of classifiers [59,60]. In this study, SMOTE has shown to outperform other sampling methods and thus, it was used to balance the datasets.

Three different machine-learning approaches were considered to develop classifiers aiming to automatically classify receptor status based on MRI phenotypes: Support Vector Machine (SVM), which belongs to a general field of kernel-based machine learning methods and is used to classify both linearly and non-linearly separable data [61]; Random Forest decision trees, an ensemble learning method for classification that operates by constructing a multitude of decision trees during training and outputting the class that is the mode of the classes (classification) [62,63]; Bayesian classifier, a family of simple "probabilistic classifiers" based on applying Bayes' theorem with strong (naïve) independence assumptions between the features [64].

Regarding model parameters, for SVM, polynomial kernel function with the degree from 1 to 5 was used. Random Forest decision trees were developed by changing confidence factor for pruning from 0.05 to 0.5 and minimum number of instances per leaf from 2 to 20. The algorithm parameters were tuned during training on folder 1. Each of those methods was used with all the combinations of relevant and non-redundant radiomic features.

The training of the machine-learning models (including classifier parameter tuning) was performed on folder 1 (around 60% of the total number of patients). Folder 1 was also employed to validate the classifier using a k-fold cross-validation technique. The 3-fold person-independent cross-validation approach was used to validate the models in folder 1 [55]. The model was then tested on folder 2 (around 40% of the total number of patients), in order to assess their ability to automatically detect the receptor status. Binary classification performance measures were adopted according to standard formulae reported in Table 2 [65].

Table 2. Binary performance measures.

Measure	Formula
Total Classification Accuracy (ACC)	$(TP + TN)/(TP + TN + FP + FN)$
Sensitivity (SEN)	$TP/(TP + FN)$
Specificity (SPE)	$TN/(FP + TN)$
Area Under the Curve (AUC)	-

True positive (TP); true negative (TN), false negative (FN); false positive (FP).

2.3.3. Best Model Selection

To evaluate the effect of normalization approaches for radiomic analysis, binary performance was calculated for each ML method across all normalization methods employed in this study. The best normalization technique for each ML model was selected as the one achieving the highest sensitivity, specificity, accuracy and area under the curve (AUC), and the classifier that employed a smaller number of radiomic features (i.e., less computational complexity model). Among the three different ML methods used to train, validate and test the classifiers (SVM, RF, BN), the best-performing model was chosen as the classifier achieving the highest AUC, which is a reliable estimator of both sensitivity and specificity rates; in case of equal AUC, the classifier with less computational complexity was chosen.

3. Results

This study was performed on 91 invasive breast cancers with radiomic imaging profiles from female patients. The patients' average age was 53.6 ± 11.5 years (range of 29–82 years). According to the clinical variables, no statistically significant differences were observed between receptor status (Table S1). For radiogenomic framework, we considered 75 matched samples of 91 invasive breast cancers.

3.1. Radiomics

A correlation analysis was run on the whole dataset to investigate the relationship between non-normalized and normalized radiomic features (i.e., Scaling, Z-Score, Robust Z-Score, Log transformation (LOG), Upper Quartile, Quantile and Whitening (WHT) methods). Spearman's rank correlation was used. Table S3 showed ρ values of the radiomic features with a p-value < 0.05. A graphical representation of the correlation results is presented in Figure 2.

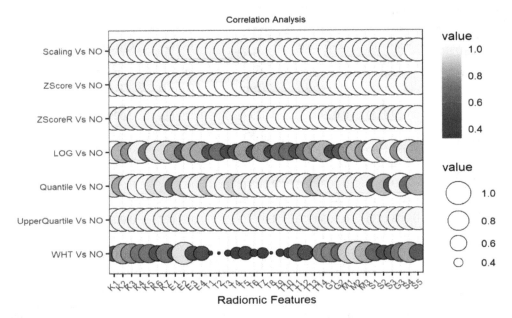

Figure 2. Correlation analysis on the whole dataset between non-normalized and normalized radiomic features. On the x-axis radiomic features are reported; on the y-axis correlation coefficients via Spearman correlation analysis are reported for each comparison between normalization methods and raw features (i.e., non-normalized radiomic features). All correlation p-values resulted less than 0.05. NO: non-normalized features; Scaling normalization method; Z-score normalization method; ZscoreR: Robust Z-score normalization method; LOG transformation; Quantile and Upper Quartile normalization method; WHT: Whitening normalization method.

As shown in Table S3 and Figure 2, non-normalized radiomic features are perfectly correlated with scaling, z-score, robust z-score and upper quartile normalized features. Between LOG transformation method and non-normalized features, only four radiomic features (E1, S1, S3, and S4) showed to be poorly correlated (ρ less than 0.8). Sixteen and thirty out of 36 radiomic features showed a very poor correlation value with the row radiomic features (i.e., non-normalized features) for the quantile and whitening normalization methods respectively.

Bland Altman analysis was also performed to visually investigate the agreement and disruption of normalized methods on the radiomic features that showed a Spearman's rank coefficient less than 0.8 with non-normalized radiomic features. Therefore, the correlation analysis was supported by the visual inspection of the Bland–Altman analysis. An increase in bias and in width of the 95% limits of agreement (LoA) was observed for the radiomic features that showed a Spearman's rank coefficient less than 0.8.

3.1.1. Statistical Analysis per Receptor Status: ER+ vs ER–

Table 3 reports the results of the statistical analysis from Wilcoxon signed-rank test indicating association between MRI phenotype and receptor status ER+ versus ER–, for each normalization method. In Table 3 the radiomic features that showed a significant p-values were reported.

As shown in Table 3 and Figure 3A, 6 out of the 36 radiomic features (T5, T11, S1, S2, S3 and G3) showed significant changes between ER– and ER+ for non-normalized, scaling, z-score, robust z-score, log-transformation and upper quartile radiomic features. Three out of these 6 features (T5, T11, G3) decreased significantly in ER– cases, while the remaining 3 features showed a significant increase trend. For quantile normalization, five features out of 36 radiomic features (T5, T11, S2, S3, and G3) changed significantly between ER– and ER+. As far as whitening normalization method is concerned, only three radiomic features (T11, S2, and G3) showed significant changes between ER– and ER+ and maintained coherent trends with the other normalization methods.

Table 3. Results from the Wilcoxon signed-rank test indicating association between MRI phenotype and molecular classification ER+ versus ER–.

Feature Names	Non-Normalized Pval (Trend)	Scaling Pval (Trend)	Z-Score Pval (Trend)	Robust Z-Score Pval (Trend)	LOG Pval (Trend)	Quantile Pval (Trend)	Upper Quartile Pval (Trend)	WHT Pval (Trend)
T5	0.029 (↓↓)	0.029 (↓↓)	0.029 (↓↓)	0.029 (↓↓)	0.029 (↓↓)	0.029 (↓↓)	0.029 (↓↓)	0.287 (↓)
T11	0.031 (↓↓)	0.031 (↓↓)	0.031 (↓↓)	0.031 (↓↓)	0.031 (↓↓)	0.031 (↓↓)	0.031 (↓↓)	0.002 (↓↓)
S1	0.003 (↑↑)	0.003 (↑↑)	0.003 (↑↑)	0.003 (↑↑)	0.003 (↑↑)	0.003 (↑↑)	0.003 (↑↑)	0.688 (↑)
S2	0.003 (↑↑)	0.003 (↑↑)	0.003 (↑↑)	0.003 (↑↑)	0.003 (↑↑)	0.003 (↑↑)	0.003 (↑↑)	0.004 (↑↑)
S3	0.011 (↑↑)	0.011 (↑↑)	0.011 (↑↑)	0.011 (↑↑)	0.011 (↑↑)	0.011 (↑↑)	0.011 (↑↑)	0.524 (↓)
G3	0.029 (↓↓)	0.029 (↓↓)	0.029 (↓↓)	0.029 (↓↓)	0.029 (↓↓)	0.029 (↓↓)	0.029 (↓↓)	0.029 (↓↓)

↓↓ (or ↑↑): used to report a significant (p-value < 0.05) decrease (or increase) of feature median in negative receptor status (ER–),↓ (or ↑) indicated a non-significant (p-value > 0.05) decrease (or increase) of a feature median in negative receptor status (ER–).

3.1.2. Statistical Analysis per Receptor Status: PR+ vs PR–

Table 4 reports the results of the statistical analysis from Wilcoxon signed-rank test indicating association between MRI phenotype and receptor status PR+ versus PR–, for each normalization method. In Table 4 the radiomic features that showed a significant p-values were reported.

As shown in Table 4 and Figure 3B, 5 out of the 36 radiomic features (E3, E4, T4, T5, and T6) showed significant changes between PR– and PR+ for non-normalized, scaling, z-score, robust z-score, log-transformation, upper quartile and quantile radiomic features. Three out of these 5 features (E3, E4, T5) showed a significantly decreased value in PR– status, while the remaining 2 features showed a significant increase. As far as whitening normalization method is concerned, only three radiomic features (T2, T5, and S2) showed significant changes between PR– and PR+. T2 and T5 showed a decreased value in PR– status, while S2 showed an increased value in PR– status.

3.1.3. Statistical Analysis per Receptor Status: HER2+ vs HER2–

Table 5 reports the results of the statistical analysis from Wilcoxon signed-rank test indicating association between MRI phenotype and receptor status HER2+ versus HER2–, for each normalization method. In Table 5 the radiomic features that showed a significant p-values were reported.

Table 4. Results from the Wilcoxon signed-rank test indicating association between MRI phenotype and molecular classification PR+ versus PR.

Feature Names	Non-Normalized Pval (Trend)	Scaling Pval (Trend)	Z-Score Pval (Trend)	Robust Z-Score Pval (Trend)	LOG Pval (Trend)	Quantile Pval (Trend)	Upper Quartile Pval (Trend)	WHT Pval (Trend)
E3	0.021 (↓↓)	0.021 (↓↓)	0.021 (↓↓)	0.021 (↓↓)	0.021 (↓↓)	0.021 (↓↓)	0.021 (↓↓)	0.418 (↑)
E4	0.038 (↓↓)	0.038 (↓↓)	0.038 (↓↓)	0.038 (↓↓)	0.038 (↓↓)	0.038 (↓↓)	0.038 (↓↓)	0.867 (↑)
T2	0.071 (↓)	0.071 (↓)	0.071 (↓)	0.071 (↓)	0.071 (↓)	0.071 (↓)	0.071 (↓)	0.046 (↓↓)
T4	0.049 (↑↑)	0.049 (↑↑)	0.049 (↑↑)	0.049 (↑↑)	0.049 (↑↑)	0.049 (↑↑)	0.049 (↑↑)	0.178 (↑)
T5	0.004 (↓↓)	0.004 (↓↓)	0.004 (↓↓)	0.004 (↓↓)	0.004 (↓↓)	0.004 (↓↓)	0.004 (↓↓)	0.02 (↓↓)
T6	0.02 (↑↑)	0.02 (↑↑)	0.02 (↑↑)	0.02 (↑↑)	0.02 (↑↑)	0.02 (↑↑)	0.02 (↑↑)	0.303 (↑)
S2	0.175 (↑)	0.175 (↑)	0.175 (↑)	0.175 (↑)	0.175 (↑)	0.175 (↑)	0.175 (↑)	0.021 (↑↑)

↓↓ (or ↑↑): used to report a significant (p-value < 0.05) decrease (or increase) of feature median in negative receptor status (PR–), ↓ (or ↑) indicated a non-significant (p-value > 0.05) decrease (or increase) of a feature median in negative receptor status (PR–).

Table 5. Results from the Wilcoxon signed-rank test indicating association between MRI phenotype and molecular classification HER2+ versus HER2–.

Feature Names	Non-Normalized Pval (Trend)	Scaling Pval (Trend)	Z-Score Pval (Trend)	Robust Z-Score Pval (Trend)	LOG Pval (Trend)	Quantile Pval (Trend)	Upper Quartile Pval (Trend)	WHT Pval (Trend)
K6	0.054 (↑)	0.054 (↑)	0.054 (↑)	0.054 (↑)	0.054 (↑)	0.054 (↑)	0.054 (↑)	0.008 (↑↑)
T8	0.414 (↑)	0.414 (↑)	0.414 (↑)	0.414 (↑)	0.414 (↑)	0.414 (↑)	0.414 (↓)	0.025 (↑↑)
M3	0.393 (↑)	0.393 (↑)	0.393 (↑)	0.393 (↑)	0.393 (↑)	0.393 (↑)	0.393 (↑)	0.048 (↑↑)

↓↓ (or ↑↑): used to report a significant (p-value<0.05) decrease (or increase) of feature median in negative receptor status (HER2+), ↓ (or ↑) indicated a non-significant (p-value > 0.05) decrease (or increase) of a feature median in negative receptor status (HER2+).

As shown in Table 5 and Figure 3C, none of 36 radiomic features showed significant changes between HER2– and HER2+ for all normalization methods but whitening transformation. As far as whitening normalization method is concerned, three radiomic features (K6, T8, and M3) showed significant changes between HER2– and HER2+. All these features showed an increased value in HER2 positive cases.

3.1.4. Statistical Analysis per Receptor Status: TN vs Others

Table 6 reports the results of the statistical analysis from Wilcoxon Rank test indicating association between MRI phenotype and receptor status TN versus Others, for each normalization method. In Table 6 the radiomic features that showed a significant p-values were reported.

As shown in Table 6 and Figure 3D, 5 out of the 36 radiomic features (E2, G2, S1, S2, and S3) showed significant changes between TN vs Others for non-normalized, scaling, z-score, robust z-score, log-transformation, upper quartile, and quantile radiomic features. All 5 features showed a significantly increased value in TN status. As far as whitening normalization method is concerned, five different radiomic features (E2, T6, T11, G2, and S2) showed significant changes between TN and Others. All features, expect T11, showed an increased value in TN status.

Table 6. Results from the Wilcoxon signed-rank test indicating association between MRI phenotype and molecular classification TN versus Others.

Feature Names	Non-Normalized Pval (Trend)	Scaling Pval (Trend)	Z-Score Pval (Trend)	Robust Z-Score Pval (Trend)	LOG Pval (Trend)	Quantile Pval (Trend)	Upper Quartile Pval (Trend)	WHT Pval (Trend)
E2	0.048 (↑↑)	0.048 (↑↑)	0.048 (↑↑)	0.048 (↑↑)	0.048 (↑↑)	0.048 (↑↑)	0.048 (↑↑)	0.035 (↑↑)
T6	0.107 (↑)	0.107 (↑)	0.107 (↑)	0.107 (↑)	0.107 (↑)	0.107 (↑)	0.107 (↑)	0.024 (↑↑)
T11	0.078 (↓)	0.078 (↓)	0.078 (↓)	0.078 (↓)	0.078 (↓)	0.078 (↓)	0.078 (↓)	0.024 (↓↓)
G2	0.048 (↑↑)	0.048 (↑↑)	0.048 (↑↑)	0.048 (↑↑)	0.048 (↑↑)	0.048 (↑↑)	0.048 (↑↑)	0.019 (↑↑)
S1	0.01 (↑↑)	0.01 (↑↑)	0.01 (↑↑)	0.01 (↑↑)	0.01 (↑↑)	0.01 (↑↑)	0.01 (↑↑)	0.458 (↑)
S2	0.01 (↑↑)	0.01 (↑↑)	0.01 (↑↑)	0.01 (↑↑)	0.01 (↑↑)	0.01 (↑↑)	0.01 (↑↑)	0.021 (↑↑)
S3	0.012 (↑↑)	0.012 (↑↑)	0.012 (↑↑)	0.012 (↑↑)	0.012 (↑↑)	0.012 (↑↑)	0.012 (↑↑)	0.259 (↑)

↓↓ (or ↑↑): used to report a significant (p-value < 0.05) decrease (or increase) of feature median in negative receptor status (TN), ↓ (or ↑) indicated a non-significant (p-value > 0.05) decrease (or increase) of a feature median in negative receptor status (TN).

3.2. Genomics

As previously shown, several MRI radiomic features showed statistically significant variations in ER, PR, HER2, and TN status across different normalization approaches.

Aberrant miRNAs expression is one of the genomic alterations occurring in breast cancer [66], which showed association with some MRI radiomic features [22] Thus, we computed miRNAs differentially expressed among TCGA breast tumor tissues with ER, PR, and HER2 receptor status annotation available. Ten differentially expressed miRNAs (DEmiRNAs, p adjusted ≤0.05), including hsa-mir-4662a, hsa-mir-486.1, hsa-mir-486.2, hsa-mir-526b(mir-515 family), hsa-mir-122, hsa-mir-653, hsa-mir-9.2, hsa-mir-135a.2, hsa-mir-184 and hsa-mir-206 (mir-1 family) were used to investigate relationship between radiomic and genomic features.

Box plots show DEmiRNAs trend as function of ER (Figure S1), PR (Figure S2), HER2 (Figure S3), and triple negative (Figure S4) receptor status, with Wilcoxon test for statistical significance (threshold p-value less than 0.05). Several DEmiRNAs showed to be statistically significant in ER receptor status (hsa-mir-122, hsa-mir-653, hsa-mir-9.2, hsa-mir-135a.2, hsa-mir-184) with a p-value < 0.05 (Figure S1). Three DEmiRNAs expression (hsa-mir-653, hsa-mir-9.2, hsa-mir-184) showed a significant p-values for PR status (Figure S2). Only two DEmiRNAs expression (hsa-mir-653, hsa-mir-135a.2) showed a significant variation in HER2 status (Figure S3). Lastly, four DEmiRNAs expression (hsa-mir-122, hsa-mir-653, hsa-mir-9.2, and hsa-mir-184) had a statistical variation in TN cases (Figure S4).

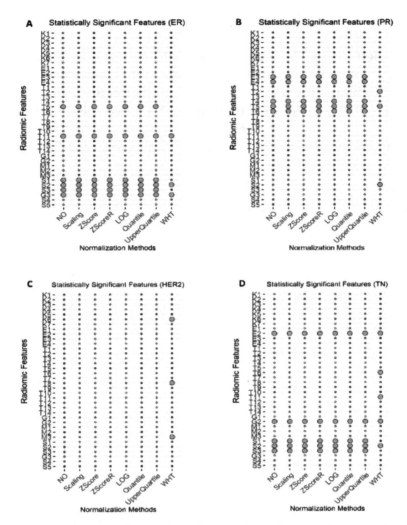

Figure 3. Statistically significant radiomic features. Statistically significant radiomic features across normalization methods are identified with a circle. (**A**) Statistically significant radiomic features for receptor status ER across normalization methods. (**B**) Statistically significant radiomic features for receptor status PR across normalization methods. (**C**) Statistically significant radiomic features for receptor status HER2 across normalization methods. (**D**) Statistically significant radiomic features for receptor status TN across normalization methods. NO: non-normalized features; Scaling normalization method; Z-score normalization method; ZscoreR: Robust Z-score normalization method; LOG transformation; Quantile and Upper Quartile normalization method; WHT: Whitening normalization method.

3.3. Radiogenomics

As shown previously, a set of statistically significant radiomic features emerged from different normalization approaches. In order to assess imaging-genomic associations, considering that the distributions of radiomic and genomic features were not normal, we carried out Spearman's correlation analysis between the statistically significant radiomic features and miRNAs differentially expressed in breast cancer.

Regarding the correlation, we chose radiomic features from two normalization methods: *i)* the upper quartile (UQ) normalized method, since the UQ method was used to normalize miRNA-seq data, and *ii)* the whitening method (WHT), because it provided statistically significant radiomic features for all receptors' status.

The samples were stratified into ER+/ER–, PR+/PR–, and HER+/HER2– and TN status. Greater attention was paid in investigating imaging-genomic associations for ER-negative, PR-negative, HER2-positive, and TN cases, which are more relevant to the clinical practise.

3.3.1. Correlation Analysis per Receptor Status: ER+ vs ER–

Spearman's correlation analysis between UQ normalized radiomic features and miRNAs, for ER negative receptor status, highlighted a statistically significant negative correlation between the shape feature G3 and hsa-mir-526b (p-value adjusted < 0.05, Table S4), representing the ratio surface area to volume based on 3D reconstruction of lesion (Figure 4A). Other correlations included the size feature S3 with hsa-mir-653 and hsa-mir-206, characterizing lesion surface area, and the enhancement texture feature T5, indicating image homogeneity, associated with hsa-mir-9.2 (Figure 4A), although these correlations were not statistically significant (Table S4).

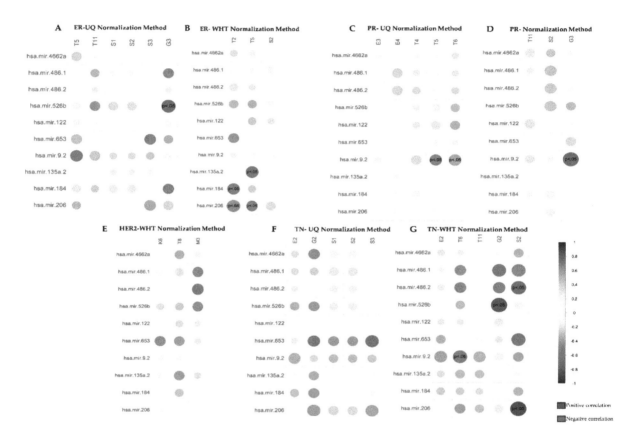

Figure 4. Spearman correlation between miRNAs expression and MRI radiomic features normalized by Upper Quartile and Whitening methods for molecular receptor status. (**A**) Correlation between ER negative breast cancer miRNAs expression and MRI radiomic features normalized by Upper Quartile (UQ) method. (**B**) Correlation between ER negative breast cancer miRNAs expression and MRI radiomic features normalized by Whitening (WHT) method. (**C**) Correlation between PR negative breast cancer miRNAs expression and MRI radiomic features normalized by Upper Quartile (UQ) method. (**D**) Correlation between PR negative breast cancer miRNAs expression and MRI radiomic features normalized by Whitening (WHT) method. (**E**) Correlation between HER2 positive breast cancer miRNAs expression and MRI radiomic features normalized by whitening methods. (**F**) Correlation between TN negative breast cancer miRNAs expression and MRI radiomic features normalized by Upper Quartile (UQ) method. (**G**) Correlation between TN negative breast cancer miRNAs expression and MRI radiomic features normalized by Whitening (WHT) method.

In contrast, when we performed Spearman's correlations for ER negative receptor status, using WHT normalized radiomic features, the shape feature G3 resulted associated with hsa-mir-9.2 (p adjusted < 0.01) in a statistically significant manner (Figure 4B, Table S4).

3.3.2. Correlation Analysis per Receptor Status: PR+ vs PR–

For PR negative receptor status, UQ normalized radiomic features T5 (angular second moment, energy) and T6 (entropy) inversely correlated with hsa-mir-9.2 (p-value adjusted < 0.05) (Figure 4C, Table S4). These enhancement texture features indicate image homogeneity and randomness of the grey levels.

Similarly, for PR negative status, WHT normalized radiomic features (T5 and T2) showed to be correlated (p-value adjusted < 0.05) with different miRNAs (hsa-mir-135a.2, hsa-mir-184, hsa-mir-206) (Figure 4D, Table S4).

3.3.3. Correlation Analysis per Receptor Status: HER2+ vs HER2–

For HER2 positive receptor status, we only performed a correlation analysis using WHT normalized radiomic features, as it was the only normalization method that identified statistically significant radiomic features. In this case, the morphological feature M3 correlated with hsa-mir-486.2, characterizing lesion enhancement structure from the central to a radial pattern, although this association was not statistically significant (Figure 4E, Table S4).

3.3.4. Correlation Analysis per Receptor Status: TN vs Others

We found interesting findings for TN receptor status, comparing UQ and WHT normalized radiomic features.

Correlation analysis of UQ normalized radiomic features highlighted that G2 and S3 were inversely correlated with hsa-mir-653 and hsa-mir-206, respectively (Figure 4F), whereas we found a positive correlation between the enhancement texture feature E2 and hsa-mir-9.2, indicating enhancement variance kinetics. However, none of these correlations were statistically significant (Table S4).

Conversely, when we used WHT normalized radiomic features, we found several statistically significant correlations. Indeed, negative correlations were found between the shape feature G2 measuring irregularity of the lesion with hsa-mir-526b (p adjusted < 0.01), hsa-mir-486-1 and hsa-mir-486-2 (both, p-adjusted n.s.) (Figure 4G, Table S4). We found positive correlations with the size feature S2 indicating effective diameter of a sphere with the same volume of the lesion with hsa-mir-206 (p-value adjusted < 0.01), hsa-mir-486-1 (p-value adjusted n.s.) and hsa-mir-486-2 (p-adjusted < 0.05) and negative correlation with hsa-mir-653 (p-adjusted n.s.) (Figure 4G, Table S4). In addition, we found positive correlations between the enhancement variance kinetics E2, enhancement texture T6 and T11 features with hsa-mir-9.2. Among these associations, only T6 was statically significant (p-value adjusted < 0.05) (Figure 4G, Table S4).

3.4. Machine Learning Per Molecular Classification

Regarding the feature selection process, all possible combinations of relevant and non-redundant radiomic features were investigated for each normalization methods employed in the study. Each machine learning method was trained and validated with all combinations of radiomic features using folder 1. The best feature combination was chosen as the one achieving the best AUC during training. The classifiers were, then, tested on folder 2.

3.4.1. Receptor Status: ER– vs ER+

Figure 5 shows the best performance of the three machine learning classifiers (SVM, RF, and NB) across all normalization methods to automatically detect ER receptor status. For each normalization approach the radiomic features chosen as the one achieving the best performance are reported along with the respective performance in Tables S5–S7.

Figure 6A shows the best classifiers for each of the machine learning methods according to the criteria defined in Section 2.3.3. The classifier achieving the best performances to detect ER– status is Random Forest using only two radiomic features (T11 and S2) normalized via whitening method.

Figure 6B shows the ROC curves for the best classifiers to automatically detect ER receptor status. Box plots of radiomic features chosen by the machine learning methods to automatically detect ER status are shown in Figure S5.

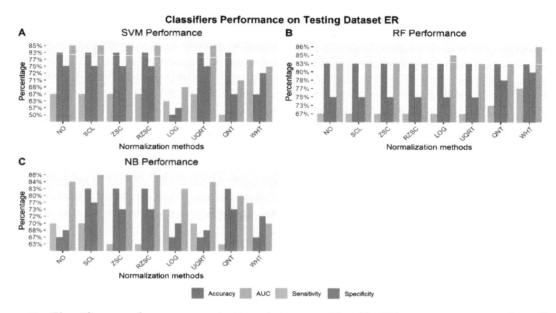

Figure 5. Classifiers performance on testing dataset to identify ER receptor status via radiomic features across normalization methods (NO: non-normalized features; SCL: Scaling normalization method; ZSC: Z-score normalization method; RZSC: Robust Z-score normalization method; LOG transformation; UPQRT: Upper Quartile normalization methods; QNT: Quantile normalization method; WHT: Whitening normalization method). **A)** Support Vector Machine (SVM) Performance on Testing dataset ER+ vs ER–. **B)** Random Forest (RF) Performance on Testing dataset ER+ vs ER–. **C)** Naïve Bayesian (NB) Performance on Testing dataset ER+ vs ER–.

A

Feature Names	Normalization Methods	ML Methods	SEN	SPE	ACC	AUC
T5, T11	NO; Scaling; Z-score; Robust Z-score; Upper Quartile.	SVM	67%	83%	75%	85%
T11, S2	WHT	RF	77%	83%	80%	86%
T5, S2, G3	Scaling	NB	70%	83%	77%	86%

NO: non-normalized features; LOG transformation method; WHT: Whitening normalization method. SVM: Support Vector Machine; RF: Random Forest; NB: Naïve Bayesian. SEN: Sensitivity; SPE: Specificity; ACC: Accuracy; AUC: Area Under the Curve; ML: Machine Learning.

B

a) Support Vector Machine (NO)   b) Random Forest (WHT)   c) Naïve Bayesian (Scaling)

Figure 6. Classifiers' performance to detect ER receptor status. (**A**) Comparison table among classifiers: ER+ vs ER–. (**B**) ROC curves for the best classifiers to automatically detect ER receptor status. a) Best classifier for Support Vector Machine Method. The normalization methods that achieved the best performance are Scaling, Z-score, Robust Z-score, Upper Quartile normalization methods. They achieved the same performance; therefore, one ROC curve with non-normalized features is reported. b) Best classifier for Random Forest Method. The normalization method that achieved the best performance is the whitening method. c) Best classifier for Naïve Bayesian Method. The normalization method that achieved the best performance is scaling method.

3.4.2. Receptor Status: PR– vs PR+

Figure 7 shows the best performance of the three machine learning classifiers (SVM, RF, and NB) across all normalization methods to automatically detect PR receptor status. For each normalization approach the radiomic features chosen as the one achieving the best performance are reported along with the respective performance in Tables S8–S10.

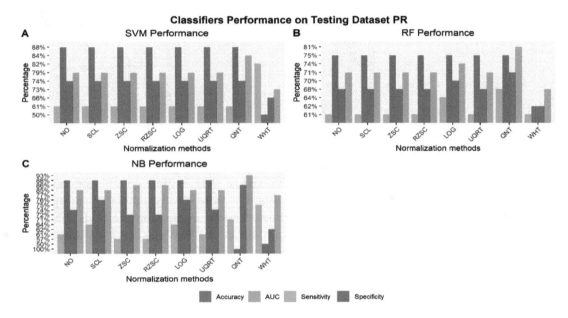

Figure 7. Classifiers performance on testing dataset to identify PR receptor status via radiomic features across normalization methods (NO: non-normalized features; SCL: Scaling normalization method; ZSC: Z-score normalization method; RZSC: Robust Z-score normalization method; LOG transformation; UPQRT: Upper Quartile normalization methods; QNT: Quantile normalization method; WHT: Whitening normalization method). A) Support Vector Machine (SVM) Performance on Testing dataset PR+ vs PR–. B) Random Forest (RF) Performance on Testing dataset PR+ vs PR–. C) Naïve Bayesian (NB) Performance on Testing dataset PR+ vs PR–.

Figure 8A shows the best classifiers for each of the machine learning methods according to the criteria defined in Section 2.3.3. The classifier achieving the best performances to detect PR negative status is Naïve Bayesian model using only two radiomic features (E4 and T5) normalized via quantile method. Figure 8B shows the ROC curves for the best classifiers to automatically detect PR receptor status. Box plots of radiomic features chosen by the machine learning methods to automatically detect PR status are shown in Figure S6.

3.4.3. Receptor Status: HER2– vs HER2+

Figure 9A shows the best classifiers for each of the machine learning methods according to the criteria defined in Section 2.3.3. The classifier achieving the best performances to detect HER2 receptor status is Random Forest model using only two radiomic features (T8 and K6) normalized via whitening normalization method. Figure 9B shows the ROC curves for the best classifiers to automatically detect HER2 receptor status. Box plots of radiomic features chosen by the machine learning methods to automatically detect HER2 status are shown in Figure S7.

3.4.4. Receptor Status: TN vs Others

Figure 10 shows the best performance of the three machine learning classifiers (SVM, RF, and NB) across all normalization methods to automatically detect TN cases. For each normalization approach the radiomic features chosen as the one achieving the best performance are reported along with the respective performance in Tables S11–S13.

A

Feature Names	Normalization Methods	ML Methods	SEN	SPE	ACC	AUC
E3, T5	Quantile	SVM	61%	88%	74%	84%
E3, T5	Quantile	RF	68%	75%	71%	81%
E4, T5	Quantile	NB	71%	99%	86%	93%

SVM: Support Vector Machine; RF: Random Forest; NB: Naïve Bayesian. SEN: Sensitivity; SPE: Specificity; ACC: Accuracy; AUC: Area Under the Curve.

B

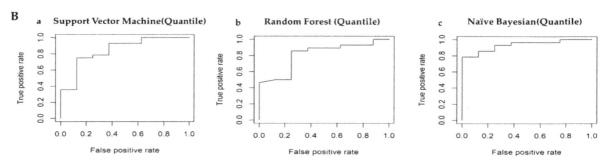

Figure 8. Classifiers' performance to detect PR receptor status. (**A**) Comparison table among classifiers: PR+ vs PR–. (**B**) ROC curves for the best classifiers to automatically detect PR receptor status. a) Best classifier for Support Vector Machine Method. The normalization methods that achieved the best performance is the quantile normalization method. b) Best classifier for Random Forest Method. The normalization method that achieved the best performance is the quantile method. c) Best classifier for Naïve Bayesian Method. The normalization method that achieved the best performance is quantile method.

A

Feature Names	Normalization Methods	ML Methods	SEN	SPE	ACC	AUC
T8, M3	WHT	SVM	40%	73%	57%	66%
T8, K6	WHT	RF	99%	76%	88%	91%
T8, M3	WHT	NB	75%	86%	81%	91%

WHT: Whitening normalization method; SVM: Support Vector Machine; RF: Random Forest; NB: Naïve Bayesian. SEN: Sensitivity; SPE: Specificity; ACC: Accuracy; AUC: Area Under the Curve.

B

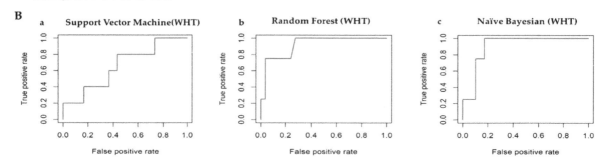

Figure 9. Classifiers' performance to detect HER2 receptor status. (**A**) Comparison table among classifiers: HER2+ vs HER2–. (**B**) ROC curves for the best classifiers to automatically detect HER2 receptor status. Radiomic Feature normalized by whitening methods were considered for the classification task. a) Best classifier for Support Vector Machine Method. b) Best classifier for Random Forest Method. c) Best classifier for Naïve Bayesian method.

Figure 11A shows the best classifiers for each of the machine learning methods according to the criteria defined in Section 2.3.3. The classifier achieving the best performances to detect TN cases is Random Forest model using only two radiomic features (T11 and G2) normalized via whitening method. Figure 11B shows the ROC curves for the best classifiers to automatically detect TN cases. Box plots of radiomic features chosen by the machine learning methods to automatically detect TN cases are shown in Figure S8.

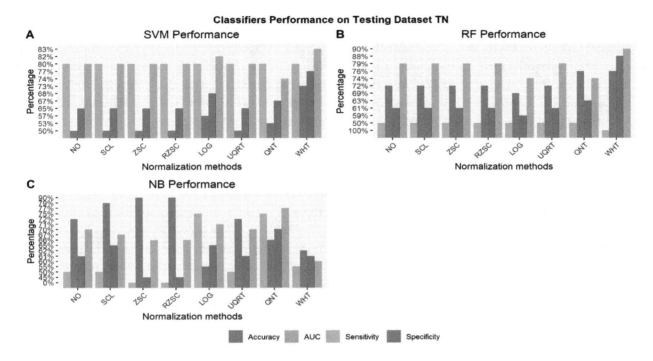

Figure 10. Classifiers performance on testing dataset to identify TN cases via radiomic features across normalization methods (NO: non-normalized features; SCL: Scaling normalization method; ZSC: Z-score normalization method; RZSC: Robust Z-score normalization method; LOG transformation; UPQRT: Upper Quartile normalization methods; QNT: Quantile normalization method; WHT: Whitening normalization method). **A**) Support Vector Machine (SVM) Performance on Testing dataset TN vs Others. **B**) Random Forest (RF) Performance on Testing dataset TN vs Others. **C**) Naïve Bayesian (NB) Performance on Testing dataset TN vs Others.

A

Feature Names	Normalization Methods	ML Methods	SEN	SPE	ACC	AUC
E2, G2	WHT	SVM	80%	73%	77%	83%
T11, G2	WHT	RF	98%	76%	88%	91%
T11, S2	WHT	NB	75%	66%	70%	77%

WHT: Whitening normalization method; SVM: Support Vector Machine; RF: Random Forest; NB: Naïve Bayesian. SEN: Sensitivity; SPE: Specificity; ACC: Accuracy; AUC: Area Under the Curve.

B

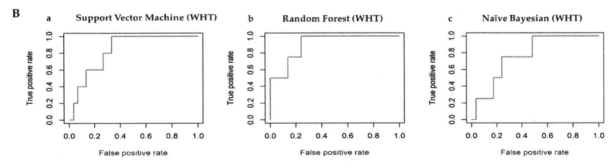

Figure 11. Classifiers' performance to detect TN receptor status. (**A**) Comparison table among classifiers: TN vs Others. (**B**) ROC curves for the best classifiers to automatically detect TN receptor status. a) Best classifier for Support Vector Machine Method. The normalization methods that achieved the best performance is the quantile normalization method. b) Best classifier for Random Forest Method. The normalization method that achieved the best performance is the quantile method. c) Best classifier for Naïve Bayesian Method. The normalization method that achieved the best performance is quantile method.

4. Discussion

The results from this study demonstrate that quantitative radiomic analysis shows potential as a means for high-throughput image-based phenotyping to automatically detect breast cancer receptor status via machine learning methods. Moreover, this study investigates the effect of normalization methods on radiomic features to automatically detect receptor status of breast cancer patients. Altogether our results suggest that quantitative radiomic analysis is influenced by normalization method choice.

The results from the correlation analysis along with visual inspection by Bland–Altman analysis, showed that all radiomic features are perfectly correlated with non-normalized radiomic features using scaling, z-score, robust z-score, and upper quartile normalization methods. Therefore, these methods help reducing bias and do not alter the information carried by the "row" radiomic features. These normalization methods, thus, result less aggressive than log-transformation, quantile, and whitening methods. In fact, four, sixteen and thirty out of 36 radiomic features showed a poorly correlation value with non-normalized radiomic features for log-transformation, quantile, and whitening normalization methods respectively. These results were expected. Log-transformation should be carefully applied to radiomic data as does not always decrease the skewness of the distribution but can make it more skewed than the raw data. Another common use of the log-transformation is to reduce the variability of data, especially in data sets including outliers, but it can often increase the variability of data. Moreover, log-transformation can only be used for positive outcomes, thus, for negative values it is common to add a small positive constant, a, to all observations before applying this transformation. Although this practice can appear quite meaningless, it can have a noticeable effect on the level of statistical significance [67]. Therefore, log-transformation should be carefully used in radiomic studies.

Quantile normalization method transforms original data to remove undesirable technical variation. Technical variation could cause apparent differences between samples. This kind of normalization is achieved by forcing the observed distributions to be the same and the average distribution, obtained by taking the average of each quantile across samples, is used as the reference. This method has worked well in practice, but important information could be wiped out and features that are not statically different across samples can be artificially induced [51]. Therefore, although it could improve the predictive power of the features, it should be used carefully.

Whitening normalization using PCA can make a more substantial normalization of the features to give it zero mean and unit covariance, so that transformed features become decorrelated [68]. One weakness of this transformation is that it can greatly exaggerate the noise in the data, since it stretches all dimensions (including noise) to be of equal size in the input. However, this method is often used as pre-processing step for machine learning models as it improves the overall performance.

Consequently, "aggressive" normalization methods should be carefully assessed based on the nature of the data and the main goal of the analysis.

Regarding the statistical analysis per receptor status, the results are in agreement with the existing literature [69].

Our results indicate that ER-negative cases may have larger volume, diameter and lesion area whereas less homogeneity and brightness than ER-positive cases. Similar observations were also reported by Chen et al. [70] in a correlation study between ER status and breast MRI radiomics and Li et al. [7] that showed an higher effective diameter, irregularity and entropy in ER-negative cases.

Different results were observed using quantile and whitening transformation methods. In fact, less features showed to be significantly different between positive and negative ER cases. One features (S1) and three features (T5, S1, S3) were not statistically significant using whitening and quantile transformation methods compared to the other investigated normalization methods. Moreover, these phenotypes captured on imaging are in agreement with prior literature showing that ER− tumors have higher microvessel density [71], higher levels of vascular endothelial growth factor [72], and higher proliferative activity [72].

Our results indicate that PR-negative cases may have lower enhancement-variance rate and homogeneity while higher entropy. PR-negative cases are also larger, more irregular in shape, more heterogeneous, and have a faster contrast uptake than PR-positive cases as also demonstrated by Li et al. [7]. These observations confirm the existing evidence that PR cancers tend to have high growth factor signaling [73]. Different results were observed using whitening-transformation method. In fact, less features showed to be significantly different between positive and negative PR cases. Three radiomic features showed significant changes between PR cases, while T5 was also captured as significant feature (p-value < 0.05) by other normalization methods, T2 and S2 were not statistically significant using other transformation methods.

As far as HER2 growth factor is concerned, none of 36 radiomic features showed significant changes between positive and negative HER2 cases except for whitening-transformation. Indeed, features normalized by whitening method showed an increased value in enhancement texture, structure and voxel for HER2 positive case.

TN cases showed to be larger, more irregular in shape, heterogeneous, and have a faster contrast uptake rate than all the other cases. Similar results were achieved by Agner et al. [28] showing more lesion heterogeneity in TN breast cancers than non-TN cancers. Li et al. [7] reported that TN cases are larger in size due to the over expression of oncogenes that favor cell proliferation defined by the absence of ER, PR, and HER2 receptors. Youk et al. [74] showed that larger tumor size was significantly associated with TN breast cancer. Using whitening transformation, different radiomic features showed statistical changes between cases but maintained the overall trends.

Overall, imaging phenotypes like enhancement texture, size features convey pathophysiologic characteristics like proliferation and angiogenesis provide clues to more accurate prognosis and optimal treatment. It is interesting to note that enhancement texture (especially heterogeneity) emerged as an important discriminatory indicator. In our study, a decrease in homogeneity was observed in ER−, PR−, and TN cancers relative to ER+, PR+, and non-TN cancers, in agreement with the exiting literature. Enhancement texture homogeneity was also found to be positively associated with tumor stage, suggesting that larger, heterogeneous tumors are potentially linked to more aggressive cancers [7] with higher probability of recurrence [41].

Moreover, we questioned whether radiomic features may be associated with aberrantly expressed breast cancer miRNAs. Thus, we evaluated the correlation degree using two different radiomic features normalization methods. In accordance with the exiting literature, breast miRNAs expression resulted associated especially to MR radiomic features such as shape and enhancement texture features [22]. However, as expected, we showed that various radiomic features normalization approaches capture different imaging-genomic associations. For example, for ER receptor status the upper quartile normalized G3 feature correlated with hsa-mir-526b whereas whitening normalized G3 feature correlated with hsa-mir-9.2. For this reason, once chosen the appropriate radiomic framework of analysis, conspicuous testing of radiomic results on external and independent image datasets are encouraged.

Using machine learning algorithms, enhancement texture features were selected as the most predictive feature for tumor receptor status. Hence, radiomic features have a high predictive power to detect clinical variables related to the genomic status of a tumor, such as ER status and PR status. The machine learning method that better performed to automatically detect ER, HER2, and TN cases is the Random Forest with an AUC of 86%, 91%, and 91% respectively. Naïve Bayesian outperformed the other methods to detect PR cases with 93% AUC.

Compared to the existing literature, the results achieved in this study via machine learning methods outperformed other studies.

Xie et al. [32] achieved an AUC of 91% via linear SVM using several whole-tumor texture features extracted from DCE and DWI-related original images, while we achieved the same AUC values using only two DCE imaging feature, reducing considerably the computational complexity of the Random Forest model. Agner et al. [28] used the morphologic and texture features extracted from the whole tumor on the early postcontrast images in conjunction with an SVM classifier, achieving a lower AUC (of 74%) to detect TN cases. Li at al. [7] also achieved a lower AUC value using quantitative imaging phenotypes of size, shape, and enhancement texture via linear discriminant analysis to predict clinical receptor status, namely ER+ vs ER– (89% AUC), PR+ vs PR– (69% AUC), HER2+ vs HER2– (65%AUC),and TN cases (67% AUC). Yoon et al. [33] used a deep learning approach utilizing imaging data from TCIA to generate prediction of clinical outcomes receptor status. They achieved lower performance to predict ER (82% AUC), PR (75% AUC), HER2 (72% AUC), but they accomplished a slightly higher AUC values using the combination of radiomics and genomics data.

Overall, in this study using robust machine learning methods and employing few radiomic feature to reduce the computational complexity of the ML models, we achieved better AUC values to discriminate clinical receptor status, paving the way to non-invasive disease monitoring using imaging features as potential surrogate markers of underlying molecular activity that may aid in clinical diagnosis and treatment planning.

Most of the radiomic features chosen by the ML methods were normalized using whitening transformation, whereas to detect PR cases the radiomic features were normalized by quantile transformation. These results were expected as quantile and whitening transformation are considered among the best normalizing transformation when compared to other alternatives in machine learning models [52,75]. Both transformation methods reduce the leverage of potentially influential points among candidate predictors and remove redundancy among them. In fact, normalization of the covariates mitigates the leverage and potential influence of these covariates to an extent, which in some cases, will allow for more robust model selection.

However, this study presents some limitations. The MR images used in this study were acquired by different institutions more than 10 years ago. These may have had different acquisition protocols, different weight-based dosing regimen for contrast agents, and different time resolution of post-contrast sequences, and therefore, these images may not reflect current MRI technology, which has advanced considerably during the past decade. Consequently, our results can only be generalized to this population. However, the bias was limited by performing several normalization methods on the extracted radiomic features. Another limitation of our study was that the patient sample was relatively small and unbalanced, but by performing a cross validation for each molecular classification assessment (e.g., between ER+ and ER– cases) and applying balancing methods (SMOTE) to the developed model, the overall bias was reduced. In addition, our study lacks further validation on internal cohort, for which patient recruitment is ongoing.

Therefore, after this pilot study, which helped us establishing a robust framework of analysis, upcoming work will include studies on a larger and more recent clinically annotated data set to verify and validate the results from this preliminary study. We will further assess the role of the MRI phenotypes in combination with genomic and clinical information to improve the prediction power of the machine learning-based models. Furthermore, molecular breast cancer intrinsic subtypes will be also investigated.

5. Conclusions

In this study, our results demonstrate that there are statistically significant associations between radiomic tumor features and breast cancer molecular receptor status. Breast tumor characterization, including the ER, PR, and HER2 molecular receptor status, represents a primary goal to direct treatment options and targeted chemotherapies. Thus, in order to achieve a more accurate and early diagnosis is relevant to identify non-invasive diagnostic imaging biomarker associated to the molecular receptor status. This study investigated several statistical approaches to identify the relationship between medical imaging quantitative descriptors of clinical phenotypes and molecular tumor characteristics. Moreover, the prediction power of each radiomic feature normalization method was assessed by three advanced machine learning algorithms. The results from this study offer a better understanding into the underlying tumor biology including tumor enhancement texture. Identifying receptor status via imaging phenotypes may aid in clinical diagnosis and treatment planning. At the same time, we aware researchers to implement in radiomic analysis framework different radiomic feature normalization approaches and standards for post-acquisition data processing, in order to ensure more robust findings.

Another important advantage of our approach is that opens the door to the identification of non-invasive in vivo imaging surrogate markers that could reflect the underlying tumor biology.

Supplementary Materials
Figure S1: Relationship between breast cancer miRNAs expression and ER receptor status; Figure S2: Relationship between breast cancer miRNAs expression and PR receptor status; Figure S3: Relationship between breast cancer miRNAs expression and HER2 receptor status; Figure S4: Relationship between breast cancer miRNAs expression and TN cases; Figure S5. Box plots of radiomic features chosen by the machine learning methods to automatically detect ER status; Figure S6: Box plots of radiomic features chosen by the machine learning methods to automatically detect PR status; Figure S7: Box plots of radiomic features chosen by the machine learning methods to automatically detect HER2 receptor; Figure S8: Box plots of radiomic features chosen by the machine learning methods to automatically detect TN cases. Table S1: Additional Clinical Parameters; Table S2: Radiomic Features; Table S3: Correlation Analysis on the Whole Dataset between Non-Normalized and Normalized Radiomic Features; Table S4: Imaging-genomic associations; Table S5: Support Vector Machine Performance on Testing dataset ER+ vs ER–; Table S6: Random Forest Performance on Testing dataset ER+ vs ER–; Table S7: Naïve Bayesian Performance on Testing dataset ER+ vs ER–; Table S8: Support Vector Machine Performance on Testing dataset PR+ vs PR–; Table S9: Random Forest Performance on Testing dataset PR+ vs PR–; Table S10: Naïve Bayesian Performance on Testing dataset PR+ vs PR–; Table S11: Support Vector Machine Performance on Testing dataset TN vs Others; Table S12: Random Forest Performance on Testing dataset TN vs Others; Table S13: Naïve Bayesian Performance on Testing dataset TN vs Others.

Author Contributions: R.C. and K.P. wrote the manuscript, designed the analysis framework for radiomics and genomics, contributing equally to this work. M.F. contributed to conception and design and supported data analysis. E.N. interpreted data and validated the results. M.S. revised the manuscript critically and approved the version to be published. All authors have read and agreed to the published version of the manuscript.

References

1. Siegel, R.; Ma, J.; Zou, Z.; Jemal, A. Cancer statistics, 2014. *CA Cancer J. Clin.* **2014**, *64*, 9–29. [CrossRef] [PubMed]
2. Fiordelisi, M.; Auletta, L.; Meomartino, L.; Basso, L.; Fatone, G.; Salvatore, M.; Mancini, M.; Greco, A. Preclinical Molecular Imaging for Precision Medicine in Breast Cancer Mouse Models. *Contrast Media Mol. Imaging* **2019**, *2019*, 8946729. [CrossRef] [PubMed]
3. Carey, L.A.; Perou, C.M.; Livasy, C.A.; Dressler, L.G.; Cowan, D.; Conway, K.; Karaca, G.; Troester, M.A.; Tse, C.K.; Edmiston, S. Race, breast cancer subtypes, and survival in the Carolina Breast Cancer Study. *JAMA* **2006**, *295*, 2492–2502. [CrossRef] [PubMed]
4. Voduc, K.D.; Cheang, M.C.; Tyldesley, S.; Gelmon, K.; Nielsen, T.O.; Kennecke, H. Breast cancer subtypes and the risk of local and regional relapse. *J. Clin. Oncol.* **2010**, *28*, 1684–1691. [CrossRef] [PubMed]
5. Metzger-Filho, O.; Sun, Z.; Viale, G.; Price, K.N.; Crivellari, D.; Snyder, R.D.; Gelber, R.D.; Castiglione-Gertsch, M.; Coates, A.S.; Goldhirsch, A. Patterns of recurrence and outcome according to breast cancer subtypes in lymph node–negative disease: Results from International Breast Cancer Study Group Trials VIII and IX. *J. Clin. Oncol.* **2013**, *31*, 3083. [CrossRef]
6. Arvold, N.D.; Taghian, A.G.; Niemierko, A.; Raad, R.F.A.; Sreedhara, M.; Nguyen, P.L.; Bellon, J.R.; Wong, J.S.; Smith, B.L.; Harris, J.R. Age, breast cancer subtype approximation, and local recurrence after breast-conserving therapy. *J. Clin. Oncol.* **2011**, *29*, 3885. [CrossRef]
7. Li, H.; Zhu, Y.; Burnside, E.S.; Huang, E.; Drukker, K.; Hoadley, K.A.; Fan, C.; Conzen, S.D.; Zuley, M.; Net, J.M. Quantitative MRI radiomics in the prediction of molecular classifications of breast cancer subtypes in the TCGA/TCIA data set. *NPJ Breast Cancer* **2016**, *2*, 16012. [CrossRef]
8. Goldhirsch, A.; Wood, W.C.; Coates, A.S.; Gelber, R.D.; Thürlimann, B.; Senn, H.-J.; Members, P. Strategies for subtypes—dealing with the diversity of breast cancer: Highlights of the St Gallen International Expert Consensus on the Primary Therapy of Early Breast Cancer 2011. *Ann. Oncol.* **2011**, *22*, 1736–1747. [CrossRef]
9. Gnant, M.; Harbeck, N.; Thomssen, C. St. Gallen/Vienna 2017: A brief summary of the consensus discussion about escalation and de-escalation of primary breast cancer treatment. *Breast Care* **2017**, *12*, 101–106. [CrossRef]
10. Aerts, H.J. The potential of radiomic-based phenotyping in precision medicine: A review. *JAMA Oncol.* **2016**, *2*, 1636–1642. [CrossRef]
11. Wu, J.; Tha, K.K.; Xing, L.; Li, R. Radiomics and radiogenomics for precision radiotherapy. In *J. Radiat. Res.*; 2018; Volume 59, (Suppl_1), pp. i25–i31.

12. Gillies, R.J.; Kinahan, P.E.; Hricak, H. Radiomics: Images are more than pictures, they are data. *Radiology* **2015**, *278*, 563–577. [CrossRef] [PubMed]

13. Wu, J.; Li, B.; Sun, X.; Cao, G.; Rubin, D.L.; Napel, S.; Ikeda, D.M.; Kurian, A.W.; Li, R. Heterogeneous enhancement patterns of tumor-adjacent parenchyma at MR imaging are associated with dysregulated signaling pathways and poor survival in breast cancer. *Radiology* **2017**, *285*, 401–413. [CrossRef] [PubMed]

14. Mazurowski, M.A. Radiogenomics: What it is and why it is important. *J. Am. Coll. Radiol.* **2015**, *12*, 862–866. [CrossRef] [PubMed]

15. Network, C.G.A. Comprehensive molecular portraits of human breast tumours. *Nature* **2012**, *490*, 61. [CrossRef] [PubMed]

16. Clark, K.; Vendt, B.; Smith, K.; Freymann, J.; Kirby, J.; Koppel, P.; Moore, S.; Phillips, S.; Maffitt, D.; Pringle, M. The Cancer Imaging Archive (TCIA): Maintaining and operating a public information repository. *J. Digit. Imag.* **2013**, *26*, 1045–1057. [CrossRef]

17. Zanfardino, M.; Pane, K.; Mirabelli, P.; Salvatore, M.; Franzese, M. TCGA-TCIA Impact on Radiogenomics Cancer Research: A Systematic Review. *Intl. J. Mol. Sci.* **2019**, *20*, 6033. [CrossRef]

18. Zanfardino, M.; Franzese, M.; Pane, K.; Cavaliere, C.; Monti, S.; Esposito, G.; Salvatore, M.; Aiello, M. Bringing radiomics into a multi-omics framework for a comprehensive genotype–phenotype characterization of oncological diseases. *J. Translat. Med.* **2019**, *17*, 337. [CrossRef]

19. Schiano, C.; Franzese, M.; Pane, K.; Garbino, N.; Soricelli, A.; Salvatore, M.; de Nigris, F.; Napoli, C. Hybrid 18F-FDG-PET/MRI Measurement of Standardized Uptake Value Coupled with Yin Yang 1 Signature in Metastatic Breast Cancer. A Preliminary Study. *Cancers* **2019**, *11*, 1444. [CrossRef]

20. Bhooshan, N.; Giger, M.L.; Jansen, S.A.; Li, H.; Lan, L.; Newstead, G.M. Cancerous breast lesions on dynamic contrast-enhanced MR images: Computerized characterization for image-based prognostic markers. *Radiology* **2010**, *254*, 680–690. [CrossRef]

21. Guo, W.; Li, H.; Zhu, Y.; Lan, L.; Yang, S.; Drukker, K.; Morris, E.A.; Burnside, E.S.; Whitman, G.J.; Giger, M.L. Prediction of clinical phenotypes in invasive breast carcinomas from the integration of radiomics and genomics data. *J. Med. Imag.* **2015**, *2*, 041007. [CrossRef]

22. Zhu, Y.; Li, H.; Guo, W.; Drukker, K.; Lan, L.; Giger, M.L.; Ji, Y. Deciphering genomic underpinnings of quantitative MRI-based radiomic phenotypes of invasive breast carcinoma. *Sci. Rep.* **2015**, *5*, 17787. [CrossRef] [PubMed]

23. Giger, M.L.; Karssemeijer, N.; Schnabel, J.A. Breast image analysis for risk assessment, detection, diagnosis, and treatment of cancer. *Annu. Rev. Biomed. Eng.* **2013**, *15*, 327–357. [CrossRef] [PubMed]

24. Bhooshan, N.; Giger, M.; Edwards, D.; Yuan, Y.; Jansen, S.; Li, H.; Lan, L.; Sattar, H.; Newstead, G. Computerized three-class classification of MRI-based prognostic markers for breast cancer. *Phys. Med. Biol.* **2011**, *56*, 5995.

25. Grimm, L.J.; Zhang, J.; Mazurowski, M.A. Computational approach to radiogenomics of breast cancer: Luminal A and luminal B molecular subtypes are associated with imaging features on routine breast MRI extracted using computer vision algorithms. *J. Magnet. Resonance Imag.* **2015**, *42*, 902–907. [CrossRef]

26. Wu, J.; Cui, Y.; Sun, X.; Cao, G.; Li, B.; Ikeda, D.M.; Kurian, A.W.; Li, R. Unsupervised clustering of quantitative image phenotypes reveals breast cancer subtypes with distinct prognoses and molecular pathways. *Clin. Cancer Res.* **2017**, *23*, 3334–3342. [CrossRef]

27. Burnside, E.S.; Drukker, K.; Li, H.; Bonaccio, E.; Zuley, M.; Ganott, M.; Net, J.M.; Sutton, E.J.; Brandt, K.R.; Whitman, G.J. Using computer-extracted image phenotypes from tumors on breast magnetic resonance imaging to predict breast cancer pathologic stage. *Cancer* **2016**, *122*, 748–757. [CrossRef]

28. Agner, S.C.; Rosen, M.A.; Englander, S.; Tomaszewski, J.E.; Feldman, M.D.; Zhang, P.; Mies, C.; Schnall, M.D.; Madabhushi, A. Computerized image analysis for identifying triple-negative breast cancers and differentiating them from other molecular subtypes of breast cancer on dynamic contrast-enhanced MR images: A feasibility study. *Radiology* **2014**, *272*, 91–99. [CrossRef]

29. Yamaguchi, K.; Abe, H.; Newstead, G.M.; Egashira, R.; Nakazono, T.; Imaizumi, T.; Irie, H. Intratumoral heterogeneity of the distribution of kinetic parameters in breast cancer: Comparison based on the molecular subtypes of invasive breast cancer. *Breast Cancer* **2015**, *22*, 496–502. [CrossRef]

30. Fiordelisi, M.F.; Cavaliere, C.; Auletta, L.; Basso, L.; Salvatore, M. Magnetic Resonance Imaging for Translational Research in Oncology. *J. Clin. Med.* **2019**, *8*, 1883. [CrossRef]

31. Blaschke, E.; Abe, H. MRI phenotype of breast cancer: Kinetic assessment for molecular subtypes. *J. Magnet. Resonance Imag.* **2015**, *42*, 920–924. [CrossRef]

32. Xie, T.; Wang, Z.; Zhao, Q.; Bai, Q.; Zhou, X.; Gu, Y.; Peng, W.; Wang, H. Machine Learning-based Analysis of MR Multiparametric Radiomics for the Subtype Classification of Breast Cancer. *Fron. Oncol.* **2019**, *9*, 505. [CrossRef] [PubMed]

33. Yoon, H.-J.; Ramanathan, A.; Alamudun, F.; Tourassi, G. Deep radiogenomics for predicting clinical phenotypes in invasive breast cancer. In In Proceedings of the 14th International Workshop on Breast Imaging (IWBI 2018), Atlanta, GA, USA, 8–11 July 2018; International Society for Optics and Photonics: Bellingham, WA, USA, 2018; p. 107181H.

34. Parmar, C.; Barry, J.D.; Hosny, A.; Quackenbush, J.; Aerts, H. Data Analysis Strategies in Medical Imaging. *Clin. Cancer Res.* **2018**, *24*, 3492–3499. [CrossRef] [PubMed]

35. Kotsiantis, S.; Kanellopoulos, D.; Pintelas, P. Data preprocessing for supervised leaning. *Intl. J. Comput. Sci.* **2006**, *1*, 111–117.

36. Rizzo, S.; Botta, F.; Raimondi, S.; Origgi, D.; Fanciullo, C.; Morganti, A.G.; Bellomi, M. Radiomics: The facts and the challenges of image analysis. *Eur. Radiol. Exp.* **2018**, *2*, 1–8. [CrossRef]

37. Madabhushi, A.; Udupa, J.K. New methods of MR image intensity standardization via generalized scale. *Med. Phys.* **2006**, *33*, 3426–3434. [CrossRef]

38. Nyúl, L.G.; Udupa, J.K. On standardizing the MR image intensity scale. *Magnet. Resonance Med.* **1999**, *42*, 1072–1081.

39. Nyúl, L.G.; Udupa, J.K.; Zhang, X. New variants of a method of MRI scale standardization. *IEEE Trans. Med. Imag.* **2000**, *19*, 143–150. [CrossRef]

40. Ge, Y.; Udupa, J.K.; Nyul, L.G.; Wei, L.; Grossman, R.I. Numerical tissue characterization in MS via standardization of the MR image intensity scale. *J. Magnet. Resonance Imag.* **2000**, *12*, 715–721. [CrossRef]

41. Li, H.; Zhu, Y.; Burnside, E.S.; Drukker, K.; Hoadley, K.A.; Fan, C.; Conzen, S.D.; Whitman, G.J.; Sutton, E.J.; Net, J.M. MR imaging radiomics signatures for predicting the risk of breast cancer recurrence as given by research versions of MammaPrint, Oncotype DX, and PAM50 gene assays. *Radiology* **2016**, *281*, 382–391. [CrossRef]

42. R Core Team. *R: A Language and Environment for Statistical Computing*; R Foundation for Statistical Computing: Vienna, Austria, 2012. Available online: http://www.R-project.org (accessed on 2 January 2020).

43. Colaprico, A.; Silva, T.C.; Olsen, C.; Garofano, L.; Cava, C.; Garolini, D.; Sabedot, T.S.; Malta, T.M.; Pagnotta, S.M.; Castiglioni, I. TCGAbiolinks: An R/Bioconductor package for integrative analysis of TCGA data. *Nucl. Acids Res.* **2015**, *44*, e71. [CrossRef]

44. Incoronato, M.; Grimaldi, A.M.; Mirabelli, P.; Cavaliere, C.; Parente, C.A.; Franzese, M.; Staibano, S.; Ilardi, G.; Russo, D.; Soricelli, A. Circulating miRNAs in Untreated Breast Cancer: An Exploratory Multimodality Morpho-Functional Study. *Cancers* **2019**, *11*, 876. [CrossRef] [PubMed]

45. Shapiro, S.S.; Wilk, M.B. An analysis of variance test for normality (complete samples). *Biometrika*, 1965; 52, 3/4, 591–611.

46. Abdi, H. Z-scores. *Encyclopedia of Measurement and Statistics* **2007**, *3*, 1055–1058.

47. Huynh, H.; Meyer, P. Use of robust z in detecting unstable items in item response theory models. *Pract. Assess. Res. Eval.* **2010**, *15*, 1–8.

48. Feng, C.; Wang, H.; Lu, N.; Tu, X.M. Log transformation: Application and interpretation in biomedical research. *Stat. Med.* **2013**, *32*, 230–239. [CrossRef] [PubMed]

49. Bullard, J.H.; Purdom, E.; Hansen, K.D.; Dudoit, S. Evaluation of statistical methods for normalization and differential expression in mRNA-Seq experiments. *BMC Bioinf.* **2010**, *11*, 94. [CrossRef]

50. Bolstad, B.M.; Irizarry, R.A.; Åstrand, M.; Speed, T.P. A comparison of normalization methods for high density oligonucleotide array data based on variance and bias. *Bioinformatics* **2003**, *19*, 185–193. [CrossRef]

51. Hicks, S.C.; Irizarry, R.A. When to use quantile normalization? *BioRxiv* **2014**, 012203.

52. Kessy, A.; Lewin, A.; Strimmer, K. Optimal whitening and decorrelation. *Am. Statist.* **2018**, *72*, 309–314. [CrossRef]

53. Bland, J.M.; Altman, D. Statistical methods for assessing agreement between two methods of clinical measurement. *Lancet* **1986**, *327*, 307–310. [CrossRef]

54. Castaldo, R.; Melillo, P.; Bracale, U.; Caserta, M.; Triassi, M.; Pecchia, L. Acute mental stress assessment via short term HRV analysis in healthy adults: A systematic review with meta-analysis. *Biomed. Signal Process. Control* **2015**, *18*, 370–377. [CrossRef]

55. Castaldo, R.; Melillo, P.; Izzo, R.; Luca, N.D.; Pecchia, L. Fall Prediction in Hypertensive Patients via Short-Term HRV Analysis. *IEEE J. Biomed. Health Inf.* **2017**, *21*, 399–406. [CrossRef] [PubMed]

56. Castaldo, R.; Montesinos, L.; Melillo, P.; James, C.; Pecchia, L. Ultra-short term HRV features as surrogates of short term HRV: A case study on mental stress detection in real life. *BMC Med. Inform. Decis. Making* **2019**, *19*, 12. [CrossRef] [PubMed]

57. Robinson, M.D.; Smyth, G.K. Moderated statistical tests for assessing differences in tag abundance. *Bioinformatics* **2007**, *23*, 2881–2887. [CrossRef] [PubMed]

58. Foster, K.R.; Koprowski, R.; Skufca, J.D. Machine learning, medical diagnosis, and biomedical engineering research-commentary. *BioMed. Eng. OnLine* **2014**, *13*, 10.1186. [CrossRef]

59. Chawla, N.V.; Bowyer, K.W.; Hall, L.O.; Kegelmeyer, W.P. SMOTE: Synthetic minority over-sampling technique. *J. Artif. Intell. Res.* **2002**, *16*, 321–357. [CrossRef]

60. Provost, F. Machine learning from imbalanced data sets 101. In *Proceedings of the AAAI'2000 Workshop on Imbalanced Data Sets*; AAAI Press: Menlo Park, CA, USA, 2000; pp. 1–3.

61. Vapnik, V.N. *Statistical Learning Theory*; Wiley: New York, NY, USA, 1998; p. 736.

62. Quinlan, J.R. *C4.5: Programs For Machine Learning*; Morgan Kaufmann Publishers: San Mateo, CA, USA, 1993.

63. Nguyen, C.; Wang, Y.; Nguyen, H.N. Random forest classifier combined with feature selection for breast cancer diagnosis and prognostic. *J. Biomed. Sci. Eng.* **2013**, *6*, 551. [CrossRef]

64. Kononenko, I. *Semi-Naive Bayesian Classifier*; European Working Session on Learning; Springer: Dordrecht, The Netherlands, 1991; pp. 206–219.

65. Kohl, M. Performance measures in binary classification. *Intl. J. Stat. Med. Res.* **2012**, *1*, 79–81. [CrossRef]

66. Loh, H.-Y.; Norman, B.P.; Lai, K.-S.; Rahman, N.M.A.N.A.; Alitheen, N.B.M.; Osman, M.A. The Regulatory Role of MicroRNAs in Breast Cancer. *Intl. J. Mol. Sci.* **2019**, *20*, 4940. [CrossRef]

67. Changyong, F.; Hongyue, W.; Naiji, L.; Tian, C.; Hua, H.; Ying, L. Log-transformation and its implications for data analysis. *Shanghai Arch. Psychiat.* **2014**, *26*, 105.

68. Haga, A.; Takahashi, W.; Aoki, S.; Nawa, K.; Yamashita, H.; Abe, O.; Nakagawa, K. Standardization of imaging features for radiomics analysis. *J. Med. Invest.* **2019**, *66*, 35–37. [CrossRef]

69. Panayides, A.S.; Pattichis, M.S.; Leandrou, S.; Pitris, C.; Constantinidou, A.; Pattichis, C.S. Radiogenomics for precision medicine with a big data analytics perspective. *IEEE J. Biomed. Health Inform.* **2018**, *23*, 2063–2079. [CrossRef] [PubMed]

70. Chen, J.H.; Baek, H.M.; Nalcioglu, O.; Su, M.Y. Estrogen receptor and breast MR imaging features: A correlation study. *J. Magnet. Resonance Imag.* **2008**, *27*, 825–833. [CrossRef]

71. Koukourakis, M.I.; Manolas, C.; Minopoulos, G.; Giatromanolaki, A.; Sivridis, E. Angiogenesis relates to estrogen receptor negativity, c-erbB-2 overexpression and early relapse in node-negative ductal carcinoma of the breast. *Intl. J. Surg. Pathol.* **2003**, *11*, 29–34. [CrossRef]

72. Fuckar, D.; Dekanic, A.; Stifter, S.; Mustac, E.; Krstulja, M.; Dobrila, F.; Jonjic, N. VEGF expression is associated with negative estrogen receptor status in patients with breast cancer. *Intl. J. Surg. Pathol.* **2006**, *14*, 49–55. [CrossRef] [PubMed]

73. Arpino, G.; Weiss, H.; Lee, A.V.; Schiff, R.; De Placido, S.; Osborne, C.K.; Elledge, R.M. Estrogen receptor–positive, progesterone receptor–negative breast cancer: Association with growth factor receptor expression and tamoxifen resistance. *J. Nat. Cancer Inst.* **2005**, *97*, 1254–1261. [CrossRef] [PubMed]

74. Youk, J.H.; Son, E.J.; Chung, J.; Kim, J.-A.; Kim, E.-k. Triple-negative invasive breast cancer on dynamic contrast-enhanced and diffusion-weighted MR imaging: Comparison with other breast cancer subtypes. *Eur. Radiol.* **2012**, *22*, 1724–1734. [CrossRef]

75. Peterson, R.A.; Cavanaugh, J.E. Ordered quantile normalization: A semiparametric transformation built for the cross-validation era. *J. Appl. Stat.* **2019**, 1–16. [CrossRef]

10

Hybrid ^{18}F-FDG-PET/MRI Measurement of Standardized Uptake Value Coupled with Yin Yang 1 Signature in Metastatic Breast Cancer

Concetta Schiano [1,*], Monica Franzese [1], Katia Pane [1], Nunzia Garbino [1], Andrea Soricelli [1,2], Marco Salvatore [1,†], Filomena de Nigris [3,†] and Claudio Napoli [1,4,†]

[1] IRCCS SDN, 80134 Naples, Italy
[2] Department of Motor Sciences and Healthiness, University of Naples Parthenope, 80134 Naples, Italy
[3] Department of Precision Medicine, University of Campania "Luigi Vanvitelli", 80138 Naples, Italy
[4] Department of Advanced Medical and Surgical Sciences, University of Campania "Luigi Vanvitelli", 80138 Naples, Italy
*   Correspondence: tina.schiano@gmail.com or cshiano@sdn-napoli.it

†   Contributed equally to the design of the study.

Abstract: Purpose: Detection of breast cancer (BC) metastasis at the early stage is important for the assessment of BC progression status. Image analysis represents a valuable tool for the management of oncological patients. Our preliminary study combined imaging parameters from hybrid ^{18}F-FDG-PET/MRI and the expression level of the transcriptional factor Yin Yang 1 (YY1) for the detection of early metastases. Methods: The study enrolled suspected $n = 217$ BC patients that underwent ^{18}F-FDG-PET/MRI scans. The analysis retrospectively included $n = 55$ subjects. $n = 40$ were BC patients and $n = 15$ imaging-negative female individuals were healthy subjects (HS). Standard radiomics parameters were extracted from PET/MRI image. RNA was obtained from peripheral blood mononuclear cells and YY1 expression level was evaluated by real time reverse transcription polymerase chain reactions (qRT-PCR). An enzyme-linked immuosorbent assay (ELISA) was used to determine the amount of YY1 serum protein. Statistical comparison between subgroups was evaluated by Mann-Whitney U and Spearman's tests. Results: Radiomics showed a significant positive correlation between Greg-level co-occurrence matrix (GLCM) and standardized uptake value maximum (SUVmax) ($r = 0.8$ and $r = 0.8$ respectively) in BC patients. YY1 level was significant overexpressed in estrogen receptor (ER)-positive/progesteron receptor-positive/human epidermal growth factor receptor2-negative (ER+/PR+/HER2-) subtype of BC patients with synchronous metastasis (SM) at primary diagnosis compared to metachronous metastasis (MM) and HS ($p < 0.001$) and correlating significantly with ^{18}F-FDG-uptake parameter (SUVmax) ($r = 0.48$). Conclusions: The combination of functional ^{18}F-FDG-PET/MRI parameters and molecular determination of YY1 could represent a novel integrated approach to predict synchronous metastatic disease with more accuracy than ^{18}F-FDG-PET/MRI alone.

Keywords: breast; imaging; marker; radiomics; Yin Yang 1

---

1. Introduction

PET and MRI scans are useful instruments to diagnose the presence of metastatic disease providing both morphological and metabolic information [1–3]. However, an exclusive use of imaging technique, has some limitations, such as high cost, sensitivity and specificity [4]. We are confident that the combination of non-invasive methods with the parameters derived from image analysis will be of great interest for clinical practice.

A growing amount of data has established that polycomb oncoprotein Yin Yang 1 (YY1) has a prognostic impact in malignancy [5–7]. YY1 is frequently overexpressed in a wide range of solid and non-solid tumors, regulating a broad class of genes involved in control of both cell cycle and apoptosis. In vitro and in vivo studies have reported the expression of YY1 has been associated with development of a malignant phenotype in some human cancers, tumor progression, metastasis formation, and correlating with poor prognosis and drug/immune resistance [8–17]. However, conflicting results have been shown when YY1 was evaluated during the progression and metastasis of breast cancer (BC). The role of YY1 in metastatic BC has recently been verified by meta-analysis showing that YY1 exhibited significantly high mRNA levels in basal-like BCs versus normal tissues [18]. In contrast, Lieberthal et al. reported an increased expression of YY1 in invasive BC cells [19]. Furthermore, recently, YY1 was reported as anti-oncogene in invasive human BC cells [20]. Specifically, three potential binding sites for YY1 were found on a lincRNA involved in occurrence and progression of human cancers [20]. Moreover, about 70%–80% of diagnosed BCs are estrogen receptor positive and treated with endocrine therapy. However, this treatment is ineffective for patients with metastatic disease [21].

This study represents the first assessment of YY1 mRNA and protein expression levels in peripheral blood from BC patients, which have been correlated with imaging parameters from hybrid ^{18}F-FDG-PET/MRI in order to improve the early detection of metastatic disease.

2. Materials and Methods

2.1. Study Cohort

The study was approved by the institutional ethics committee (IRCCS Fondazione SDN) in accordance with the ethical standard of the Declaration of Helsinki. A written informed consent was obtained from all subjects enrolled (healthy subjects (HS) and BC patients). All clinical-pathological characteristics are reported in Table 1. Exclusion criteria included age <18 years, pregnancy, different cancer detection, and general contraindications for contrast agent injection. All eligible patients had ^{18}F-FDG-PET/MRI scans between 2014 and 2018. Our retrospective study enrolled consecutive suspected $n = 217$ oncological patients that underwent ^{18}F-FDG-PET/MRI scans. Individuals with negative imaging were considered HS ($n = 15$) (Figure 1) [22].

Table 1. Patient clinical-pathological characteristics.

	Number or Values
Total Cohort	52
Healthy Subjects "Control group"	15
Breast cancer group "Synchronous metastasis" (SM)	11
Breast cancer group "Metachronous metastasis" (MM)	26
Mean age (years)	57
Range (min–max)	32–88
TNM	13
T0	1
T1	2
T2	7
T3	3
NA	24

Table 1. *Cont.*

	Number or Values
Tumor Grade	10
G2	8
G3	2
NA	27
Ki 67 Status [a]	12
Low	4
High	8
NA	25
ER Status	15
Negative	3
Positive	12
NA	22
PR Status	15
Negative	3
Positive	12
NA	22
Her2 Status [b]	13
Negative	9
Positive	3
NA	24

[a] Ki67 $\geq$ 20% was considered High. [b] one Her2 Status was equivocal. NA = Not available.

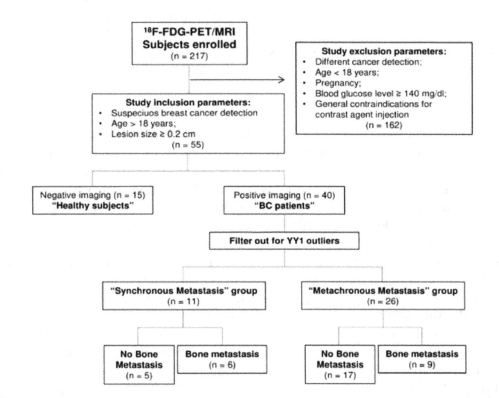

Figure 1. Eligible patients included in the study. Subject flow chart describing inclusion and exclusion criteria for the selection of the patients.

2.2. Sample Collection

Peripheral blood mononuclear cells (PBMCs) and serum aliquots were isolated as previously described [23]. Briefly, PBMCs were isolated by density gradient centrifugation on Histopaque-10771

(Sigma-Aldrich). After centrifugation, white blood cells were recovered and washed twice with phosphate-buffered saline (PBS) pH7.4 (Gibco; Life Technologies/Gibco, Italy). White cells and serum aliquots were frozen at −80 °C at the IRCCS SDN Biobank [24].

2.3. RNA Extraction and Real-Time Quantitative Reverse Transcription Polymerase Chain Reaction (qRT-PCR) Assay

Total RNAs were extracted using Trizol solution (Life Technologies/Gibco, Italy), according to the manufacturer's instructions. The specificity of oligonucleotide pair used was verified with the Basic Local Alignment Search Tool (BLAST), NCBI program and through in-silico polymerase chain reaction (PCR) analysis by UCSC (Genome Browser website) [23]. Primers were designed by Primer 3 software (http://bioinfo.ut.ee/primer3-0.4.0/) and synthesized by Life Technologies [23]. Quantitative real-time PCR was performed according to the supplier protocols (BioRad). Melt curve analysis was performed to verify a single product species. Selective primer sequences used for YY1 (NM_003403) were 5′-CAAAACTAAAACGACACCAAC-3′ (Forward) and 5′-TGAAGTCCAGTGAAAAGCGT-3′ (Reverse). Ribosomal protein S18 (RPS18; NM_022551) was used as housekeeping gene [23]. All reactions were carried out at least in triplicate for every cDNA template and qRT-PCR data were analyzed by Ct (threshold cycle) approach. The expression levels of the target gene normalized with the internal housekeeping gene were presented as delta-Ct (ΔCt), calculation [23]. The relative expression was estimated among groups considered.

2.4. YY1 Enzyme-Linked Immunosorbent Assay (ELISA) Test

Prior analysis, serum samples were stored at -80 °C. All samples were thawed only once prior to use. For the detection and quantification of our antigen of interest, enzyme-linked immunosorbent assay (ELISA) was used, according to the manufacturer's instructions with signals detection at 450 nm (Biocompare, Italy Cat. number ABIN4973888). Kit detection range was 0.156–10 ng/mL with sensitivity <0.059 ng/mL.

2.5. Hybrid ^{18}F-FDG-PET/MRI Technique

All patients were acquired on both a PET/CT device and on a 3T hybrid PET/MRI system (mMR Biograph; Siemens, Erlangen, Germany, with system sensitivity of 13.2 cps/kBq, transverse resolution of 4.4 mm and axial resolution of 4.5 mm) equipped with a dedicated breast coil, according to previously described acquisition protocols [25,26]. After fasting for 8 hours, patients were administered about 401 ± 32 MBq (mean ± standard deviation) of ^{18}F-FDG was administered to the patients, through an antecubital catheter. ^{18}F-FDG-PET/MRI images were performed concurrently after an uptake period of more than 60 minutes. The protocol was optimized for accurate detection and staging as previously described [25,27], briefly: an axial T2 turbo spin echo sequence; axial and coronal T2 turbo inversion recovery; diffusion weighted imaging (DWI), considered the most specific technique for the breast study. To investigate both morphological and dynamic breast parameters, all patients were injected with gadolinium diethylene triamine pentacetate (GD-DTPA; Magnevist) at 0.1 mmol/kg body weight, The dynamic study provides six axial spoiled gradient echo (SPGRE) 3D VIBE sequence before, during and after injection of contrast agent with variable flip-angle thus making a fat suppression. The attenuation correction is given by the segmentation (DIXON) in tissue classes, obtaining both water and fat maps. PET data are related only to these specific elements. Considering the PET data, the process of image reconstruction is done through an iterative algorithm called OSEM composed by three iterations on a matrix 172 × 172. Its main feature is the noise reduction in regions of low absorption. Image noise control is obtained by dividing data into 21 subsets analyzed cyclically.

2.6. Image Analysis

This study enrolled consecutive n. 217 subjects, of whom n. 15 HS and n. 202 oncological patients that underwent PET/MRI scans (Figure 1). After screening criteria, n. 52 female subjects were retrospectively available for analysis; in detail, 37 were BC patients and 15 HS (Figure 1). BC primary lesions were classified according to the American Joint Committee on Cancer Disease (AJCC) [28]. BC histology was confirmed by immunohistochemistry (IHC) analysis only for few patients diagnosed. Quantitative analysis was performed using PMOD (Version 3.8; PMOD Technologies, Switzerland), which consists of a complete set of tools, able to extrapolate quantitative parameters from the image. After importing all the ^{18}F-FDG-PET/MRI examinations into the PMOD software, the breast lesion automatic segmentation was done on the PET image. A reference cut-off of 41% of the standardized uptake value maximum (SUVmax) and volume of interest (VOI) were reported also on MRI images. Axial T2, DWI, apparent diffusion coefficient (ADC) and post administration 3D VIBE sequence were analyzed. One representative patient case was shown in Figure 2. For all subjects, we considered the following parameters: VOI, SUVmax and standardized uptake value minimum (SUVmin), average, standard deviation (SD), number of pixels and hot average (mean of pixels that presents higher values) of SUV body-weighted (SUVbw) and of SUV lean body mass (SUVlbm). SUVbw was expressed like c(t)/(Injected dose/body weight), where c(t) is tissue radioactivity concentration at time t. While SUVlbm referred to the value of standardized lean body mass absorption. Some texture indices referred to the histogram pixel within a VOI, and others based on to the gray-level co-occurrence matrix (GLCM). This latter matrix is defined as the distribution of co-occurring pixel values (grayscale values, or colors) at a given offset. In this stud, texture indices were: GLCM contrast (measure of the contrast intensity between pixels and its close over the entire image); Statistic Energy (the sum of the squared elements in the GLCM); GLCM sum variance (heterogeneity measure on close pixels).

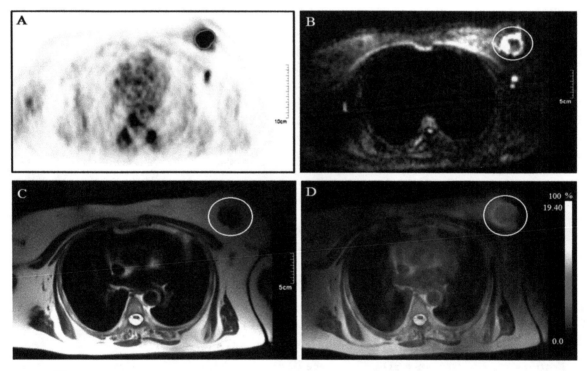

Figure 2. ^{18}F-FDG-PET/MRI scan Images of a 57-year-old patient with a breast heteroplasia with lymph node and bone metastases. The yellow circle indicates the lesion located on the left breast: (**A**) PET image showing uptake after 60 minutes of a segmented lesion (pink depicted); (**B**) Lesion revealed on T2 weighted image acquired on the axial plane; (**C**) hyperintensity of the lesion on diffusion-weighted magnetic resonance imaging; (**D**) ^{18}F-FDG-PET/MRI fusion image.

2.7. Statistical Analysis

Statistical analyses were performed using R environment (http://www.R-project.org). The distribution of biomedical imaging data (PET and MRI) was tested by Shapiro–Wilk test normality. The correlation between the statistical and textural parameters mostly used for breast lesions was evaluated using (Spearman's correlation test). In addition, the Wilcoxon–Mann–Whitney test was used to establish the statistical significance of molecular signature between the different BC groups and HS. To compare different hormone receptor subtypes, Kruskal–Wallis test was performed. For all tests a p value was considered for statistical significance when $p \leq 0.05$ and most significant when $p \leq 0.01$. Spearman's correlation was calculated to compare values of SUV max and YY1 levels.

3. Results

3.1. Study Population and Imaging Features

The mean age of all subject enrolled was 50 ± 4.6 years in HS compared to 53 ± 2.8 years in BC patients.

Moreover, within the metastatic BC cancer patients, we had patients with primary metastases (synchronous disease) and patients who developed metastases during follow-up (metachronous disease),.Thus, the cohort was divided in three groups: (i) "Healthy Subjects" (HS) ($n = 15$); (ii) "Synchronous Metastasis" (SM), which includes BC patients with one or multiple metastases at primary diagnosis ($n = 11$); and (iii) "Metachronous Metastasis" (MM), including BC patients who developed metastasis at follow up ($n = 26$). The metastasis were localized in bone ($n = 9$) and in different site, such as liver, uterus, lung, thyroid, and axillar and thoracic lymph nodes ($n = 17$).

Several features were extrapolated in order to investigate the sensitivity, specificity, and accuracy of ^{18}F-FDG-PET/MRI technique. By integration of high sensitivity of PET with the high spatial and temporal resolution of MRI we obtained information and characterized on the tumor malignancy (Figure 2) and detect small metastasis present in the body (Tumor Volume ≥ 1.2 cm^3 and GLCM_contrast_T2 ≥ 0.002). All features were related to the media pixel histogram within a VOI and to the GLCM, as highlighted by PET and MRI images as reported in Tables 2 and 3.

Table 2. Descriptive statistics of features extracted from PET images.

Synchronous Metastasis Group					
Features	**Mean ± SD**	**Median**	**Min**	**Max**	**Range**
Volume	9.54 ± 7.06	8.73	1.91	23.30	21.39
SUV_max	5.16 ± 4.19	3.78	1.33	13.24	11.91
n_voxels	721.86 ± 1247.68	247.00	54.00	3516.00	3462.00
Statistic_Energy	1.01 ± 0.01	0.01	0.01	0.01	0.00
GLCM_contrast	0.04 ± 0.03	0.03	0.00	0.09	0.09
Metachronous Metastasis Group					
Features	**Mean ± SD**	**Median**	**Min**	**Max**	**Range**
Volume	27.76 ± 40.35	7.21	2.86	122.19	119.33
SUV_max	5.26 ± 4.88	2.54	1.19	15.14	13.95
n_voxels	945.78 ± 1617.10	142.00	81.00	4998.00	4917.00
Statistic_Energy	1.01 ± 0.01	0.01	0.01	0.01	0.01
GLCM_contrast	0.03 ± 0.03	0.02	0.00	0.10	0.09

Table 3. Descriptive statistics of features extracted from MRI images.

Synchronous Metastasis Group					
Features	Mean ± SD	Median	Min	Max	Range
Volume	9.33 ± 6.40	8.73	1.56	23.30	21.75
T2_mean	8.72 ± 8.22	6.58	0.16	24.81	24.65
GLCM_contrast_T2	1.87 ± 2.45	0.03	0.00	7.39	7.39
GLCM_entropy_T2	1.87 ± 1.72	0.39	0.06	5.47	5.41
B_value	5.75 ± 4.71	4.42	0.02	14.54	14.52
ADC_mean	5.94 ± 5.06	5.29	0.82	16.23	15.40
GLCM_contrast_ADC	1.01 ± 0.02	0.02	0.00	0.07	0.06
GLCM_entropy_ADC	1.34 ± 0.06	0.37	0.25	0.40	0.15
Metachronous Metastasis Group					
Features	Mean ± SD	Median	Min	Max	Range
Volume	17.15 ± 22.04	5.02	2.86	54.53	51.67
T2_mean	5.16 ± 5.71	2.09	1.18	15.74	14.56
GLCM_contrast_T2	1.01 ± 0.03	0.01	0.00	0.09	0.08
GLCM_entropy_T2	1.35 ± 0.03	0.36	0.31	0.41	0.10
B_value	4.07 ± 4.14	1.88	1.44	11.58	10.14
ADC_mean	2.97 ± 2.94	1.53	0.45	8.50	8.04
GLCM_contrast_ADC	1.07 ± 0.15	0.01	0.00	0.41	0.40
GLCM_entropy_ADC	0.32 ± 0.13	0.37	0.04	0.38	0.34

3.2. YY1 Molecular Expression in Breast Cancer (BC) Patient

In order to analyze the expression level of YY1, from all patients PBMCs were recovered and total RNAs were extracted. Gene YY1 expression was evaluated in BC patients compared to control samples by real time RT-PCR. Same amount of YY1 has been shown in the MM group compared HS group. Conversely, in the SM group showed a 20-fold increase of YY1 mRNA compared with the HS group and 19-fold increase compared with the MM group ($p \leq 0.01$) using the non-parametric Wilcoxon test (Figure 3A). Moreover, the expression levels of YY1 (mRNA) were compared between MM and SM groups also considering the bone and no bone metastasis, respectively (Figure 3B). In contrast, YY1 protein level, dosed with ELISA assay, showed a significant increase in BC patients (MM and SM respectively, $p < 0.01$; $p < 0.01$). Differently from the expression trend, protein level of YY1 marker was higher into MM compared with HS group, although we did not know the underlying mechanism (Figure 4A,B).

Up-regulation of YY1 has been shown in estrogen receptor-positive (ER+) BCs [29] however, the regulatory mechanisms are still unknown. In our preliminary analysis, we also found YY1 overexpression in ER+ compared to ER- tumors, taking into account a total of $n = 15$ patients (see Table 1). Interestingly, we observed that YY1 mRNA specifically increased in (ER)-positive/- progesteron receptor-positive (PR+)/-human epidermal growth factor receptor2-negative (HER2-) (ER+/PR+/HER2-) compared to the "triple negative" (ER-/PR-/HER2-) and "triple positive" (ER+/PR+/HER2+) BC subtypes ($p = 0.27$, Kruskal-Wallis test) (Figure 5). Therefore, these data needs to be further elucidated, taking into account larger cohort including also different HER2+ and HER2- combinations such as ER-/PR-/HER2+, not diagnosed in our cases.

3.3. Correlation Between YY1 and FDG-PET/MRI in BC Patients

In order to select ^{18}F-FDG-PET/MRI parameters to correlate with YY1, first we evaluated the association between all imaging features by Spearman correlation test [30]. As shown in Figure 6, a significant positive correlation was observed between textural parameters: GLCM_contrast, SUVmin and SUVmax ($r = 0.8$; $r = 0.8$ respectively) (Table 2, Table 3 and Supplementary Materials Table S1) [30]. Subsequently, the Spearman test significantly correlated YY1 mRNA level (-ΔCt values) and

^{18}F-FDG-uptake (SUVmax) ($r = 0.48$) in SM patients with invasive BC cancer (Figure 7A,B). As reported in Figure 7B, pink color indicates that there was a negative correlation between YY1 expression reported as ΔCt values and ^{18}F-FDG-uptake. However, considering that small ΔCt values correspond to high gene expression, our preliminary results showed that YY1 mRNA expression and SUVmax reported the same trend (Figure 7B). Instead, no correlation was observed between YY1 protein and ^{18}F-FDG-PET/MRI parameters (data not shown). Overall, our study is the first attempts to evaluate the potential of combining imaging differences between SM and MM breast patient subgroups and YY1 gene expression, for a better diagnostic analysis of tumor metastasis (see Discussion).

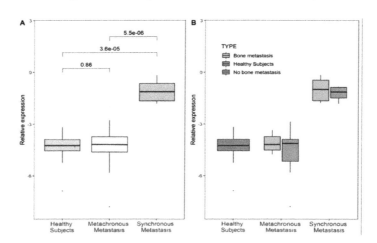

Figure 3. YY1 mRNA level and metastatic breast cancer. Expression level of YY1 in BC patients clustered into "Healthy Subjects" (HS), "Metachronous Metastasis" (MM) and "Synchronous Metastasis" (SM) group. (**A**) YY1 mRNA level in PBMCs from BC patients ($n = 11$ SM and $n = 26$ MM) and HS patients ($n = 15$). Data are reported as (-ΔCt). Each group was compared. (**B**) BC patients for SM and MM group were classified in two categories: no bone metastasis ($n = $ SM and $n = $ MM, respectively) and bone metastasis ($n = 5$ SM and $n = 17$ MM, respectively); the distribution did not show statistically significant difference between two categories included in each group. Statistical analysis was performed by the Wilcoxon test, and p value < 0.05 was considered significant.

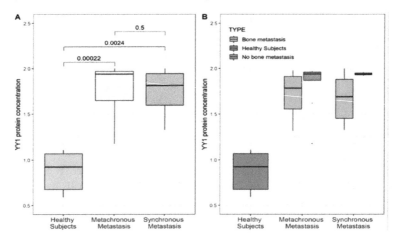

Figure 4. YY1 protein level and metastatic breast cancer. Serum protein level of YY1 in BC patients grouped as "Healthy Subjects" (HS), "Metachronous Metastasis" (MM) and "Synchronous Metastasis" (SM) group. (**A**) Comparison of YY1 protein level between BC patients ($n = 11$ SM and $n = 26$ MM) and HS patients ($n = 15$). Protein concentration is reported as ng/mL. Enzyme-linked immunosorbent assay (ELISA) YY1 protein level in BC patient sera indicated a media concentration of 1.8 ± 0.3 ng/ml in MM and 1.7 ± 0.3 ng/ml in SM patients compared to 0.8 ± 0.3 ng/ml in HS ($p < 0.01$; $p < 0.01$). (**B**) Comparison of YY1 protein level in SM and MM patients subgrouped as: no bone metastasis ($n = 5$ SM and $n = 17$ MM, respectively) and bone metastasis ($n = 5$ SM and $n = 17$ MM, respectively); Statistical significance was determined by Wilcoxon test, p value < 0.05 was considered significant.

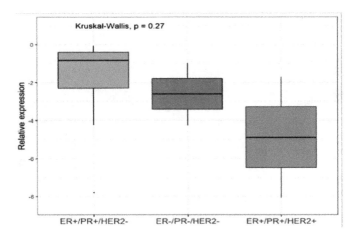

Figure 5. YY1 levels and receptor status in metastatic breast cancer. Comparison of YY1 mRNA level between estrogen receptor -positive/progesteron receptor-positive/human epidermal growth factor receptor2-negative (ER+/PR+/HER2-) compared to the "triple positive" (ER+/PR+/HER2+) and "triple negative" (ER-/PR-/HER2-) BC receptor status. Relative expression is reported as (-ΔCt). Statistical significance was determined by Kruskal-Wallis test, p value <0.05 was considered significant.

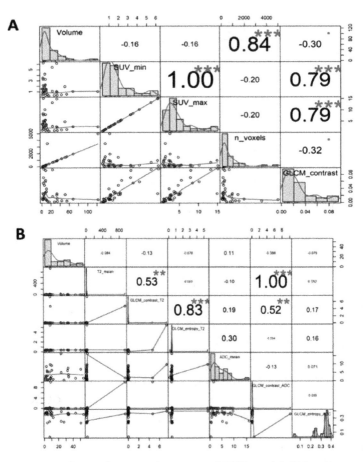

Figure 6. Correlation matrix for radiomics features of PET and MRI images. Correlation charts represent the correlation matrix between the statistical and textural parameters extracted from PET images (**A**) and MRI images (**B**) mostly used for breast lesions. The distribution of each variable is shown on the diagonal. On the bottom of the diagonal: the bivariate scatter plots with a fitted line are displayed. On the top of the diagonal: the value of the correlation plus the significance level as stars. Each significance level is associated to a symbol: p values 0.001; 0.01; 0.05; with symbols "***"; "**"; "*" respectively.

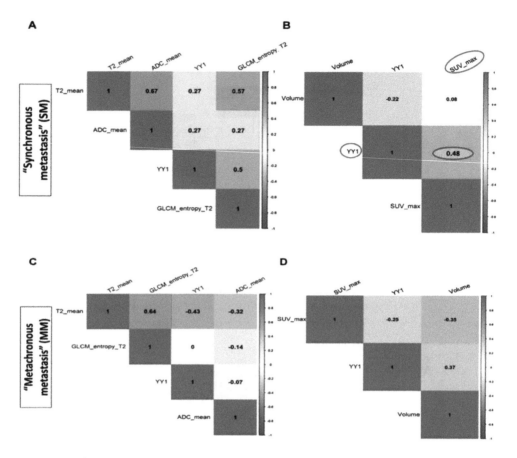

Figure 7. Radiomic features and YY1 molecular analysis. Correlation plot illustrates the Spearman test coefficient between YY1 expression level and PET/RMI parameters across "Synchronous Metatstasis" (SM) (**A,B**) and "Metachronous Metatstasis" (MM) BC patients (**C,D**). Color scale bar shows the positive correlation in blue and the negative correlation in pink; color intensity represents the strength of the correlation coefficient. Data indicated a statistical significant correlation between YY1mRNA and SUVmax in patients with SM ρ = 0.48. In the Supplementary Materials Table S1 are reported all analyzed findings for each patient at primary diagnosis.

4. Discussion and Conclusions

This preliminary study evaluated the feasibility of using diagnostic imaging and blood circulating level of YY1 as prospective tool to assess the presence of metastasis and tumor grade at diagnosis. The combination of imaging parameters and molecular biomarkers to improve the sensitive and specificity of primary tumor and metastatic lesions diagnosis it is of great interest for both better clinical decision-making and treatment management. To date, an accurate diagnosis of BC patients is difficult due to the tumor heterogeneity of clinical presentation and the co-presence of almost undetectable micro-metastasis. Moreover, based on the expression of hormone receptors in tumor tissues, approximately 70%–80% of BC is ER+ [31–34].

The multifunctional factor YY1 is overexpressed in many types of cancer, including BC [14,35–40] with potential clinical significance [6–10], although Lieberthal et al. reported that a decreased YY1 expression might contribute to the invasive phenotype of metastatic BC cells [19]. However, other authors also previously reported that the YY1 protein level is lower in BC tissue than in the normal breast tissues [29,41,42]. Clearly, more intensive studies are needed to clarify the role of YY1 and its molecular mechanism in BC. Our preliminary data indicated that YY1 transcript in PBMCs of BC subjects showed a significant increase in patients with metastasis at primary diagnosis than the "Healthy Subjects" group. We indicated this group as "Synchronous Metastasis". Interestingly, YY1 was particularly higher in patients BC with bone metastasis although not statistically significant.

In our analysis, we included SM patients with specific BC receptor status; indeed our cohort included about 80% of ER+ tumors, which reflects the recurrence of the majority of breast cancer. As well-known, hormone receptor status is crucial for medical decision-making since strongly related to hormone therapy response. Preliminary data indicated that YY1 might play an important role in ER+ compared to ER- tumors in according to other receptors. Prompted by Lieberthal et al. results on BC model cell lines [19] we evaluated YY1 mRNA level in PBMCs from patients stratified as ER/PR-positive tumors with respect to triple negative (ER-/PR-/HER2-) and triple positive receptor status (ER+/PR+/HER2+). In particular, we observed that YY1 mRNA specifically increased in hormone receptor positive BCs (ER+/PR+/HER2-) compared to the "triple positive" (ER+/PR+/HER2+) and "triple negative" (ER-/PR-/HER2-) subtypes although not statistically significant.

^{18}F-FDG-PET is the gold standard for in vivo evaluation of tumor glucose metabolism and ^{18}F-FDG uptake. In particular, post-contrast MR images were highly correlated to the molecular subtypes of BC, such as normal-like, luminal A and B, HER2-enriched, and basal-like [43]. Additionally, several radiomics features, such as GLCM textural features and SUVs are currently used to classify BC tumor grade [44–46]. In particular, SUVmax is common feature of ^{18}F-FDG-PET that potentially reflects the tumor biology, prognosis and response to treatment [44–46]. Here, we reported for the first time, a correlation of ^{18}F-FDG-PET parameters with YY1 molecular marker. We showed that SUVmax were statistically correlated with blood circulating YY1 mRNAs in a small number of BC patients ($r = 0.48$), suggesting that at higher tumor uptake correspond to high blood level of YY1 (mRNAs). In summary, our study attempts to include another layer of information, which is imaging "phenotype" to tumor metastasis diagnosis. However, imaging phenotype differences between the BC synchronous (SM) and metachronous metastasis (MM) groups, have been so far poorly investigated [47–49]. We assessed if the addition of imaging layer could contribute to better discriminate SM and MM BC subgroups in combination with YY1 gene expression.

Our results, showed a quite weak correlation between imaging and molecular features, although other information could be useful for further consideration. For instance, we found a positive correlation between YY1 expression (mRNA) and SUVmax for SM rather than MM subgroups. SUVmax is routinely used imaging diagnostic parameter [50]. In BC studies, it usually indicates the degree of tumor metabolism and hence can predict its behavior and prognosis [51].

In spite of our observations, the pathogenic role, the release mechanism and cell origin of circulating YY1 in blood remain unknown.

Furthermore, the present study has some limitations, which probably affected also our correlation analysis. It was a retrospective study performed at a single institution with a relatively small number of patients, and recurrence was documented in very few subjects. Moreover, we were unable to analyze overall survival because there were no disease-related deaths among the study population. In detail, in our study, the ROI segmentation was performed automatically. Maybe a manual segmentation could provide more accurate data. Furthermore, the knowledge of the tumor status for each patient would allow a potential correlation between YY1 with the invasiveness of BC. Surely, a larger number of subjects with the same characteristics could improve data sensitivity and specificity. In addition, the data could not be validated internally. Finally, an external validation of our findings would allow us to generalize the results and discriminate YY1 trend in all BC subtypes.

Nevertheless, although there are all the previous limitations and further multicenter studies are needed to confirm our results, all the preliminary data reported above are promising and suggest that a combined approach between different technologies for the clinical diagnosis of BC can provide more differentiated information related to the detection of metastases for treatment decision.

Author Contributions: Data curation, M.F., K.P. and F.d.N.; Formal analysis, A.S. and M.S.; Methodology, C.S.; Resources, C.N.; Software, M.F., K.P. and N.G.; Supervision, A.S., M.S. and C.N.; Validation, M.F., K.P. and F.d.N.; Writing—original draft, C.S.; Writing—review and editing, F.d.N. and C.N.

Acknowledgments: We thank Teresa Infante, for collaborating to initial sets of YY1 experiments.

Abbreviations

ADC	Apparent Diffusion Coefficient
BC	Breast cancer
DWI	Diffusion Weighted Imaging
ELISA	Enzyme-Linked Immunosorbent Assay
ER	Estrogen Receptor
^{18}F-FDG-PET/MRI	Fluorine-18-fluorodeoxyglucose Positron Emission Tomography/ Magnetic Risonance Imaging
GLCM	Gray Level Co-occurrence Matrix
HER2	Human Epidermal Growth Factor Receptor 2
HS	Healthy subjects
IHC	Immunohistochemistry
MM	Metachronous Metastasis
PBMCs	Peripheral blood mononuclear cells
PET/CT	Positron Emission Tomography/ Computed Tomography
PR	Progesteron Receptor
RT-PCR	Reverse Transcription Polymerase Chain Reaction
SM	Synchronous Metastasis
SUV	Standardized Uptake Value
VOI	Volume of interest
YY1	YY1 Transcription Factor

References

1. Schiano, C.; Soricelli, A.; De Nigris, F.; Napoli, C. New challenges in integrated diagnosis by imaging and osteo-immunology in bone lesions. *Expert Rev. Clin. Immunol.* **2018**, *15*, 289–301. [CrossRef] [PubMed]

2. Werner, M.K.; Schmidt, H.; Schwenzer, N.F. MR/PET: A New Challenge in Hybrid Imaging. *Am. J. Roentgenol.* **2012**, *199*, 272–277. [CrossRef] [PubMed]

3. Schlemmer, H.P.; Pichler, B.J.; Krieg, R.; Heiss, W.D. An integrated MR/PET system: prospective applications. *Abdom. Imaging* **2009**, *34*, 668–674. [CrossRef] [PubMed]

4. Alcantara, D.; Leal, M.P.; Garcia-Bocanegra, I.; Garcia-Martin, M.L.; García-Bocanegra, I.; García-Martín, M.L. Molecular imaging of breast cancer: present and future directions. *Front. Chem.* **2014**, *2*, 112. [CrossRef] [PubMed]

5. Nicholson, S.; Whitehouse, H.; Naidoo, K.; Byers, R. Yin Yang 1 in human cancer. *Crit. Rev. Oncog.* **2011**, *16*, 245–260. [CrossRef] [PubMed]

6. Zaravinos, A.; Spandidos, D.A. Yin Yang 1 expression in human tumors. *Cell Cycle* **2010**, *9*, 512–522. [CrossRef] [PubMed]

7. Zhang, Q.; Stovall, D.B.; Inoue, K.; Sui, G. The oncogenic role of Yin Yang 1. *Crit. Rev. Oncog.* **2011**, *16*, 163–197. [CrossRef]

8. Castellano, G.; Torrisi, E.; Ligresti, G.; Malaponte, G.; McCubrey, J.A.; Nicoletti, F.; Travali, S.; Canevari, S.; Libra, M. Yin Yang 1 overexpression in diffuse large B-cell lymphoma is associated with B-cell transformation and tumor progression. *Cell Cycle* **2010**, *9*, 557–563. [CrossRef]

9. Baritaki, S.; Huerta-Yepez, S.; Sakai, T.; Spandidos, D.A.; Bonavida, B. Chemotherapeutic drugs sensitize cancer cells to TRAIL-mediated apoptosis: up-regulation of DR5 and inhibition of Yin Yang 1. *Mol. Cancer Ther.* **2007**, *6*, 1387–1399. [CrossRef]

10. De Nigris, F.; Zanella, L.; Cacciatore, F.; De Chiara, A.; Fazioli, F.; Chiappetta, G.; Apice, G.; Infante, T.; Monaco, M.; Rossiello, R.; et al. YY1 overexpression is associated with poor prognosis and metastasis-free survival in patients suffering osteosarcoma. *BMC Cancer* **2011**, *11*, 472. [CrossRef]

11. Seligson, D.; Horvath, S.; Huerta-Yepez, S.; Hanna, S.; Garban, H.; Roberts, A.; Shi, T.; Liu, X.; Chia, D.; Goodglick, L.; et al. Expression of transcription factor Yin Yang 1 in prostate cancer. *Int. J. Oncol.* **2005**, *27*, 131–141. [CrossRef]

12. De Nigris, F.; Rossiello, R.; Schiano, C.; Arra, C.; Williams-Ignarro, S.; Barbieri, A.; Lanza, A.; Balestrieri, A.; Giuliano, M.T.; Ignarro, L.J.; et al. Deletion of Yin Yang 1 protein in osteosarcoma cells on cell invasion and CXCR4/angiogenesis and metastasis. *Cancer Res.* **2008**, *68*, 1797–1808. [CrossRef]

13. De Nigris, F.; Botti, C.; de Chiara, A.; Rossiello, R.; Apice, G.; Fazioli, F.; Fiorito, C.; Sica, V.; Napoli, C. Expression of transcription factor Yin Yang 1 in human osteosarcomas. *Eur. J. Cancer* **2006**, *42*, 2420–2424. [CrossRef]

14. Chinnappan, D.; Ratnasari, A.; Andry, C.; King, T.C.; Xiao, D.; Weber, H.C. Transcription factor YY1 expression in human gastrointestinal cancer cells. *Int. J. Oncol.* **2009**, *34*, 1417–1423. [PubMed]

15. Allouche, A.; Nolens, G.; Tancredi, A.; Delacroix, L.; Mardaga, J.; Fridman, V.; Winkler, R.; Boniver, J.; Delvenne, P.; Begon, D.Y. The combined immunodetection of AP-2alpha and YY1 transcription factors is associated with ERBB2 gene overexpression in primary breast tumors. *Breast Cancer Res.* **2008**, *10*, R9. [CrossRef]

16. Begon, D.Y.; Delacroix, L.; Vernimmen, D.; Jackers, P.; Winkler, R. Yin Yang 1 Cooperates with Activator Protein 2 to StimulateERBB2Gene Expression in Mammary Cancer Cells. *J. Biol. Chem.* **2005**, *280*, 24428–24434. [CrossRef] [PubMed]

17. Wu, F.; Lee, A.S. YY1 as a regulator of replication-dependent hamster histone H3.2 promoter and an interactive partner of AP-2. *J. Biol. Chem.* **2001**, *276*, 28–34. [CrossRef]

18. Thomassen, M.; Tan, Q.; Kruse, T.A. Gene expression meta-analysis identifies metastatic pathways and transcription factors in breast cancer. *BMC Cancer* **2008**, *8*, 394. [CrossRef]

19. Lieberthal, J.G.; Kaminsky, M.; Parkhurst, C.N.; Tanese, N. The role of YY1 in reduced HP1alpha gene expression in invasive human breast cancer cells. *Breast Cancer Res.* **2009**, *11*, 42. [CrossRef]

20. Shen, X.; Zhong, J.; Yu, P.; Zhao, Q.; Huang, T. YY1-regulated LINC00152 promotes triple negative breast cancer progression by affecting on stability of PTEN protein. *Biochem. Biophys. Res. Commun.* **2019**, *509*, 448–454. [CrossRef]

21. Hoefnagel, L.D.; Moelans, C.B.; Meijer, S.L.; van Slooten, H.J.; Wesseling, P.; Wesseling, J.; Westenend, P.J.; Bart, J.; Seldenrijk, C.A.; Nagtegaal, I.D.; et al. Prognostic value of estrogen receptor alpha and progesterone receptor conversion in distant breast cancer metastases. *Cancer* **2012**, *118*, 4929–4935. [CrossRef]

22. American Joint Committee on Cancer. *Breast Cancer Staging*, 7th ed.; American Joint Committee on Cancer: Chicago, IL, USA, 2009.

23. Rienzo, M.; Schiano, C.; Casamassimi, A.; Grimaldi, V.; Infante, T.; Napoli, C. Identification of valid reference housekeeping genes for gene expression analysis in tumor neovascularization studies. *Clin. Transl. Oncol.* **2013**, *15*, 211–218. [CrossRef]

24. Mirabelli, P.; Incoronato, M.; Coppola, L.; Infante, T.; Parente, C.A.; Nicolai, E.; Soricelli, A.; Salvatore, M. SDN Biobank: Bioresource of Human Samples Associated with Functional and/or Morphological Bioimaging Results for the Study of Oncological, Cardiological, Neurological, and Metabolic Diseases. *Open J. Bioresour.* **2017**, *4*, 356. [CrossRef]

25. Daye, D.; Signore, A.; Iannace, C.; Vangel, M.; Luongo, A.; Filomena, M.; Mansi, L.; Salvatore, M.; Fuin, N.; Catana, C.; et al. Staging performance of whole-body DWI, PET/CT and PET/MRI in invasive ductal carcinoma of the breast. *Int. J. Oncol.* **2017**, *51*, 281–288.

26. Pace, L.; Nicolai, E.; Luongo, A.; Aiello, M.; Catalano, O.A.; Soricelli, A.; Salvatore, M. Comparison of whole-body PET/CT and PET/MRI in breast cancer patients: Lesion detection and quantitation of 18F-deoxyglucose uptake in lesions and in normal organ tissues. *Eur. J. Radiol.* **2014**, *83*, 289–296. [CrossRef]

27. Catalano, O.A.; Nicolai, E.; Rosen, B.R.; Luongo, A.; Catalano, M.; Iannace, C.; Guimarães, A.; Vangel, M.G.; Mahmood, U.; Soricelli, A.; et al. Comparison of CE-FDG-PET/CT with CE-FDG-PET/MR in the evaluation of osseous metastases in breast cancer patients. *Br. J. Cancer* **2015**, *112*, 1452–1460. [CrossRef]

28. Ehinger, A.; Malmström, P.; Bendahl, P.O.; Elston, C.W.; Falck, A.K.; Forsare, C.; Grabau, D.; Rydén, L.; Stål, O.; Fernö, M.; et al. Histological grade provides significant prognostic information in addition to breast cancer subtypes defined according to St Gallen 2013. *Acta Oncol.* **2017**, *56*, 68–74. [CrossRef]

29. Lee, M.H.; Lahusen, T.; Wang, R.H.; Xiao, C.; Xu, X.; Hwang, Y.S.; He, W.W.; Shi, Y.; Deng, C.X. Yin Yang 1 positively regulates BRCA1 and inhibits mammary cancer formation. *Oncogene* **2012**, *31*, 116–127. [CrossRef]

30. Groheux, D.; Giacchetti, S.; Moretti, J.L.; Porcher, R.; Espié, M.; Lehmann-Che, J.; de Roquancourt, A.; Hamy, A.S.; Cuvier, C.; Vercellino, L.; et al. Correlation of high 18F-FDG uptake to clinical, pathological and biological prognostic factors in breast cancer. *Eur. J. Nucl. Med. Mol. Imaging* **2011**, *38*, 426–435. [CrossRef]

31. Wang, M.Y.; Huang, H.Y.; Kuo, Y.L.; Lo, C.; Sun, H.Y.; Lyu, Y.J.; Chen, B.R.; Li, J.N.; Chen, P.S. TARBP2-Enhanced Resistance during Tamoxifen Treatment in Breast Cancer. *Cancers* **2019**, *11*, 210. [CrossRef]

32. Bray, F.; Ferlay, J.; Soerjomataram, I.; Siegel, R.L.; Torre, L.A.; Jemal, A. Global cancer statistics 2018: GLOBOCAN estimates of incidence and mortality worldwide for 36 cancers in 185 countries. *CA Cancer J. Clin.* **2018**, *68*, 394–424. [CrossRef]

33. Perou, C.M.; Sørlie, T.; Eisen, M.B.; Van De Rijn, M.; Jeffrey, S.S.; Rees, C.A.; Pollack, J.R.; Ross, D.T.;

Johnsen, H.; Akslen, L.A.; et al. Molecular portraits of human breast tumours. *Nature* **2000**, *406*, 747–752. [CrossRef]

34. Howlader, N.; Altekruse, S.F.; Li, C.I.; Chen, V.W.; Clarke, C.A.; Ries, L.A.G.; Cronin, K.A. US Incidence of Breast Cancer Subtypes Defined by Joint Hormone Receptor and HER2 Status. *J. Natl. Cancer Inst.* **2014**, *106*. [CrossRef]

35. Wan, M.; Huang, W.; Kute, T.E.; Miller, L.D.; Zhang, Q.; Hatcher, H.; Wang, J.; Stovall, D.B.; Russell, G.B.; Cao, P.D.; et al. Yin Yang 1 plays an essential role in breast cancer and negatively regulates p27. *Am. J. Pathol.* **2012**, *180*, 2120–2133. [CrossRef]

36. Wang, A.M.; Huang, T.T.; Hsu, K.W.; Huang, K.H.; Fang, W.L.; Yang, M.H.; Lo, S.S.; Chi, C.W.; Lin, J.J.; Yeh, T.S. Yin Yang 1 is a target of microRNA-34 family and contributes to gastric carcinogenesis. *Oncotarget* **2014**, *5*, 5002–5016. [CrossRef]

37. Kang, W.; Tong, J.H.; Chan, A.W.; Zhao, J.; Dong, Y.; Wang, S.; Yang, W.; Mc Sin, F.; Ng, S.S.; Yu, J.; et al. Yin Yang 1 contributes to gastric carcinogenesis and its nuclear expression correlates with shorter survival in patients with early stage gastric adenocarcinoma. *J. Transl. Med.* **2014**, *12*, 80. [CrossRef]

38. Bonavida, B.; Kaufhold, S. Prognostic significance of YY1 protein expression and mRNA levels by bioinformatics analysis in human cancers: A therapeutic target. *Pharmacol. Ther.* **2015**, *150*, 149–168. [CrossRef]

39. Shi, J.; Hao, A.; Zhang, Q.; Sui, G. The role of YY1 in oncogenesis and its potential as a drug target in cancer therapies. *Curr. Cancer Drug Targets* **2015**, *15*, 145–157. [CrossRef]

40. Yang, W.; Feng, B.; Meng, Y.; Wang, J.; Geng, B.; Cui, Q.; Zhang, H.; Yang, Y.; Yang, J. FAM3C-YY1 axis is essential for TGFβ-promoted proliferation and migration of human breast cancer MDA-MB-231 cells via the activation of HSF1. *J. Cell. Mol. Med.* **2019**, *23*, 3464–3475. [CrossRef]

41. Zhang, Z.; Zhu, Y.; Wang, Z.; Zhang, T.; Wu, P.; Huang, J. Yin-yang effect of tumor infiltrating B cells in breast cancer: From mechanism to immunotherapy. *Cancer Lett.* **2017**, *393*, 1–7. [CrossRef]

42. Powe, D.G.; Akhtar, G.; Habashy, H.O.; Abdel-Fatah, T.M.; Rakha, E.A.; Green, A.R.; O Ellis, I. Investigating AP-2 and YY1 protein expression as a cause of high HER2 gene transcription in breast cancers with discordant HER2 gene amplification. *Breast Cancer Res.* **2009**, *11*, R90. [CrossRef]

43. Li, H.; Zhu, Y.; Burnside, E.S.; Huang, E.; Drukker, K.; Hoadley, K.A.; Fan, C.; Conzen, S.D.; Zuley, M.; Net, J.M.; et al. Quantitative MRI radiomics in the prediction of molecular classifications of breast cancer subtypes in the TCGA/TCIA data set. *NPJ Breast Cancer* **2016**, *2*, 16012. [CrossRef]

44. Grueneisen, J.; Sawicki, L.M.; Wetter, A.; Kirchner, J.; Kinner, S.; Aktas, B.; Forsting, M.; Ruhlmann, V.; Umutlu, L. Evaluation of PET and MR datasets in integrated ^{18}F-FDG PET/MRI: A comparison of different MR sequences for whole-body restaging of breast cancer patients. *Eur. J. Radiol.* **2017**, *89*, 14–19. [CrossRef]

45. Rahim, M.K.; Kim, S.E.; So, H.; Kim, H.J.; Cheon, G.J.; Lee, E.S.; Kang, K.W.; Lee, D.S. Recent Trends in PET Image Interpretations Using Volumetric and Texture-based Quantification Methods in Nuclear Oncology. *Nucl. Med. Mol. Imaging* **2014**, *48*, 1–15. [CrossRef]

46. Chang, C.C.; Cho, S.F.; Chen, Y.W.; Tu, H.P.; Lin, C.Y.; Chang, C.S. SUV on Dual-Phase FDG PET/CT Correlates With the Ki-67 Proliferation Index in Patients With Newly Diagnosed Non-Hodgkin Lymphoma. *Clin. Nucl. Med.* **2012**, *37*, e189–e195. [CrossRef]

47. Güth, U.; Magaton, I.; Huang, D.J.; Fisher, R.; Schötzau, A.; Vetter, M. Primary and secondary distant metastatic breast cancer: Two sides of the same coin. *Breast* **2014**, *23*, 26–32. [CrossRef]

48. Gerratana, L.; Fanotto, V.; Bonotto, M.; Bolzonello, S.; Minisini, A.M.; Fasola, G.; Puglisi, F. Pattern of metastasis and outcome in patients with breast cancer. *Clin. Exp. Metastasis* **2015**, *32*, 125–133. [CrossRef]

49. Kast, K.; Link, T.; Friedrich, K.; Petzold, A.; Niedostatek, A.; Schoffer, O.; Werner, C.; Klug, S.J.; Werner, A.; Gatzweiler, A.; et al. Impact of breast cancer subtypes and patterns of metastasis on outcome. *Breast Cancer Res. Treat.* **2015**, *150*, 621–629. [CrossRef]

50. Bailly, C.; Bodet-Milin, C.; Bourgeois, M.; Gouard, S.; Ansquer, C.; Barbaud, M.; Sébille, J.C.; Chérel, M.; Kraeber-Bodéré, F.; Carlier, T. Exploring Tumor Heterogeneity Using PET Imaging: The Big Picture. *Cancers* **2019**, *11*, 1282. [CrossRef]

51. Jain, A.; Dubey, I.; Chauhan, M.; Kumar, R.; Agarwal, S.; Kishore, B.; Vishnoi, M.; Paliwal, D.; John, A.; Kumar, N.; et al. Tumor characteristics and metabolic quantification in carcinoma breast: An institutional experience. *Indian J. Cancer* **2017**, *54*, 333. [CrossRef]

11

In Vivo Assessment of VCAM-1 Expression by SPECT/CT Imaging in Mice Models of Human Triple Negative Breast Cancer

Christopher Montemagno [1], Laurent Dumas [1,2], Pierre Cavaillès [3], Mitra Ahmadi [1], Sandrine Bacot [1], Marlène Debiossat [1], Audrey Soubies [1], Loic Djaïleb [1], Julien Leenhardt [1], Nicolas De Leiris [1], Maeva Dufies [4], Gilles Pagès [4,5], Sophie Hernot [6], Nick Devoogdt [6], Pascale Perret [1], Laurent Riou [1], Daniel Fagret [1], Catherine Ghezzi [1,†] and Alexis Broisat [1,*,†]

[1] Laboratory of Bioclinical Radiopharmaceutics, Universite Grenoble Alpes, Inserm, CHU Grenoble Alpes, LRB, 38000 Grenoble, France
[2] Advanced Accelator Applications, 01630 Saint-Genis-Pouilly, France
[3] Natural Barriers and Infectiosity, Universite Grenoble Alpes, CNRS, CHU Grenoble Alpes, TIMC-IMAG, 38000 Grenoble, France
[4] Biomedical Department, Centre Scientifique de Monaco, 980000 Monaco, Monaco
[5] Institute for Research on Cancer and Aging of Nice, Universite Cote d'Azur, CNRS UMR 7284, INSERM U1081, Centre Antoine Lacassagne, 061489 Nice, France
[6] Laboratory of In Vivo Cellular and Molecular Imaging, ICMI-BEFY, Vrije Universiteit Brussel, Laarbeeklan 103, B-1090 Brussels, Belgium
*   Correspondence: alexis.broisat@inserm.fr
†   Contributed equally to this work.

Abstract: Recent progress in breast cancer research has led to the identification of Vascular Cell Adhesion Molecule-1 (VCAM-1) as a key actor of metastatic colonization. VCAM-1 promotes lung-metastases and is associated with clinical early recurrence and poor outcome in triple negative breast cancer (TNBC). Our objective was to perform the in vivo imaging of VCAM-1 in mice models of TNBC. The Cancer Genomic Atlas (TCGA) database was analyzed to evaluate the prognostic role of VCAM-1 in TNBC. MDA-MB-231 (VCAM-1+) and control HCC70 (VCAM-1-) TNBC cells were subcutaneously xenografted in mice and VCAM-1 expression was assessed in vivo by single-photon emission computed tomography (SPECT) imaging using ^{99m}Tc-cAbVCAM1-5. Then, MDA-MB-231 cells were intravenously injected in mice and VCAM-1 expression in lung metastasis was assessed by SPECT imaging after 8 weeks. TCGA analysis showed that VCAM-1 is associated with a poor prognosis in TNBC patients. In subcutaneous tumor models, ^{99m}Tc-cAbVCAM1-5 uptake was 2-fold higher in MDA-MB-231 than in HCC70 ($p < 0.01$), and 4-fold higher than that of the irrelevant control ($p < 0.01$). Moreover, ^{99m}Tc-cAbVCAM1-5 uptake in MDA-MB-231 lung metastases was also higher than that of ^{99m}Tc-Ctl ($p < 0.05$). ^{99m}Tc-cAbVCAM1-5 is therefore a suitable tool to evaluate the role of VCAM-1 as a marker of tumor aggressiveness of TNBC.

Keywords: triple negative breast cancer; VCAM-1; SPECT imaging; sdAbs

1. Introduction

Breast cancer (BC) is the most common female malignancy, accounting for more than 30% of all malignant tumors in women [1]. Breast cancer is a heterogeneous disease consisting of various subtypes with distinct molecular and pathological profiles [2,3]. Triple Negative Breast Cancer (TNBC) subtypes represent 10% to 20% of BC and are characterized by the lack of progesterone receptor, estrogen receptor and human epidermal growth factor receptor 2 expression [4]. TNBC are mostly associated with poor clinical outcome and high rate of metastasis and relapse following treatment [5,6]. Lung, bones, brain and liver are the most common sites of distant metastasis. Despite intense clinical research efforts, only limited advances have been obtained in the management of BC metastases.

Recent studies have led to the identification of new genes and mechanisms that mediate metastatic colonization [7]. Among them, Vascular Cell Adhesion Molecule-1 (VCAM-1) plays a key role in BC progression and metastatic processes [8,9]. VCAM-1 belongs to the immunoglobulin super family group of adhesion molecules. It is a 110 kDa glycoprotein mainly expressed at the endothelial cells surface during inflammation, but also by macrophages and dendritic cells [10]. The ability of VCAM-1 expressed by endothelial cells to bind tumor cells suggest that it could contribute to metastatic spread. Indeed, VCAM-1 expression on endothelial cells plays a key role in angiogenesis, in tumor cell transmigration, and therefore promotes tumor development and dissemination of tumor cells [11].

In the last few years, a growing interest into VCAM-1 expression on tumor cells has emerged. In BC, the overexpression of VCAM-1 on tumor cells correlates with early relapse and poor patient outcome [12,13]. The direct interaction of VCAM-1 with its ligand Very-Late Antigen -4 (VLA-4) expressed on leukocytes allows tumor cell survival in lungs and consequently lung metastasis [14]. Moreover, VCAM-1 is involved in the transition from dormant micro-metastases to overt macro-metastases in bones, a turning point in BC progression [13,15]. Inhibition of the VCAM-1 and VLA-4 interaction impairs bone metastasis progression and lung colonization [13,14,16]. VCAM-1 is also involved into chemoresistance and tumor immune escape [17–19]. Therefore, VCAM-1 is a key player with multiple functionalities in directing the metastatic spread. VCAM-1 expression could be induced by pro-inflammatory cytokines, such as Tumor Necrosis Factor-α (TNF-α), IL-1 or IL-6, major mediators of tumor progression [19].

To assess the role of VCAM-1 in the metastatic phenotype of BC, nuclear imaging may represent a powerful tool. We recently developed a single domain antibody (sdAb)-based radiotracer targeting VCAM-1 called [99m]Technetium-cAbVCAM1-5 (^{99m}Tc-cAbVCAM1-5), which is ongoing clinical transfer for detection of inflamed atherosclerosis lesions [20,21]. The aim of the present study was to assess VCAM-1 expression using ^{99m}Tc-cAbVCAM1-5 in subcutaneous and lung metastasis mice models of TNBC.

2. Results

2.1. VCAM-1 Is Overexpressed in TNBC and Associated with Decreased OS

980 breast cancer patients of The Cancer Genomic Atlas (TCGA) were analyzed for VCAM-1 mRNA levels and subsequent overall survival (OS) follow-up (Figure 1). VCAM-1 expression was higher in TNBC ($n = 114$) as compared to non-TNBC patients ($n = 866$) ($p < 0.001$, Figure 1A). High VCAM-1 expression was associated with decreased OS in TNBC but not in non-TNBC patients (respectively $p = 0.035$ and $p = 0.6886$, Figure 1B,C). TNF-α mRNA expression is overexpressed in TNBC as compared to non-TNBC patients ($p < 0.001$, Figure 1A).

2.2. MDA-MB-231 Cells Overexpress VCAM-1 mRNA and Protein

The expression of VCAM-1 was first assessed on two TNBC cell lines. VCAM-1 mRNA levels were undetectable at the basal level or following TNF-α stimulation in HCC70 cells. However, MDA-MB-231 cells expressed VCAM-1 mRNA basal levels. They were induced by a 3.5-fold upon TNF-α stimulation (1.0 ± 0.1 vs. 3.5 ± 1.3, $p < 0.05$, Figure 2A). Consistently, VCAM-1 protein was undetectable in HCC70 cells whereas MDA-MB-231 expressed basal VCAM-1 protein levels and TNF-α induced a 3.5-fold increase of these basal levels (Figure 2B,C, Figure S1).

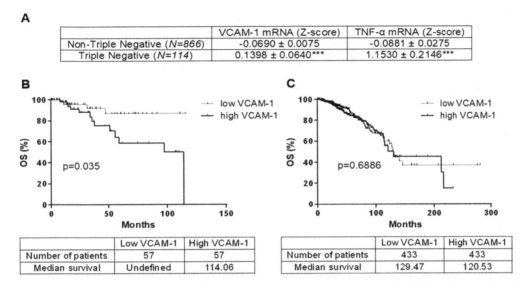

Figure 1. VCAM-1 is overexpressed in Triple-Negative Breast Cancer (TNBC) and associated with a decrease of overall survival. (**A**) Expression of VCAM-1 and TNF-α in TNBC and Non-TNBC were compared in TCGA datasets for breast cancer. Values represent the z scores for $\log_2$-transformed normalized RNA-seq read counts. (**B,C**) Kaplan-Meier analysis of OS of TNBC (**B**) and Non-TNBC (**C**) patients. OS (months) were calculated from patient subgroups with VCAM-1 mRNA levels that were less or greater than the median value. Statistical significance (*p*-value) is indicated. *** $p < 0.001$. Nb: Number.

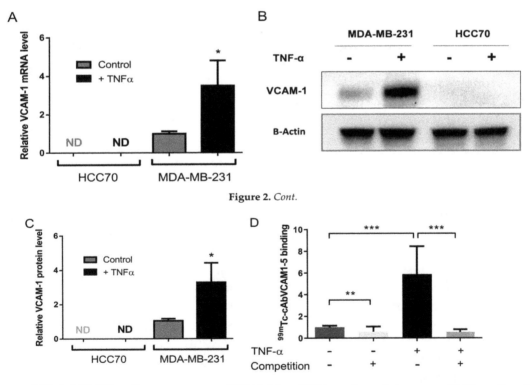

Figure 2. *Cont.*

Figure 2. MDA-MB-231 cells overexpress VCAM-1 mRNA and protein upon TNF-α stimulation. MDA-MB-231 and HCC70 cells were treated or not for 18 h with TNF-α (50 ng/mL) and VCAM-1 expression was assessed by RT-qPCR (**A**) and WB (**B**). (**C**) Bands of WB were quantified using ImageJ software. (**D**) ^{99m}Tc-AbVCAM1-5 binding was performed on MDA-MB-231 cells stimulated or not with TNF-α, in the presence or absence of a 100-fold excess of unlabeled cAbVCAM1-5. Unspecific binding was estimated by ^{99m}Tc-AbVCAM1-5 incubation on HCC70 cells. Results are expressed in fold-change vs. untreated and unstimulated MDA-MB-231 $N = 6$ per condition. * $p < 0.05$; ** $p < 0.01$; *** $p < 0.001$; ND, not detected.

2.3. ^{99m}Tc-cAbVCAM1-5 Binds Specifically to VCAM-1 Expressing TNBC Cells

Unlabeled cAbVCAM1-5 bound to VCAM-1-positive MDA-MB-231 but not to VCAM-1-negative HCC70 cells (Figure S2). ^{99m}Tc-cAbVCAM1-5 affinity was evaluated on both mouse and human recombinant protein and found to be in the nanomolar range scale (Kd = 12.5 ± 3.6 nM for mVCAM-1 and 36.3 ± 7.0 nM for hVCAM-1) (Figure S3). To further demonstrate the specificity of the binding on MDA-MB-231 cells, in vitro competition studies were then performed to determine the ability of the radiolabeled ^{99m}Tc-cAbVCAM1-5 to bind specifically to MDA-MB-231 (Figure 2D). ^{99m}Tc-cAbVCAM1-5 binding to TNF- α stimulated cells was 5-fold higher than to unstimulated cells (5.8 ± 2.6 vs. 1.0 ± 0.2, respectively, $p < 0.001$). Moreover, the addition of an excess of unlabeled cAbVCAM1-5 significantly decreased ^{99m}Tc-cAbVCAM1-5 binding on unstimulated and on stimulated MDA-MB-231 cells by 42% ($p < 0.01$) and 90% ($p < 0.001$), respectively. These results demonstrated that ^{99m}Tc-cAbVCAM1-5 binds specifically to VCAM-1 expressing cells.

2.4. SPECT/CT Imaging of VCAM-1 in Subcutaneous Tumor Model

^{99m}Tc-cAbVCAM1-5 potential to perform in vivo imaging of VCAM-1-expressing tumors was then evaluated. Whole-body SPECT/CT images of mice subcutaneously implanted with MDA-MB-231 and HCC70 tumors are presented in Figure 3A and in Figure S4. ^{99m}Tc-cAbVCAM1-5 uptake was readily detectable in MDA-MB-231 tumors, whereas a weak signal was detectable from HCC70 tumor and from MDA-MB-231 or HCC70 tumors using the irrelevant ^{99m}Tc-Ctl (Figure 3A). Quantification of SPECT images confirmed that ^{99m}Tc-cAbVCAM1-5 uptake in MDA-MB-231 tumors (1.7 ± 0.5% ID/cm^3) was significantly higher than in HCC70 tumors (0.9 ± 0.2% ID/cm^3, $p < 0.01$), whereas ^{99m}Tc-Ctl uptake was similar in HCC70 and in MDA-MB-231 tumors (0.6 ± 0.1 vs. 0.6 ± 0.2% ID/cm^3, respectively) (Figure 3B) and significantly lower than ^{99m}Tc-cAbVCAM1-5 tumor uptake in MDA-MB-231 ($p < 0.01$) and HCC70 tumors ($p < 0.05$). The biodistribution of ^{99m}Tc-cAbVCAM1-5 and ^{99m}Tc-Ctl determined ex vivo by gamma-well counting was in accordance with that obtained following SPECT image quantification, thereby demonstrating the accuracy of the method (Figure 3C and Figure S5). Specific ^{99m}Tc-cAbVCAM1-5 uptake in lymphoid organs was observed which was consistent with VCAM-1 expression (Table S1).

2.5. Ex Vivo Assessment of VCAM-1 Expression in Subcutaneous Tumors

Since VCAM-1 is also involved in inflammatory and angiogenic processes, we next determined which part of its expression was attributable to tumor cells (human VCAM-1), or to the inflammatory and endothelial cells (mouse VCAM-1) using RT-qPCR (Figure 4). Consistently with in vitro results, hVCAM-1 mRNA was expressed by MDA-MD-231 but was not detectable in HCC70 tumors. Moreover, hVCAM-1 expression was nearly 4-fold higher than that of mVCAM-1 in MDA-MB-231 xenograft tumors ($p < 0.001$), suggesting that the hVCAM-1 expression by tumor cells was the predominant form present in MDA-MB-231 subcutaneous xenografts. Interestingly, no significant difference was observed in mVCAM-1 mRNA expression between HCC70 and MDA-MB-231 tumors (1.6 ± 1.0 vs. 1.0 ± 0.1). This results strongly suggests that the signal obtained on SPECT/CT images reflects VCAM-1-expressing tumor cells.

2.6. SPECT/CT Imaging of VCAM-1 in an Experimental Metastasis Model

Because VCAM-1 is involved in lung colonization we next investigated the ability of ^{99m}Tc-cAbVCAM1-5 to perform its imaging in an experimental metastasis model. Representative SPECT/CT images are presented in Figure 5A and in Figure S6.

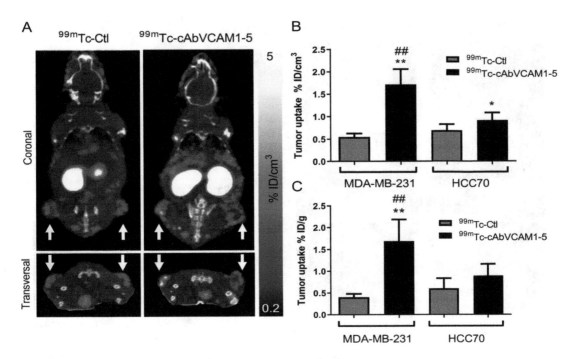

Figure 3. In vivo biodistribution of ^{99m}Tc-cAbVCAM1-5 in mice bearing HCC70 and MDA-MB-231 tumor xenografts. (**A**) Representative coronal and transversal views of fused SPECT/CT images of HCC70 (right hind limb, white arrow) and MDA-MB-231 (left hind limb, yellow arrow) tumor-bearing mice at 1 h after i.v injection of ^{99m}Tc-cAbVCA1M-5 or ^{99m}Tc-Ctl. (**B**) In vivo quantification of ^{99m}Tc-cAbVCAM1-5 and ^{99m}Tc-Ctl tumor uptake from SPECT images. (**C**) Ex vivo quantification of ^{99m}Tc-cAbVCAM1-5 and ^{99m}Tc-Ctl tumor uptake from post-mortem biodistribution studies. Results were expressed as % ID/cm^3 (imaging) and % ID/g (ex vivo) of tumor. Statistics: * $p < 0.05$, ** $p < 0.01$ vs. ^{99m}Tc-Ctl; ## $p < 0.01$ vs. HCC70.

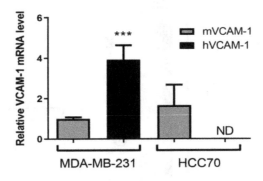

Figure 4. Ex vivo assessment of VCAM-1 expression by RT-qPCR. 50 mg of MDA-MB-231 and HCC70 xenografts were harvested and tested for human and mice VCAM-1 expression by RT-qPCR. *** $p < 0.001$ vs. MDA-MB-231 mVCAM-1.

^{99m}Tc-cAbVCAM1-5 lung uptake was readily observable, whereas a weak signal was obtained with ^{99m}Tc-Ctl (Figure 5A). Quantification of SPECT/CT images confirmed that the lung uptake was 2.5-fold higher with ^{99m}Tc-cAbVCAM1-5 than ^{99m}Tc-Ctl (1.7 ± 0.4 vs. 0.7 ± 0.1% ID/cm^3, $p < 0.05$, Figure 5B). When performing image quantification of pulmonary activity, the volume of interest contains a mixture of tissue and air, thereby leading to an underestimation of the uptake. ^{99m}Tc-cAbVCAM1-5 lung uptake was therefore further evaluated using ex vivo gamma-well counting (Figure 5C) and autoradiography (Figure 6A,B). Using these two technics, ^{99m}Tc-cAbVCAM1-5 uptake was found to represent ~3% ID/g and 4–5 fold-higher value than that obtained with ^{99m}Tc- Ctl ($p < 0.05$ for both technics). ^{99m}Tc-cAbVCAM1-5 uptake was also evaluated in lung-metastasis free mice and found to be 3-fold lower than lung-metastasis bearing mice ($p < 0.05$, Figure S7).

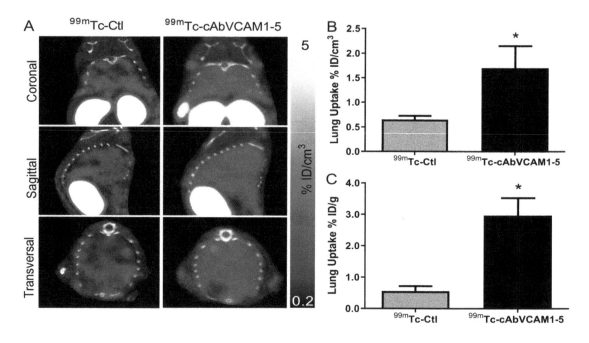

Figure 5. In vivo biodistribution of ^{99m}Tc-cAbVCAM1-5 in a pulmonary experimental metastasis model. (**A**) Representative coronal and transversal views of fused SPECT/CT images of MDA-MB-231 lung metastases at 1 h after i.v. injection of ^{99m}Tc-cAbVCAM1-5 or ^{99m}Tc-Ctl. (**B**) In vivo quantification of ^{99m}Tc-cAbVCAM1-5 and ^{99m}Tc-Ctl lung uptake from SPECT images. (**C**) Ex vivo quantification of ^{99m}Tc-cAbVCAM1-5 and ^{99m}Tc-Ctl lung uptake from post-mortem biodistribution studies. Results were expressed as % ID/cm^3 (imaging) and % ID/g (ex vivo) of tumor. Statistics: * $p < 0.05$ vs. ^{99m}Tc-Ctl.

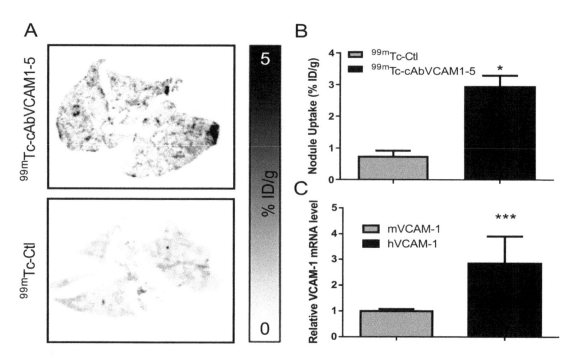

Figure 6. Ex vivo assessment of ^{99m}Tc-cAbVCAM1-5 uptake in metastatic nodules and assessment of VCAM-1 expression by RT-qPCR. (**A**) Autoradiography on 20 μm metastasis-containing lung slices. (**B**) Autoradiographic image quantification of ^{99m}Tc-cAbVCAM1-5 and ^{99m}Tc-Ctl uptake in MDA-MB-231 metastatic nodules. * $p < 0.05$ vs. ^{99m}Tc-Ctl. (**C**) 50 mg of lung containing metastases (MDA-MB-231) were harvested and tested for human and mice VCAM-1 expression by RT-qPCR. *** $p < 0.001$ vs. MDA-MB-231 mVCAM-1.

2.7. Ex Vivo Assessment of VCAM-1 Expression in the Experimental Metastasis Model

As in the subcutaneous xenograft study, VCAM-1 lung expression was assessed by RT-qPCR (Figure 6C). Both mVCAM-1 and hVCAM-1 mRNA were expressed, with the predominant expression of hVCAM-1 in tumors. Indeed, hVCAM-1 was nearly 3-fold more expressed than mVCAM-1 (2.8 ± 1.1 vs. 1.0 ± 0.1, $p < 0.001$). This results strongly suggests that the ^{99m}Tc-cAbVCAM1-5 imaging reflects VCAM-1 tumor cells expression in this model.

3. Discussion

Despite major advances in fundamental knowledge and therapeutic opportunities, BC remains the leading form of malignancy among women [1]. If the 5-year relative survival of BC is almost 100% when the cancer is restricted to the breast, the prognosis of patients with metastatic BC is unfavorable with a 5-year survival rate of 25% [22]. Moreover, among women initially diagnosed without metastasis, 20 to 25% will develop a metastatic disease in the next 5 years [23]. Despite intense clinical research efforts, there is still a strong need for novel molecular target and therapies to improve management of BC metastases [24]. The identification of genes and mechanisms involved in metastatic processes and the development of effective treatments against metastatic BC are outstanding challenges in current experimental and clinical research. In the past few years, growing interest into tumorigenicity and metastatic processes has led to the identification of VCAM-1 as a key actor for tumor growth, metastasis and angiogenesis [25].

In BC, VCAM-1 expression on tumor cells is an important actor for metastatic colonization of lungs and bones [9]. In the lungs VCAM-1 binds to $\alpha4\beta1$ integrin expressed on macrophages triggering the activation of the PI3K/Akt survival pathway in cancer cells [14]. In bone, VCAM-1 expressing tumor cells binds to $\alpha4\beta1$ integrin-expressing osteoclast progenitors to mediate osteolytic metastasis [13]. Moreover, VCAM-1 expression seems to be correlated to poor outcome in BC [12]. The results provided by the TCGA analysis showed that VCAM-1 is overexpressed in TNBC in comparison to Non-TNBC. Moreover, VCAM-1 expression is associated with a poor prognosis only in TNBC patients. In addition to BC, VCAM-1 increased expression has also been described in other cancer types such as glioblastoma, gastric and ovarian cancer. In these cancers, VCAM-1 expression correlated with the tumor grade [26–28]. Considering the role of VCAM-1 in directing the metastatic spread, VCAM-1 imaging agents could be used to (1) understand the biological role of VCAM-1 in metastatic processes and (2) to evaluate the prognostic value of VCAM-1 expression in clinical practice. Therefore, radiotracers have been developed for VCAM-1 imaging in tumors [29,30].

Our group recently developed ^{99m}Tc-cAbVCAM1-5, a radiotracer targeting VCAM-1 which is ongoing clinical transfer for the detection of inflamed atherosclerotic lesions [20,21,31]. The purpose of the present study was to evaluate this new tool for the pre-clinical nuclear imaging of VCAM-1 in TNBC. Two TNBC cell lines were employed, MDA-MB-231 and HCC70. The MDA-MB-231 cell line is highly metastatic whereas few results were available on HCC70. In vitro experiments demonstrated that MDA-MB-231 expressed hVCAM-1 mRNA and protein, and that expression was increased after TNF-α stimulation which is consistent with previous studies [19]. TNF-α is a key activator of VCAM-1 through NF-κB signaling [32]. A bundle of evidences links TNF-α and NF-κB pathway to tumor survival, growth and invasion [33,34]. The results provided by the TCGA showed higher TNF-α expression in TNBC in comparison to Non-TNBC tumors. These results suggest that the TNF-α/VCAM-1 axis is a relevant target in TNBC. As demonstrated by in vitro competition studies, the ^{99m}Tc-cAbVCAM1-5 tracer specifically binds human VCAM-1. Using this imaging agent, subcutaneous MDA-MB-231 tumors were successfully visualized by SPECT/CT imaging, whereas significantly lower signals were found in HCC70 tumors (which do not express hVCAM-1 mRNA and protein) or using the negative irrelevant control sdAb, thereby indicating that the signal was specific and predominantly attributable to tumor cell expressing VCAM-1 rather than murine endothelial or inflammatory cells. These results were in agreement with the level of murine and human VCAM-1 mRNA determined in tumor biopsies by RT-qPCR. Additional studies are however warranted in order to investigate if, similarly to that has been observed in vitro, in vivo hVCAM-1 expression in MDA-MB-231 tumor cells can be increased by TNF-α or other cytokines present in the microenvironment, leading to increased ^{99m}Tc-cAbVCAM1-5 uptake.

Therefore, ^{99m}Tc-cAbVCAM1-5 is a validated tool to investigate the role of VCAM-1 in metastatic processes. However our results support that using VCAM-1 as a tumor inflammatory marker should be carefully considered due to the potential expression of VCAM-1 by tumor cells themselves.

Because of VCAM-1 is aberrantly expressed in BC cells and mediates lung metastasis, ^{99m}Tc-cAbVCAM1-5 imaging was further studied in an experimental lung metastasis model with MDA-MB-231 cells. According to SPECT/CT quantifications, ^{99m}Tc-cAbVCAM1-5 lung uptake was 3-fold higher than that of ^{99m}Tc-Ctl whereas it was found to be 5-fold higher by ex vivo gamma-well counting. This difference can be attributed to the fact that when performing in vivo lung imaging quantification, the volume of interest contains a mixture of tissue and air, thereby leading to underestimation of the uptake.

Autoradiography further confirmed that ^{99m}Tc-cAbVCAM1-5 uptake was localized in metastatic nodules, and RT-qPCR showed that, in the whole lung, hVCAM-1 expression was found to be 3-fold higher than mVCAM-1 indicating that ^{99m}Tc-cAbVCAM1-5 uptake highlights presence of tumor cells rather than inflammatory processes. This result is consistent with a previous study demonstrating VCAM-1 tumor expression rather than endothelial cells one in lung metastasis of BC patients [14]. ^{99m}Tc-cAbVCAM-1 is therefore a validate tool to study the prognostic value of VCAM-1 in the metastatic disease.

Other VCAM-1-targeting radiotracers have been developed. ^{99m}Tc-cAbVCAM1-5 tumor uptake was comparable to that obtained by Scalici et al. using ^{111}In-tVCAM-4, an indium-111 labeled peptide targeting VCAM-1 [30]. Indeed, in an experimental mouse model of metastatic ovarian cancer, ^{111}In-tVCAM-4 uptake in tumor was of ~2% ID/g at 4 h post-injection. Using a ^{68}Ga-labeled Single Chain Variable Fragment, Zhang et al. obtained a ~5% ID/g tumor uptake in a mouse model of melanoma. Nevertheless, due to the fast blood clearance of sdAbs-based imaging agents, ^{99m}Tc-cAbVCAM1-5 tumor-to-blood ratio (5 at 2 h) favorably compared to that of this imaging agent (2 at 3 h) [29].

4. Materials and Methods

4.1. Patients—Online Data

Normalized RNA sequencing (RNA-Seq) data of The Cancer Genome Atlas (TCGA) were downloaded from cBioportal (Breast Invasive Carcinoma—TCGA Provisional; RNA-Seq V2) [35]. Data were available for 980 BC tumor samples (866 Non-TNBC and 114 TNBC). The results published here are based upon data generated by the TCGA Research Network [36,37].

4.2. Cell Lines and Culture Conditions

MDA-MB-231 cells were cultured with Dulbecco's Modified Eagle's Medium supplemented with 10% fetal bovine serum and 1% penicillin-streptomycin. HCC70 cells were cultured using Roswell Park Memorial Institute-1640 medium, supplemented with 10% fetal bovine serum and 1% penicillin-streptomycin.

4.3. RT-qPCR Assay

HCC70 and MDA-MB-231 cells were stimulated or not with Tumor Necrosis Factor-α (TNF-α, 50 ng/mL, Peprotech®, Rocky Hill, NJ, USA) for 18 h. Cell lysis and extraction of total RNA from cell lines were performed using PureLink[TM] RNA Mini Kit (ThermoFisher Scientific, Illkirch, France) according to the manufacturer's protocol. Reverse transcription (RT) was performed using an iScript Reverse transcription kit (iScript RT supermix; BioRad, Hercules, CA, USA). The reaction mixtures were incubated at 25 °C for 5 min, 46 °C for 20 min, 95 °C for 1 min and held at 4 °C. For the assessment of VCAM-1 expression in xenograft tumors and in metastatic nodules, 20–50 mg of tissue was ground (PureLink^{TM} RNA Mini Kit; ThermoFisher Scientific), and the same protocol as for the in vitro assay was applied. Quantitative Polymerase Chain Reaction (qPCR) was performed on the resulting cDNA with the Fast SYBR Green Master Mix (ThermoFisher Scientific, Illkirch, France), using a Real Time PCR system (Applied Biosystem StepOne Plus; ThermoFisher Scientific). The primer sequences were as follows: human VCAM-1 (hVCAM-1) Forward, 5'-AGTTGAAGGATGCGGGAGTA-3', Reverse 5'-ACCCCTTCAT GTTGGCTTTTC-3'; murine VCAM-1 (mVCAM-1) Forward, 5'- GCCACCCTCACCTTAATTGC -3', Reverse 5'- TCAGAACAACCGAATCCCCA-3'. The expression levels of mRNAs were normalized to the endogenous control actin, and were calculated with the formula $2^{-\Delta\Delta CT}$. The primer sequence for actin was as follows: Forward, 5'-CTCCTGAGCGCAAGTACTCC-3', Reverse 5'-TGTTTTCT GCGCAAGTTAGG-3'.

4.4. Western Blot Assay

HCC70 and MDA-MB-231 cells were treated or not with TNF-α (50 ng/mL) for 18 h. Total proteins were extracted with RIPA buffer. Proteins were separated by 7.5% denaturing SDS-PAGE and transferred onto a nitrocellulose membrane. The membrane was incubated with the anti-VCAM-1 antibody (1/2000; Rabbit anti-VCAM-1, ab134047 Abcam®, Cambridge, UK). As a loading control, the membrane was probed with an anti-β-actin antibody (1/10,000; Beckton Dickinson). Revelation was assessed using the chemiluminescence ECL kit (BioRad). Bands were quantified by densitometry using ImageJ software.

4.5. Flow Cytometry

MDA-MB-231 and HCC70 cells (200.000) treated or not with TNF-α (50 ng/mL) for 18 h were collected and washed with phosphate buffered saline solution (PBS). Cells were incubated with cAbVCAM1-5 (10 µg/mL) and then with an anti-poly histidine antibody (anti-6x His tag antibody, ab9108 Abcam), followed by a AlexaFluor®488-anti-Rabbit-IgG (Goat anti-Rabbit IgG H&L, AlexaFluor®488, ab150077 Abcam). Binding was measured on a FACS Accuri C6 analyzer (BD Biosciences, San Jose, CA, USA). Background fluorescence was determined by measuring the fluorescent signal from cells stained with the irrelevant control sdAb.

4.6. Saturation Binding Experiments and In Vitro Competition Studies

Saturation binding experiments was determined on 96-well plates coated with mouse or human recombinant VCAM-1 protein (100 ng/well; R&D Systems, Minneapolis, MN, USA). Serial dilutions of ^{99m}Tc-cAbVCAM1-5 were incubated for 1 h at room temperature before being washed 5 times with PBS-polysorbate 0.1%. The radioactivity in each well was then determined using a γ-counter (Wizard^2; Perkin Elmer, Courtaboeuf, France) and corrected for unspecific binding. Binding curves were fitted using a non linear regression equation (specific binding: $y = B_{max} \times x/(K_D + x)$, with x being the radioligand concentration, K_D being the dissociation constant, and B_{max} being the maximum number of binding sites, or receptor density) (GraphPad Prism, version 6, software, San Diego, CA, USA), to determine K_D values.

For in vitro competition studies, 12,000 HCC70 and MDA-MB-231 cells were coated in 96-well plates (Stripwell^{TM} Plate, Corning®, Corning, NY, USA) in their respective culture medium. After 24 h, cells were treated with 50 ng/mL of TNF-α for 18 h. Then, cells were rinsed with PBS and fixed with paraformaldehyde (PFA) 4% for 10 min. Following 1 h of saturation with PBS-BSA 1%, cells were incubated with 30 nM of ^{99m}Tc-cAbVCAM1-5 in the absence or presence of a 100-fold excess of unlabeled cAbVCAM1-5 at room temperature for 1 h before being washed 5 times with PBS-Tween 0.05%. Bound activity was determined using a gamma-counter (Wizard^2, Perkin Elmer) and results were corrected from nonspecific binding determined on HCC70 cells.

4.7. Tumor Models

All animal procedures conformed to French government guidelines (Articles R214-87 to R214-126; European directive 2010/63/UE). They were performed in an approved facility (C385161 0005) under permit APAFIS#3690-2016011916045217 v4 and APAFIS#8683-2017012611031820 v3 from the French Ministry of Research. To evaluate ^{99m}Tc-cAbVCAM1-5 biodistribution and tumor uptake, 12 female BALB/c nu/nu mice (5 weeks old) were subcutaneously inoculated into the left flank with MDA-MB-231 (3×10^6) and into the right flank with HCC70 (3×10^6), in a 2:1 PBS/Matrigel® (Corning) mixture. The tumors were allowed to grow for 3 weeks to reach ~150–200 mm^3. For the experimental metastasis model, 9 female C.B17 SCID (Severe Combined ImmunoDeficient) mice (5 weeks old) were intravenously injected with MDA-MB-231 cells (1 M in 150 μL) in PBS. Eight weeks later, SPECT/CT imaging and biodistribution studies were performed.

4.8. SPECT/CT Imaging

For the subcutaneous xenograft study, mice were divided in 2 groups: tumor bearing mice injected with (i) the human/mouse cross-reactive sdAb ^{99m}Tc-cAbVCAM1-5 ($n = 6$) or (ii) with the irrelevant control sdAb, ^{99m}Tc-Ctl ($n = 6$). The previously described BcII10a control sdAb was used in this study (20). SPECT/CT acquisitions were performed 1 hour after intravenous injection of 57.6 ± 9.8 MBq of ^{99m}Tc-cAbVCAM1-5 or ^{99m}Tc-Ctl. The cAbVCAM1-5 and control sdAbs were radiolabeled as previously described using the tricarbonyl method [20]. Whole body SPECT/CT acquisitions were performed using a dedicated system (nanoSPECT-CT; Mediso, Budapest, Hungary). For the experimental metastasis study, mice were injected with 61.9 ± 16.2 MBq of ^{99m}Tc-cAbVCAM1-5 ($n = 5$) or the irrelevant ^{99m}Tc-Ctl ($n = 4$). Biodistributions were also performed on healthy mice ($n = 4$). SPECT/CT acquisition was centered on the thoracic region. CT and SPECT acquisitions were reconstructed and fused using Nucline software (Mediso), and SPECT quantification based on CT was performed using VivoQuant™ (InviCRO, Boston, MA, USA). For the xenograft tumor model, a 50 mm^3 sphere was drawn at the center of the tumor on the basis of the CT image. For the metastasis assay, total quantification of pulmonary tracer uptake based on the CT image was performed. ^{99m}Tc-sdAbs activity was expressed as a percentage of the injected dose per cm^3 (% ID/cm^3).

4.9. Post-Mortem Analysis

Two hours after injection and immediately following SPECT/CT image acquisitions, anesthetized mice were euthanized using CO_2 and tumors (either subcutaneous or the whole lungs with metastasis) were harvested along with other organs. Samples were weighed and their radioactivity determined with a γ-counter (Wizard^2, PerkinElmer, Courtaboeuf, France). Results were corrected for decay, injected dose and organ weight and expressed as % ID/g. Subcutaneous tumors were then immediately frozen in −40 °C isopentane, whereas metastatic lungs were inflated with a 1:1 mixture of PBS/Optimal Cutting Temperature prior being frozen. In order to investigate whether the VCAM-1 expression status determined in vitro on HCC70 and MDA-MB-231 cells was preserved in vivo, RT-qPCR was performed on HCC70 and MDA-MB-231 subcutaneous tumor slices and tissue samples. Moreover, due to the fact that ex vivo counting on lung with metastases reflects a mixture of healthy tissue and tumor uptake, lung autoradiography was performed to precisely evaluate the tumor uptake. To that purpose, 20 μm-thick lung slices, together with reference organs of known activities, were exposed overnight on an autoradiographic film which was then scanned using a phosphoimager (Fujifilm BAS-5000, FUJIFILM, Montigny, France). Slices were then stained with hematoxylin-eosin and regions of interest were delineated on tumor nodules, thereby allowing the quantification of ^{99m}Tc-cAbVCAM1-5 or ^{99m}Tc-Ctl uptake as a percentage of injected dose per gram (% ID/g).

4.10. Statistics

For the in vitro and mice experiments: Data were expressed as mean ± standard deviation and analyzed using an unpaired Mann Whitney test for inter group analysis. Significance of linear correlations was assessed with a Pearson's test. p values < 0.05 were considered significant. Data were analyzed with Prism 7.0 (GraphPad Software).

For patients: The Student's t-test was used to compare continuous variables. Overall survival (OS) was defined as the time between surgery and the date of death from any cause. The Kaplan-Meier method was used to produce survival curves and analyses of censored data were performed using Cox models. Data were analyzed with Prism 7.0 (GraphPad Software).

5. Conclusions

In the two mouse models of TNBC, SPECT imaging of VCAM-1 was successfully performed and the signal originated from the tumor was found to reflect hVCAM-1 expression by cancer cells rather than mVCAM-1 expression by the tumor stroma. ^{99m}Tc-cAbVCAM1-5 can therefore be used as a preclinical tool to evaluate the role of VCAM-1 expression by tumor cells in tumor development and metastasis. In clinical practice, VCAM-1 expression has been reported to be correlated with poorer outcome in TNBC but also in other cancer type such as glioblastoma and ovarian cancer, and VCAM-1 imaging has been proposed as a tool for the assessment of tumor aggressiveness. Further studies will however be necessary to evaluate the prognostic value of ^{99m}Tc-cAbVCAM1-5 tumor imaging in clinical practice.

Author Contributions: Conceptualization, C.M., A.B., C.G., D.F; methodology, C.M., P.C., A.B., C.G., D.F; formal analysis, C.M., L.D., P.C., M.A., S.B., M.D., A.S., L.D., J.L., N.L., M.D., G.P., S.H., N.D., P.P., L.R., A.B., C.G., D.F; investigation, C.M., L.D., P.C., M.A., S.B., M.D., A.S., L.D., J.L., N.L., M.D., G.P., S.H., N.D., P.P., L.R; resources, C.M., L.D., P.C., M.A., S.B., M.D., A.S., L.D., J.L., N.L., M.D., G.P., A.B., C.G., D.F.; writing—original draft preparation, C.M, A.B, C.G; writing—review and editing, C.M., L.D., P.C., M.A., S.B., M.D., A.S., L.D., J.L., N.L., M.D., G.P., S.H., N.D., P.P., L.R., A.B., C.G., D.F; visualization, C.M., A.B., C.G., D.F; supervision, A.B, D.F., C.G.; funding acquisition, A.B., C.G., D.F.

Acknowledgments: This work was partly funded by France Life Imaging, grant "ANR-11-INBS-0006".

References

1. Ferlay, J.; Steliarova-Foucher, E.; Lortet-Tieulent, J.; Rosso, S.; Coebergh, J.W.W.; Comber, H.; Forman, D.; Bray, F. Cancer incidence and mortality patterns in Europe: Estimates for 40 countries in 2012. *Eur. J. Cancer* **2013**, *49*, 1374–1403. [CrossRef] [PubMed]

2. Perou, C.M.; Sorlie, T.B.; Eisen, C.; Van De Rijn, M.; Jeffrey, S.S.; Rees, C.A.; Pollack, J.R.; Ross, D.T.; Johnsen, H.; Akslen, L.A.; et al. Molecular portraits of human breast tumours. *Nature* **2000**, 747–752. [CrossRef] [PubMed]

3. Sorlie, T.; Tibshirani, R.; Parker, J.; Hastie, T.; Marron, J.S.; Nobel, A.; Deng, S.; Johnsen, H.; Pesich, R.; Geisler, S.; et al. Repeated observation of breast tumor subtypes in independent gene expression data sets. *Proc. Natl. Acad. Sci. USA* **2003**, *100*, 8418–8423. [CrossRef] [PubMed]

4. Reis-Filho, J.S.; Tutt, A.N.J. Triple negative tumours: A critical review: Triple negative tumours. *Histopathology* **2007**, *52*, 108–118. [CrossRef] [PubMed]

5. Dent, R.; Trudeau, M.; Pritchard, K.I.; Hanna, W.M.; Kahn, H.K.; Sawka, C.A.; Lickley, L.A.; Rawlinson, E.; Sun, P.; Narod, S.A. Triple-Negative Breast Cancer: Clinical Features and Patterns of Recurrence. *Clin. Cancer Res.* **2007**, *13*, 4429–4434. [CrossRef] [PubMed]

6. Haffty, B.G.; Yang, Q.; Reiss, M.; Kearney, T.; Higgins, S.A.; Weidhaas, J.; Harris, L.; Hait, W.; Toppmeyer, D. Locoregional Relapse and Distant Metastasis in Conservatively Managed Triple Negative Early-Stage Breast Cancer. *J. Clin. Oncol.* **2006**, *24*, 5652–5657. [CrossRef] [PubMed]

7. Lorusso, G.; Rüegg, C. New insights into the mechanisms of organ-specific breast cancer metastasis. *Semin. Cancer Biol.* **2012**, *22*, 226–233. [CrossRef]

8. Minn, A.J.; Gupta, G.P.; Siegel, P.M.; Bos, P.D.; Shu, W.; Giri, D.D.; Viale, A.; Olshen, A.B.; Gerald, W.L.; Massagué, J. Genes that mediate breast cancer metastasis to lung. *Nature* **2005**, *436*, 518. [CrossRef]

9. Chen, Q.; Massague, J. Molecular Pathways: VCAM-1 as a Potential Therapeutic Target in Metastasis. *Clin. Cancer Res.* **2012**, *18*, 5520–5525. [CrossRef]

10. Cook-Mills, J.M.; Marchese, M.E.; Abdala-Valencia, H. Vascular cell adhesion molecule-1 expression and signaling during disease: Regulation by reactive oxygen species and antioxidants. *Antioxid. Redox Signal.* **2011**, *15*, 1607–1638. [CrossRef]

11. Schlesinger, M.; Bendas, G. Vascular cell adhesion molecule-1 (VCAM-1)-An increasing insight into its role in tumorigenicity and metastasis: VCAM-1 in tumorigenicity. *Int. J. Cancer* **2015**, *136*, 2504–2514. [CrossRef] [PubMed]

12. Maimaiti, Y.; Wang, C.; Mushajiang, M.; Tan, J.; Huang, B.; Zhou, J.; Huang, T. Overexpression of VCAM-1 is correlated with poor survival of patients with breast cancer. *Int. J. Clin. Exp. Pathol.* **2016**, *9*, 7451–7457.

13. Lu, X.; Mu, E.; Wei, Y.; Riethdorf, S.; Yang, Q.; Yuan, M.; Yan, J.; Hua, Y.; Tiede, B.J.; Lu, X.; et al. VCAM-1 Promotes Osteolytic Expansion of Indolent Bone Micrometastasis of Breast Cancer by Engaging α4β1-Positive Osteoclast Progenitors. *Cancer Cell* **2011**, *20*, 701–714. [CrossRef] [PubMed]

14. Chen, Q.; Zhang, X.H.-F.; Massagué, J. Macrophage Binding to Receptor VCAM-1 Transmits Survival Signals in Breast Cancer Cells that Invade the Lungs. *Cancer Cell* **2011**, *20*, 538–549. [CrossRef] [PubMed]

15. Kang, Y. Dissecting Tumor-Stromal Interactions in Breast Cancer Bone Metastasis. *Endocrinol. Metab.* **2016**, *31*, 206. [CrossRef] [PubMed]

16. Cao, H.; Zhang, Z.; Zhao, S.; He, X.; Yu, H.; Yin, Q.; Zhang, Z.; Gu, W.; Chen, L.; Li, Y. Hydrophobic interaction mediating self-assembled nanoparticles of succinobucol suppress lung metastasis of breast cancer by inhibition of VCAM-1 expression. *J. Control. Release* **2015**, *205*, 162–171. [CrossRef] [PubMed]

17. Wu, T.-C. The Role of Vascular Cell Adhesion Molecule-1 in Tumor Immune Evasion. *Cancer Res.* **2007**, *67*, 6003–6006. [CrossRef] [PubMed]

18. Lin, K.-Y.; Lu, D.; Hung, C.-F.; Peng, S.; Huang, L.; Jie, C.; Murillo, F.; Rowley, J.; Tsai, Y.-C.; He, L.; et al. Ectopic Expression of Vascular Cell Adhesion Molecule-1 as a New Mechanism for Tumor Immune Evasion. *Cancer Res.* **2007**, *67*, 1832–1841. [CrossRef]

19. Wang, P.-C.; Weng, C.-C.; Hou, Y.-S.; Jian, S.-F.; Fang, K.-T.; Hou, M.-F.; Cheng, K.-H. Activation of VCAM-1 and Its Associated Molecule CD44 Leads to Increased Malignant Potential of Breast Cancer Cells. *Int. J. Mol. Sci.* **2014**, *15*, 3560–3579. [CrossRef]

20. Broisat, A.; Hernot, S.; Toczek, J.; De Vos, J.; Riou, L.M.; Martin, S.; Ahmadi, M.; Thielens, N.; Wernery, U.; Caveliers, V.; et al. Nanobodies Targeting Mouse/Human VCAM1 for the Nuclear Imaging of Atherosclerotic Lesions. *Circ. Res.* **2012**, *30*, 927–937. [CrossRef]

21. Dumas, L.S.; Briand, F.; Clerc, R.; Brousseau, E.; Montemagno, C.; Ahmadi, M.; Bacot, S.; Soubies, A.; Perret, P.; Riou, L.M.; et al. Evaluation of Antiatherogenic Properties of Ezetimibe Using ^{3}H-Labeled Low-Density-Lipoprotein Cholesterol and ^{99m}Tc-cAbVCAM1–5 SPECT in ApoE$^{-/-}$ Mice Fed the Paigen Diet. *J. Nucl. Med.* **2017**, *58*, 1088–1093. [CrossRef] [PubMed]

22. Mariotto, A.B.; Etzioni, R.; Hurlbert, M.; Penberthy, L.; Mayer, M. Estimation of the Number of Women Living with Metastatic Breast Cancer in the United States. *Cancer Epidemiol. Biomark. Prev.* **2017**, *26*, 809–815. [CrossRef] [PubMed]

23. Group EBCTC. Effects of chemotherapy and hormonal therapy for early breast cancer on recurrence and 15-year survival: An overview of the randomised trials. *Lancet* **2005**, *365*, 1687–1717. [CrossRef]

24. Eckhardt, B.L.; Francis, P.A.; Parker, B.S.; Anderson, R.L. Strategies for the discovery and development of therapies for metastatic breast cancer. *Nat. Rev. Drug Discov.* **2012**, *11*, 479–497. [CrossRef] [PubMed]

25. Sharma, R.; Sharma, R.; Khaket, T.P.; Dutta, C.; Chakraborty, B.; Mukherjee, T.K. Breast cancer metastasis: Putative therapeutic role of vascular cell adhesion molecule-1. *Cell Oncol.* **2017**, *40*, 199–208. [CrossRef] [PubMed]

26. Ding, Y.-B.; Chen, G.-Y.; Xia, J.-G.; Zang, X.-W.; Yang, H.-Y.; Yang, L. Association of VCAM-1 overexpression with oncogenesis, tumor angiogenesis and metastasis of gastric carcinoma. *World J. Gastroenterol.* **2003**, *9*, 1409. [CrossRef] [PubMed]

27. Liu, Y.-S.; Lin, H.-Y.; Lai, S.-W.; Huang, C.-Y.; Huang, B.-R.; Chen, P.-Y.; Wei, K.-C.; Lu, D.-Y. MiR-181b modulates EGFR-dependent VCAM-1 expression and monocyte adhesion in glioblastoma. *Oncogene* **2017**, *36*, 5006–5022. [CrossRef]

28. Huang, J.; Zhang, J.; Li, H.; Lu, Z.; Shan, W.; Mercado-Uribe, I.; Liu, J. VCAM1 expression correlated with tumorigenesis and poor prognosis in high grade serous ovarian cancer. *Am. J. Transl. Res.* **2013**, *5*, 336.

29. Zhang, X.; Liu, C.; Hu, F.; Zhang, Y.; Wang, J.; Gao, Y.; Jiang, Y.; Zhang, Y.; Lan, X. PET Imaging of VCAM-1 Expression and Monitoring Therapy Response in Tumor with a ^{68}Ga-Labeled Single Chain Variable Fragment. *Mol. Pharm.* **2018**, *15*, 609–618. [CrossRef]

30. Scalici, J.M.; Thomas, S.; Harrer, C.; Raines, T.A.; Curran, J.; Atkins, K.A.; Conaway, M.R.; Duska, L.; Kelly, K.A.; Slack-Davis, J.K. Imaging VCAM-1 as an Indicator of Treatment Efficacy in Metastatic Ovarian Cancer. *J. Nucl. Med.* **2013**, *54*, 1883–1889. [CrossRef]

31. Broisat, A.; Toczek, J.; Dumas, L.S.; Ahmadi, M.; Bacot, S.; Perret, P.; Slimani, L.; Barone-Rochette, G.; Soubies, A.; Devoogdt, N.; et al. 99mTc-cAbVCAM1-5 Imaging Is a Sensitive and Reproducible Tool for the Detection of Inflamed Atherosclerotic Lesions in Mice. *J. Nucl. Med.* **2014**, *55*, 1678–1684. [CrossRef] [PubMed]

32. Rajan, S.; Ye, J.; Bai, S.; Huang, F.; Guo, Y.-L. NF-κB, but not p38 MAP Kinase, is required for TNF-α-induced expression of cell adhesion molecules in endothelial cells. *J. Cell. Biochem.* **2008**, *105*, 477–486. [CrossRef] [PubMed]

33. Li, B.; Vincent, A.; Cates, J.; Brantley-Sieders, D.M.; Polk, D.B.; Young, P.P. Low Levels of Tumor Necrosis Factor Increase Tumor Growth by Inducing an Endothelial Phenotype of Monocytes Recruited to the Tumor Site. *Cancer Res.* **2009**, *69*, 338–348. [CrossRef] [PubMed]

34. Cai, X.; Cao, C.; Li, J.; Chen, F.; Zhang, S.; Liu, B.; Zhang, W.; Zhang, X.; Ye, L. Inflammatory factor TNF-alpha promotes the growth of breast cancer via the positive feedback loop of TNFR1/NF-κB (and/or p38)/p-STAT3/HBXIP/TNFR1. *Oncotarget* **2017**, *8*, 58338–58352. [PubMed]

35. The cBioPortal for Cancer Genomics. Available online: https://www.cbioportal.org/study/summary?id=brca_tcga (accessed on 19 July 2019).

36. Cerami, E.; Gao, J.; Dogrusoz, U.; Gross, B.E.; Sumer, S.O.; Aksoy, B.A.; Jacobsen, A.; Byrne, C.J.; Heuer, M.L.; Larsson, E.; et al. The *cBio Cancer* Genomics Portal: An Open Platform for Exploring Multidimensional Cancer Genomics Data: Figure 1. *Cancer Discov.* **2012**, *2*, 401–404. [CrossRef] [PubMed]

37. Gao, J.; Aksoy, B.A.; Dogrusoz, U.; Dresdner, G.; Gross, B.; Sumer, S.O.; Sun, Y.; Jacobsen, A.; Sinha, R.; Larsson, E.; et al. Integrative Analysis of Complex Cancer Genomics and Clinical Profiles Using the cBioPortal. *Sci. Signal.* **2013**, *6*, pl1. [CrossRef]

12

Predictive Role of MRI and ^{18}F-FDG PET Response to Concurrent Chemoradiation in T2b Cervical Cancer on Clinical Outcome

Anna Myriam Perrone [1,2,*], Giulia Dondi [1,2], Manuela Coe [3], Martina Ferioli [4], Silvi Telo [5], Andrea Galuppi [2,4], Eugenia De Crescenzo [1], Marco Tesei [1,2], Paolo Castellucci [5], Cristina Nanni [5], Stefano Fanti [2,5], Alessio G. Morganti [2,4] and Pierandrea De Iaco [1,2]

[1] Gynecologic Oncology Unit, Sant'Orsola-Malpighi Hospital, 40138 Bologna, Italy; giulia.dondi@gmail.com (G.D.); eugeniadecrescenzo@gmail.com (E.D.C.); marco.tesei2@gmail.com (M.T.); pierandrea.deiaco@unibo.it (P.D.I.)

[2] Centro di Studio e Ricerca delle Neoplasie Ginecologiche (CSR) University of Bologna, 40138 Bologna, Italy; andrea.galuppi@aosp.bo.it (A.G.); stefano.fanti@aosp.bo.it (S.F.); alessio.morganti2@unibo.it (A.G.M.)

[3] Department of Specialized, Diagnostic, and Experimental Medicine, Sant'Orsola-Malpighi Hospital, 40138 Bologna, Italy; manuela.coe@aosp.bo.it

[4] Radiotherapy Unit, Sant'Orsola-Malpighi Hospital, 40138 Bologna, Italy; m.ferioli88@gmail.com

[5] Nuclear Medicine Unit, Sant'Orsola-Malpighi Hospital, 40138 Bologna, Italy; silvi.telo@gmail.com (S.T.); paolo.castellucci@aosp.bo.it (P.C.); cristina.nanni@aosp.bo.it (C.N.)

* Correspondence: myriam.perrone@aosp.bo.it

Abstract: Tumor response in locally advanced cervical cancer (LACC) is generally evaluated with MRI and PET, but this strategy is not supported by the literature. Therefore, we compared the diagnostic performance of these two techniques in the response evaluation to concurrent chemoradiotherapy (CCRT) in LACC. Patients with cervical cancer (CC) stage T2b treated with CCRT and submitted to MRI and PET/CT before and after treatment were enrolled in the study. All clinical, pathological, therapeutic, radiologic and follow-up data were collected and examined. The radiological response was analyzed and compared to the follow-up data. Data of 40 patients with LACC were analyzed. Agreement between MRI and PET/CT in the evaluation response to therapy was observed in 31/40 (77.5%) of cases. The agreement between MRI, PET/CT and follow-up data showed a Cohen kappa coefficient of 0.59 (95% CI = 0.267–0.913) and of 0.84 (95% CI = 0.636–1.00), respectively. Considering the evaluation of primary tumor response, PET/CT was correct in 97.5% of cases, and MRI in 92.5% of cases; no false negative cases were observed. These results suggest the use of PET/CT as a unique diagnostic imaging tool after CCRT, to correctly assess residual and progression disease.

Keywords: locally advanced cervical cancer; PET/CT; MRI; concurrent chemoradiotherapy; treatment response; follow up

1. Introduction

Cervical carcinoma (CC) is the third commonest gynecological cancer in women worldwide [1,2]. In the past, CC was routinely staged with the clinical FIGO system but the new ESGO guidelines introduced and recommended a TNM classification with a FIGO staging, too [3–5]. Early CC and locally advanced CC (LACC) represent two different realities with distinct therapeutic approaches and prognosis. Surgery is the preferred approach in the early stage while concurrent chemoradiation (CCRT) is the standard treatment option in LACC [3,6–8]. The target of the external beam radiation therapy

(EBRT) includes the pelvic lymph nodes, but the irradiation field can be extended to the common iliac and para-aortic region in patients with nodal involvement [9,10]. The residual macroscopic tumor is then boosted with brachytherapy (BRT). CCRT allows local control of the disease in 70%–80% of patients, with 66% and 58% 5-year overall survival (OS) and disease-free survival (DFS) rates, respectively [11,12]. Recurrences occur in 22%–41% of patients, mostly within the first two years after the end of treatment. The recurrence site is more frequently loco-regional while distant metastases are rare [13]. Treatment response is evaluated 3-6 months after the end of CCRT, clinically and by imaging techniques [14]. Currently there is no agreement on the gold standard imaging technique to evaluate a tumor's response. Data in the literature are lacking and contradictory. MRI and PET/CT represent the most used imaging techniques [15,16] with different purposes: the assessment of response in the primary tumor (T) performed by MRI and assessment of response of the metastases performed by PET/CT [17,18]. In daily practice, usually MRI represents the first imaging method to evaluate response to therapy and PET/CT is mostly performed only if residual disease is suspected by MRI [3]. However, since clear and reliable data in this field are missing and there is no consensus on which technique should be used, the National Comprehensive Cancer Network (NCCN) [10] recommend both MRI and PET/CT as a post-treatment assessment of tumor response in LACC after CCRT [19].

Considering the uncertainty of current evidence, we retrospectively compared the diagnostic performance of ^{18}F-FDG PET/CT and MRI in the response evaluation after CCRT in LACC stage T2b.

2. Materials and Methods

2.1. Population

The clinical data of all patients with CC referred to our Unit of Gynecologic Oncology of Sant'Orsola Hospital of Bologna (Italy) between June 2007 and January 2017 were retrospectively analyzed. Among these we selected patients with stage T2b treated with CCRT.

Inclusion criteria were (a) histologically proven squamous cell cervical cancer and adenocarcinoma performed by biopsy or cone according to the WHO criteria [20]; (b) clinical stage T2b; c) treatment with CCRT; d) a pre-treatment pelvic MRI and total body ^{18}F-FDG PET/CT and post-treatment pelvic MRI and total body ^{18}F-FDG PET/CT performed in the radiologic service of our institution; and e) adequate follow-up over 24 months.

Exclusion criteria were (a) patients younger than 18 years old; (b) rare (other than squamous or adenocarcinoma) histological type; (c) a previous history of cancer in the last 5 years; (d) other stages different from T2b; (e) previous surgery or chemotherapy; and (f) pre- or post-treatment pelvic MRI and/or total body ^{18}F-FDG PET/CT performed in other centers.

All clinical and pathological data were collected and examined, including age, body mass index (BMI), histological type, TNM staging system [5], radiotherapy and chemotherapy administration.

2.2. Concurrent Chemo-Radiotherapy Scheme

All patients underwent pelvic 3-dimensional conformal EBRT. In patients with para-aortic lymph node metastases, detected by ^{18}F-FDG-PET/CT, the fields were extended up to the level of the renal vessels or even more cranially based on the positive node site. In case of large lymphadenopathy (short axis greater than one centimeter) with high ^{18}F-FDG uptake ($SUV_{max} > 3$), a highly conformed EBRT boost was prescribed.

Cisplatin (40 mg/m^2) was administered intravenously once a week concurrently with EBRT. After radio-chemotherapy, all patients underwent a BRT boost, using the high dose rate (HDR) or pulsed dose rate (PDR) technique. The EBRT and BRT doses were prescribed according to the International Commission on Radiation Units and Measurements Reports 62 and 38, respectively [21].

2.3. Pelvic MRI Image Analysis

A baseline pelvic MRI was performed before the beginning of the treatment. An area with a high signal intensity in the cervix compared to the cervical stroma on the T2-weighted image with enhancement was considered neoplastic tissue in the pelvic MRI. Images were obtained with a high field magnet 1.5 T MRI system (GE, SIGNA LX HD-xt) using phase arrayed body coils. T2-weighted FSE images were obtained in sagittal, axial and oblique, perpendicular to the axis of the uterine cervix, and coronal with a 3–4 mm thickness and interslice gaps of 0.3/0.4 mm (matrix 320 × 224, FOV 28–32, 4NEX, TE 100, TR 3400) planes. LAVA 3D T1-weighted sequences were obtained before and after the intravenous (i.v.) injection of gadolinium contrast medium. Vaginal distension with aqueous gel (60 cc) was used in order to improve evaluation of the vaginal walls. Patients fasted for 4–6 h before the examination in order to reduce bowel motion artefacts and the bladder must be half full.

2.4. Total Body ^{18}F-FDG PET/CT Image Analysis

Whole body PET and low-dose CT scans were obtained one hour after the i.v. injection of 3.5 MBq/Kg of ^{18}F-FDG (PET scanner Discovery PET-CT 710, GE, Boston, Massachusetts, United States). A low dose Computed Tomography (CT) scan was performed both for attenuation correction and to provide an anatomical map. The CT parameters were 120KV, 80mA and 0.8 s for rotation, and a thickness of 3.75 mm. An iterative 3-D ordered subsets expectation maximization method with two iterations and 20 subsets, followed by smoothing (with a 6-mm 3-D gaussian kernel) with CT-based attenuation, scatter and random coincidence event correction, was used to reconstruct the PET images.

Patients fasted for 6 h and eventual insulin therapy was interrupted at least 6 h before the examination. All patients were positioned supine on the imaging table, arms above, and acquired from the base of the skull to the mid thighs. All ^{18}F-FDG PET/CT scans were reviewed by two expert nuclear medicine physicians with more than ten years of experience and a specific interest in gynecological malignancies. Discrepancies have been solved by consensus. For each scan, together with a visual assessment, a maximum standardized uptake value (SUV_{max}) was measured for every area of the focal uptake higher than the background and suspected to be a metastasis based on qualitative interpretation according to the location, the size and the intensity of the ^{18}F-FDG uptake.

2.5. Evaluation of the Response to CCRT

All patients were studied at baseline with pelvic MRI and total body ^{18}F-FDG PET/CT and treatment response was performed 6 months after the end of CCRT in the same tomographs. All radiological images were reviewed by M.C. for MRI and C.N. and P.C. for PET. Response to treatment was defined as complete response (CR), partial response (PR), progressive disease (PD) and stable disease (SD) according to RECIST criteria for the pelvic MRI and EORTC criteria for the ^{18}F-FDG PET/CT [22,23].

2.6. Follow Up

Patients defined as CR by both imaging techniques (^{18}F-FDG PET/CT and MRI) had a follow-up gynecological examination every 4 months in the first 2 years and every 6 months for 3 years. A chest–abdomen CT scan was performed every 12 months or in case of clinical suspicion of a relapse.

Patients defined not complete responders (PR, SD, PD) by one or both techniques were treated according to the localization of the residual or progressive disease (surgery or chemotherapy) or observed periodically with subsequent clinical or instrumental investigations in case of doubt.

Progression-free survival (PFS) was calculated from the first diagnosis to recurrence and overall survival (OS) was obtained from diagnosis to the last follow up or death.

The study was performed according to Helsinki declaration 2013, and all patients signed an informed consent and the local ethical committee of Sant'Orsola-Malpighi Hospital—Bologna approved this study (CE 322/2019/Oss/AUOBo).

2.7. Statistical Analysis

The software IBM SPSS ® 20.0, 2012 (Statistical Package for Social Science), was used for statistical data analysis and a *p*-value < 0.05 was considered statistically significant. Continuous variables were expressed as mean ± SD and categorical variables as percentages. Survival curves were calculated using the Kaplan–Meier method. Cohen's kappa was used to compare the two imaging techniques.

3. Results

3.1. Population

The flow chart of the recruitment is showed in Figure 1. In total, 40 patients met the inclusion criteria (patients with histologically proven squamous cell cervical cancer and adenocarcinoma stage T2b treated with CCRT with a pre-treatment pelvic MRI and total body ^{18}F-FDG PET/CT and post-treatment pelvic MRI and total body ^{18}F-FDG PET/CT performed in the radiologic service of our institution, and with adequate follow-up over 24 months) and were enrolled in the study. The patients' characteristics are reported in Table 1.

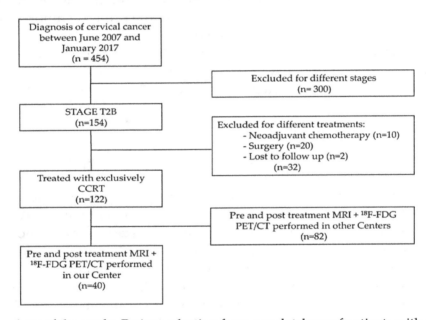

Figure 1. Flow chart of the study. Patient selection from our database of patients with cervical cancer.

Table 1. The population's characteristics.

Characteristics	Values
N	40
Age, years (mean ± SD)	61 ± 16
Mean age at diagnosis (mean ± SD)	55 ± 15
BMI mean (mean ± SD)	24.5 ± 4.2
Histotype	
Squamous *n* (%)	32 (80%)
Adenocarcinoma *n* (%)	8 (20%)
Stage TNM	
T2b	40 (100%)
N0	23 (57%)
N1	17 (43%)
M 0	40 (100%)

Note: *n*: number of patients; BMI: body mass index; T: primary tumor; N: nodes; M: metastases.

The mean EBRT total dose was 45 ± 1 Gy, eight patients (20%) needed extended-field pelvic and para-aortic radiotherapy and the mean dose of the boost on the positive nodes was 15.1 ± 6.2 Gy. All patients received weekly Cisplatin at the dose of 40 mg/sm. Eight out of 40 patients (20%) received four cycles, 27/40 (67.5%) patients received five cycles and 5/40 (12.5%) patients received six cycles. All patients received a BRT boost with a mean dose of 28.7 ± 6.3 Gy.

3.2. MRI Parameters

The mean pre-treatment maximum tumor diameter measured by MRI was 45.5 ± 14.4 mm (mean ± SD). In six patients (15%) MRI detected nodal involvement and the mean node short-axis length was 19.5 ± 8.9 mm (mean ± SD). After treatment, a complete response of the primary cervical tumor was recorded in 32 (80%) patients, while residual disease was observed in eight (20%) patients. Only one metastatic lymph node was still present (2.5%) with a short-axis length of 15 mm.

3.3. ^{18}F-FDG PET/CT Parameters

Pathological uptake was present in all primary tumors and lymph node involvement was detected in 17/40 patients (43%). The mean pre-treatment SUV$_{max}$ of the primary tumor was 14.2 ± 5.6 (mean ± SD) and the mean SUV$_{max}$ of pathologic lymph nodes was 6.2 ± 2.6 (mean ± SD). After CCRT in 35 target lesions (87.5%) the uptake of ^{18}F-FDG was normalized and the SUV$_{max}$ of the residual lesions was 9.7 ± 5.6 (mean ± SD). After the CCRT persistence, increased SUV$_{max}$ in the lymph nodes was detected in five patients (12.5%), showing a mean SUV$_{max}$ of 7.5 ± 5.1 (mean ± SD).

3.4. Agreement between MRI and ^{18}F-FDG PET/TC

Agreement between MRI and ^{18}F-FDG PET/CT in the evaluation response to therapy was observed in 31/40 (77.5%) of cases (Table 2 and Figure 2A,B). In these cases, a CR was observed in 28/31 patients (90.3%) and follow-up data showed a strong correlation with the response to therapy. In fact, only five out of 28 patients (18%) with CR experienced a subsequent treatment failure: Two local recurrences after 63 months and 64 months, respectively; one lung metastasis after 15 months; one vertebral metastasis after 24 months; and one patient showed lung and cerebellar metastases after 75 months. A PR was seen in 2/31 (6.5%) of the patients, who underwent rescue therapies. One of them underwent radical surgery and the histological exam confirmed residual disease in the cervix and in pelvic lymph nodes. The second one received palliative treatment because of severe comorbidities. Both patients died due to progressive disease after 12 and 18 months, respectively. One patient showed PD (1/31, 3.2%), and underwent a posterior exenteration (radical hysterectomy, bilateral salpingectomy, total colpectomy, pelvic and para-aortic lymphadenectomy, rectal resection with colorectal termino-terminal anastomosis and ileostomy). The patient died after 18 months.

Table 2. Concordance between MRI and FDG-PET/CT after CCRT.

MRI	^{18}F-FDG PET/CT				
	CR	PR	SD	PD	Total
CR	28	2	0	2	32
PR	3	2	0	2	7
SD	0	0	0	0	0
PD	0	0	0	1	1
Total	31	4	0	5	40

Note: CCRT: concomitant chemo-radiotherapy; CR: complete response; PR: partial response; SD: stable disease; PD: progression disease.

3.5. Disagreement between MRI and ^{18}F-FDG PET/CT

In 9/40 (22.5%) cases, MRI and ^{18}F-FDG PET/CT showed different results in terms of response (Tables 2 and 3). In Cases #1 and #2, MRI showed a CR, while ^{18}F-FDG PET/CT showed a PD due to the detection of distant metastasis in the lung and in a supraclavicular node, respectively. Both patients died after 47 and 33 months.

In Case #3 and #4, MRI showed a PR while ^{18}F-FDG PET/CT showed a PD. In particular, in Case #3 the MRI showed a PR while the ^{18}F-FDG PET/CT showed a CR of the primary lesion but also a vertebral metastasis. The patient underwent chemotherapy and died after 33 months. In Case #4, both imaging techniques showed a PR at the level of the cervical lesion but ^{18}F-FDG PET/CT detected also a common iliac lymph node metastasis. The patient underwent anterior exenteration (radical hysterectomy, bilateral salpingo-oophorectomy, total colpectomy, pelvic and para-aortic lymphadenectomy and total cystectomy with Indiana pouch neobladder reconstruction) followed by chemotherapy. The patient is still alive after 102 months of follow-up with no evidence of disease. The pathological evaluation confirmed the ^{18}F-FDG PET/CT findings.

In Cases #5 (Figure 2C,D), #6 and # 7, MRI showed a PR while the ^{18}F-FDG PET/CT showed a CR. Patients #5 and #6 are alive after 48 and 67 months of follow-up, respectively, without evidence of disease and patient # 7 died due to unrelated reasons (hearth attack).

In Case #8 both techniques reported CR in the pelvis but a glucose uptake near to the spleen was observed. The patient underwent surgery in order to remove the upper abdominal lesion and the pathological examination showed a desmoids tumor unrelated to CC. The patient is alive after 49 months of follow-up without evidence of disease.

In Case #9, ^{18}F-FDG PET/CT showed a borderline increase uptake in the primary tumor (SUV_{max} was 3.2), interpreted as a suspicious persistence of disease (PR), although MRI showed no sign of disease (CR); the patient is alive after 79 months of follow-up without evidence of disease.

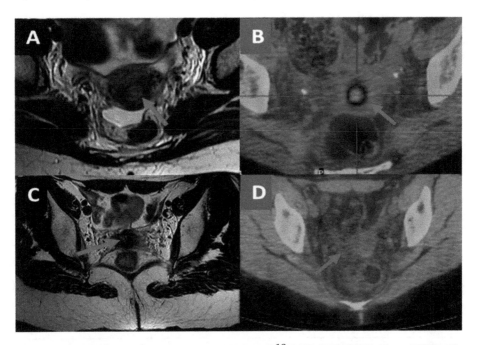

Figure 2. (**A**) and (**B**) show agreement between MRI and ^{18}F-FDG PET/CT after CCRT. The red arrows indicate the residual tumor (partial response). (**C**) and (**D**) show disagreement between MRI and ^{18}F-FDG PET/CT after CCRT. In panel (**C**) the red arrow indicates the residual tumor (partial response) and in (**D**) the red arrow indicates the absence of a tumor (complete response) in MRI and ^{18}F-FDG PET/CT, respectively.

Table 3. Details of discordant cases.

Case	^{18}F-FDG PET/CT	MRI	FU	Localization of Disease and Treatment	Status to the Last FU
1	PD	CR	PD	Lung metastasis (PET) → chemotherapy	DOD
2	PD	CR	PD	Supraclavicular node metastasis (PET) → chemotherapy	DOD
3	PD	PR	PD	Vertebral metastasis (PET) → chemotherapy	DOD
4	PD	PR	PD	Common iliac lymph node metastasis (PET) → anterior pelvectomy and chemotherapy	NED
5	CR	PR	CR	Follow up → no disease	NED
6	CR	PR	CR	Follow up → no disease	NED
7	CR	PR	CR	Follow up → Died for hearth attack	DOC
8	PR	CR	CR	Uptake near the spleen→ Abdominal surgery: desmoid tumor. Follow up → no disease	NED
9	PR	CR	CR	Follow up → no disease	NED

Note: CCRT = concomitant chemo-radiotherapy; CR = complete response; PR = partial response; SD = stable disease; PD = progressive disease; DOD = Died of disease; DOC = Died of other causes; NED = no evidence of disease; FU = follow up.

3.6. Follow-Up Outcomes

According to follow-up data we divided patients in 33 responders (82.5%) and seven non-responders (17.5%) (Table 4). Considering local control and distant metastasis, the number of false positive findings were one for ^{18}F-FDG PET/CT (Case #9) and three for pelvic MRI (Cases #5, #6 and #7). The number of false negative findings were two (Cases #1 and #2) for pelvic MRI and none for ^{18}F-FDG PET/CT.

The agreement between pelvic MRI, ^{18}F-FDG PET/CT and follow-up data showed a Cohen kappa coefficient of 0.59 (95% CI = 0.267–0.913) and of 0.84 (95% CI = 0.636–1.00), respectively.

Considering the evaluation of primary tumor response, ^{18}F-FDG PET/CT was correct in 97.5% of cases and MRI in 92.5% of cases; no false negative cases were observed with both methods.
The 5-year PFS and OS rates were, respectively, 78% and 88% (Figures 3 and 4).

Table 4. Accuracy in the treatment response evaluation of MRI and FDG-PET/CT compared to the follow-up data.

Response	FU data	^{18}F-FDG PET/CT	MRI
Responders (CR)	33 (82.5%)	31 (77.5%)	32 (80%)
Non-responders (PR + SD + PD)	7 (17.5%)	9 (22.5%)	8 (20%)
False Positive Findings	-	1	3
False Negative Findings	-	0	2

Note: CCRT: concomitant chemo-radiation therapy; CR: complete response; PR: partial response; SD: stable disease; PD: progressive disease; FU: follow up.

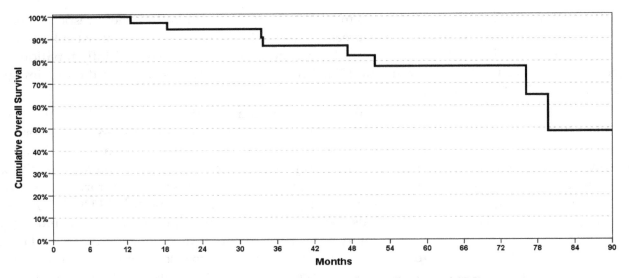

Figure 3. Kaplan–Mayer analysis of overall survival (OS).

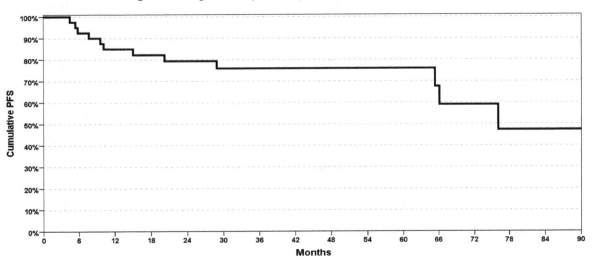

Figure 4. Kaplan–Mayer analysis of progression-free survival (PFS).

4. Discussion

Our retrospective study showed a better correspondence with the follow-up data of ^{18}F-FDG-PET/CT (0.84) with respect to MRI (0.59) in the evaluation of the response to CCR for primary tumor and distant metastasis in T2b CC.

T2b CC represents 38% of CC with the possibility of salvage surgery and complete response to therapy higher than other LACC stages. The persistence of disease in T2b tumors is important to plan salvage surgery. The surgeon's aim is to exclude the diagnosis of disease progression rather than macroscopic parametrial invasion since the therapy is not selective on the parametria but is represented by an exenteration surgery. In the literature, the role of MRI and ^{18}F-FDG-PET/CT before treatment in CC seems well defined. MRI is superior for the assessment of parametrial, vaginal, cervical, bladder and rectum involvement [24,25]. ^{18}F-FDG-PET/CT, instead, is more sensitive in detecting lymph node metastases (pelvic, paraaortic, inguinal and supraclavicular) and peritoneum, mesentery, gastrointestinal tract, pleura and mediastinal involvement [26]. Therefore, both exams are useful in the treatment choice (surgery or CCRT), and in RT planning [27,28]. However, evidence on the evaluation of response to CCRT are weak, although this assessment has a crucial role to decide subsequent treatments [29–32]. To detect residual disease, both clinical and radiological competences are needed. Unfortunately, gynecologic examination after RT is difficult to perform. Indeed, vaginal adhesions and post-RT fibrosis interfere with an accurate visualization of the cervix and with a thorough evaluation of the parametria [33]. Post-RT MRI scans may not optimally evaluate treatment response due to edema/inflammation in T2W hyperintense areas, as well as heterogeneous Gd-contrast enhancement from the main lesion [34]. On the other hand, post radiotherapy necrosis and inflammation may interfere with ^{18}F-FDG-PET/CT evaluation [35]. Therefore, well-defined roles of the two imaging techniques after CCRT are lacking.

In the assessment of primary tumor response, our data found that ^{18}F-FDG-PET/CT is more sensitive (100% versus 80%) and specific (97% versus 89%) than MRI. In fact, three cases correctly diagnosed by PET as CR were false positive using MRI (#5, #6 and #7). When we analyzed the false positive cases found with MRI, we found that probably they were due to the residual fibrosis subsequent to RT as reported in literature [36]. Based on these data, if we had performed only MRI, 20% of our patients would have received an incorrect diagnosis, while with ^{18}F-FDG-PET/CT this percentage would have been of only 3%. False positive results are an important issue: it could require subsequent exams, biopsies and the possibility of over-treatments and complications. These data are supported by a study concluding that MRI accuracy is not enough to select patients who can benefit from completion surgery if residual disease is suspected due to the high false positive rate [37]. In our experience, residual disease with MRI or ^{18}F-FDG-PET/CT after CCRT must be carefully considered before proceeding with further invasive investigations. Instead, in case of negative imaging, no doubt must arise because no false negative cases were observed with both techniques.

The incidence of metastatic progression of disease in LACC is not negligible, particularly in the upper abdomen and chest, even in patients with primary tumor controlled by CCRT. Indeed, in our series, in 10% of cases ^{18}F-FDG PET/CT showed distant metastases (PD) not detectable by pelvic MRI. In our experience, sensitivity and specificity of ^{18}F-FDG PET/CT when we considered distant metastasis was 100% and 97%, respectively; these values were higher than for MRI (71% and 91%, respectively). These values are similar to data from studies reporting 82%–100% and 78%–100% sensitivity and specificity rates for MRI, respectively, and 83%–100% and 50%–100% for ^{18}F-FDG PET/CT, respectively [38,39]. The sensitivity and specificity of PET increases for distant metastases (86% and 100%, respectively). These data highlighted the high diagnostic value of ^{18}F-FDG PET/CT and the importance of a total body evaluation in order to exclude progressive disease even if local control is achieved.

Based on this retrospective analysis we suggest that, after CCRT, ^{18}F-FDG PET/CT is effective in response evaluation and that MRI should only be reserved for special cases. It is not easy to compare the results of our study with those of the literature. To our knowledge there is a lack of studies that focused on the direct comparison between 18F-FDG PET/CT and MRI in in the response evaluation after CCRT in LACC stage T2b.

Waldestrom et al. examined 25 LACC patients (stages IB2–IIIB) with both MRI and ^{18}F-FDG PET/CT before and after CCRT and found that in almost half of the patients the ^{18}F-FDG-PET/CT before treatment provided additional diagnostic information leading to changes in treatment planning compared to information from MRI. MRI, instead, detected pelvic tumor spread not seen on the ^{18}F-FDG-PET/CT in 2/24 patients. [40]. On the contrary, a metanalysis of 15 studies of Maeds et al. evaluated the diagnostic accuracy of additional whole body ^{18}F-FDG PET/CT compared with conventional imaging in women with suspected recurrent/persistent cervical cancer, concluding that the use of ^{18}F-FDG PET/CT in recurrent cervical cancer and its endorsement by national guidelines is not supported by the literature. However, none of the studies included in this metanalysis directly compared additional PET–CT with MRI or CT separately, and the included populations were very heterogeneous and often follow-up periods were short. [41].

The results of other studies are generally based on the analysis of a single imaging technique, ^{18}F-FDG PET/CT [42,43] or CT/MRI [44], or reported that the addition of ^{18}F-FDG PET/CT to other imaging techniques increases the sensitivity and specificity [45]. Finally, no studies compared ^{18}F-FDG PET/CT with MRI and all studies had a short follow-up period. This fact represents an evident problem considering that follow-up accuracy and duration are important to confirm the radiological results, being a pathological response not available in case of CCRT. On the contrary, our study is supported by long-term follow up of 50 ± 26 months (mean ± SD), with overall survival results (Figure 3) consistent with data in the literature.

Some considerations about false positive of ^{18}F-FDG PET/CT are required. Case #8 developed a new and benign tumor, not related to the LACC. We considered this case as FP but probably it should be better considered as a concomitant disease. Case #9 was a borderline glucose case, which was not considered as a positive lesion and therefore the patient received no subsequent treatments.

Limitations of our study were the retrospective nature of the analysis and the small sample size, while strengths of the study could be considered the prolonged follow-up and the well-defined setting of patients. Further studies are needed to confirm our findings in a prospective setting.

5. Conclusions

In conclusion, ^{18}F-FDG PET/CT seems to be superior to pelvic MRI in the evaluation of the treatment response to CCRT in T2b CC. In addition, in some cases ^{18}F-FDG PET/CT detected distant metastasis resulting in a change in the therapeutic strategy. Further studies are needed to confirm that ^{18}F-FDG PET/CT should be the standard option, almost six months after the end of CCRT in LACC, to evaluate the treatment response. These results may suggest that ^{18}F-FDG-PET/CT is a unique diagnostic imaging tool to use after CCRT in order to correctly assess residual and progression disease.

Author Contributions: Conceptualization, A.M.P. and P.D.I.; methodology, S.F. and A.G.M.; software, M.T. and M.F.; validation, A.G. and M.F.; formal analysis, A.M.P and G.D.; investigation, A.M.P and P.D.I.; resources, M.C., P.C. and C.N.; data curation, G.D. and E.D.C.; writing—original draft preparation, A.M.P.; writing—review and editing, G.D. and S.T.; visualization, M.C., C.N. and P.C.; supervision, A.G.M. and S.F.; project administration, P.D.I. All authors have read and agreed to the published version of the manuscript.

Acknowledgments: The authors are grateful to Stefano Friso for data collection and statistical analysis.

References

1. Jemal, A.; Siegel, R.; Ward, E.; Hao, Y.; Xu, J.; Thun, M.J. Cancer statistics. *CA Cancer J. Clin.* **2009**, *59*, 225–249. [CrossRef] [PubMed]

2. Ries, L.A.G.; Melbert, D.; Krapcho, M.; Stinchcomb, D.G.; Howlader, N.; Horner, M.J.; Mariotto, A.; Miller, B.A.; Feuer, E.J.; Altekruse, S.F.; et al. *SEER Cancer Statistics Review, 1975–2005*; National Cancer Institute: Bethesda, MD, USA, 2008.

3. Cibula, D.; Pötter, R.; Planchamp, F.; Åvall-Lundqvist, E.; Fischerova, D.; Meder, C.H.; Köhler, C.; Landoni, F.; Lax, S.; Lindegaard, J.C.; et al. The European Society of Gynaecological Oncology/European Society for Radiotherapy and Oncology/European Society of Pathology Guidelines for the Management of Patients with Cervical Cancer. *Int. J. Gynecol. Cancer* **2018**, *28*, 641–655. [CrossRef] [PubMed]

4. Bhatla, N.; Berek, J.S.; Fredes, M.C.; Denny, L.A.; Grenman, S.; Karunaratne, K.; Kehoe, S.T.; Konishi, I.; Olawaiye, A.B.; Prat, J.; et al. Revised FIGO staging for carcinoma of the cervix uteri. *Int. J. Gynecol. Obstet.* **2019**, *145*, 129–135. [CrossRef] [PubMed]

5. Brierley, J.; Gospodarowicz, M.K.; Wittekind, C. *TNM Classification of Malignant Tumours*; Wiley: Chichester, UK, 2017.

6. Marth, C.; Landoni, F.; Mahner, S.; McCormack, M.; Gonzalez-Martin, A.; Colombo, N. Cervical cancer: ESMO Clinical Practice Guidelines for diagnosis, treatment and follow-up. *Ann. Oncol.* **2017**, *28*, iv72–iv83. [CrossRef]

7. Fagotti, A.; Anchora, L.P.; Conte, C.; Chiantera, V.; Vizza, E.; Tortorella, L.; Surico, D.; De Iaco, P.; Corrado, G.; Fanfani, F.; et al. Beyond sentinel node algorithm. Toward a more tailored surgery for cervical cancer patients. *Cancer Med.* **2016**, *5*, 1725–1730. [CrossRef]

8. Fanfani, F.; Vizza, E.; Landoni, F.; De Iaco, P.; Ferrandina, G.; Corrado, G.; Gallotta, V.; Gambacorta, M.A.; Fagotti, A.; Monterossi, G.; et al. Radical hysterectomy after chemoradiation in FIGO stage III cervical cancer patients versus chemoradiation and brachytherapy: Complications and 3-years survival. *Eur. J. Surg. Oncol.* **2016**, *42*, 1519–1525. [CrossRef]

9.   Ferrandina, G.; Anchora, L.P.; Gallotta, V.; Fagotti, A.; Vizza, E.; Chiantera, V.; De Iaco, P.; Ercoli, A.; Corrado, G.; Bottoni, C.; et al. Can We Define the Risk of Lymph Node Metastasis in Early-Stage Cervical Cancer Patients? A Large-Scale, Retrospective Study. *Ann. Surg. Oncol.* **2017**, *24*, 2311–2318. [CrossRef]

10.   Koh, W.-J.; Abu-Rustum, N.R.; Bean, S.; Bradley, K.; Campos, S.M.; Cho, K.R.; Chon, H.S.; Chu, C.; Clark, R.; Cohn, D.; et al. Cervical Cancer, Version 3.2019, NCCN Clinical Practice Guidelines in Oncology. *J. Natl. Compr. Cancer Netw.* **2019**, *17*, 64–84. [CrossRef]

11.   Chemoradiotherapy for Cervical Cancer Meta-Analysis Collaboration (CCCMAC) Reducing uncertainties about the effects of chemoradiotherapy for cervical cancer: Individual patient data meta-analysis. *Cochrane Database Syst. Rev.* **2010**, 008285.

12.   Onal, C.; Reyhan, M.; Guler, O.C.; Yapar, A.F. Treatment outcomes of patients with cervical cancer with complete metabolic responses after definitive chemoradiotherapy. *Eur. J. Nucl. Med. Mol. Imaging* **2014**, *41*, 1336–1342. [CrossRef]

13.   Quinn, M.; Benedet, J.; Odicino, F.; Maisonneuve, P.; Beller, U.; Creasman, W.T.; Heintz, A.; Ngan, H.; Pecorelli, S. Carcinoma of the Cervix Uteri. *Int. J. Gynecol. Obstet.* **2006**, *95*, S43–S103. [CrossRef]

14.   Herrera, F.G.; Prior, J.O. The role of PET/CT in cervical cancer. *Front. Oncol.* **2013**, *3*. [CrossRef] [PubMed]

15.   Schwarz, J.K.; Siegel, B.A.; Dehdashti, F.; Schwarz, J.K. Association of Posttherapy Positron Emission Tomography with Tumor Response and Survival in Cervical Carcinoma. *JAMA* **2007**, *298*, 2289. [CrossRef] [PubMed]

16.   Hricak, H. Cancer of the uterus: The value of mri pre- and post-irradiation. *Int. J. Radiat. Oncol.* **1991**, *21*, 1089–1094. [CrossRef]

17.   Saida, T.; Tanaka, Y.O.; Ohara, K.; Oki, A.; Sato, T.; Yoshikawa, H.; Minami, M. Can MRI predict local control rate of uterine cervical cancer immediately after radiation therapy? *Magn. Reson. Med Sci.* **2010**, *9*, 141–148. [CrossRef] [PubMed]

18.   Salani, R.; Khanna, N.; Frimer, M.; Bristow, R.E.; Chen, L.-M. An update on post-treatment surveillance and diagnosis of recurrence in women with gynecologic malignancies: Society of Gynecologic Oncology (SGO) recommendations. *Gynecol. Oncol.* **2017**, *146*, 3–10. [CrossRef]

19.   Hequet, D.; Marchand, E.; Place, V.; Fourchotte, V.; De La Rochefordière, A.; Dridi, S.; Coutant, C.; Lécuru, F.; Bats, A.-S.; Koskas, M.; et al. Evaluation and impact of residual disease in locally advanced cervical cancer after concurrent chemoradiation therapy: Results of a multicenter study. *Eur. J. Surg. Oncol.* **2013**, *39*, 1428–1434. [CrossRef]

20.   Kurman, R.J. World Health Organization Classification of Tumours of Female Reproductive Organs. In *World Health Organization Classification of Tumours*, 4th ed.; International Agency for Research on Cancer: Lyon, France, 2014.

21.   International Commission on Radiation Units and Measurements. *Dose and Volume Specification for Reporting Intracavitary Brachytherapy in Gynecology*; (ICRU) Report 38; The Commission: Bethesda, MD, USA, 1985.

22.   Eisenhauer, E.A.; Therasse, P.; Bogaerts, J.; Schwartz, L.; Sargent, D.; Ford, R.; Dancey, J.; Arbuck, S.; Gwyther, S.; Mooney, M.; et al. New response evaluation criteria in solid tumours: Revised RECIST guideline (version 1.1). *Eur. J. Cancer* **2009**, *45*, 228–247. [CrossRef]

23.   Young, H.; Baum, R.; Cremerius, U.; Herholz, K.; Hoekstra, O.; Lammertsma, A.A.; Pruim, J.; Price, P. Measurement of clinical and subclinical tumour response using [18F]-fluorodeoxyglucose and positron emission tomography: Review and 1999 EORTC recommendations. *Eur. J. Cancer* **1999**, *35*, 1773–1782. [CrossRef]

24.   Park, J.J.; Kim, C.K.; Park, B.K. Prediction of disease progression following concurrent chemoradiotherapy for uterine cervical cancer: Value of post-treatment diffusion-weighted imaging. *Eur. Radiol.* **2015**, *26*, 3272–3279. [CrossRef]

25.   Freeman, S.; Aly, A.M.; Kataoka, M.Y.; Addley, H.C.; Reinhold, C.; Sala, E. The Revised FIGO Staging System for Uterine Malignancies: Implications for MR Imaging. *Radiographics* **2012**, *32*, 1805–1827. [CrossRef] [PubMed]

26.   Yen, T.-C.; Ng, K.-K.; Ma, S.-Y.; Chou, H.-H.; Tsai, C.-S.; Hsueh, S.; Chang, T.-C.; Hong, J.-H.; See, L.-C.; Lin, W.-J.; et al. Value of Dual-Phase 2-Fluoro-2-Deoxy-d-Glucose Positron Emission Tomography in Cervical Cancer. *J. Clin. Oncol.* **2003**, *21*, 3651–3658. [CrossRef] [PubMed]

27.   Kusmirek, J.; Robbins, J.; Allen, H.; Barroilhet, L.; Anderson, B.; Sadowski, E. PET/CT and MRI in the imaging assessment of cervical cancer. *Abdom. Imaging* **2015**, *40*, 2486–2511. [CrossRef] [PubMed]

28. Cima, S.; Perrone, A.M.; Castellucci, P.; Macchia, G.; Buwenge, M.; Cammelli, S.; Cilla, S.; Ferioli, M.; Ferrandina, G.; Galuppi, A.; et al. Prognostic Impact of Pretreatment Fluorodeoxyglucose Positron Emission Tomography/Computed Tomography SUVmax in Patients with Locally Advanced Cervical Cancer. *Int. J. Gynecol. Cancer* **2018**, *28*, 575–580. [CrossRef] [PubMed]

29. Lima, G.M.; Matti, A.; Vara, G.; Dondi, G.; Naselli, N.; De Crescenzo, E.M.; Morganti, A.; Perrone, A.M.; De Iaco, P.; Nanni, C.; et al. Prognostic value of posttreatment 18F-FDG PET/CT and predictors of metabolic response to therapy in patients with locally advanced cervical cancer treated with concomitant chemoradiation therapy: An analysis of intensity- and volume-based PET parameters. *Eur. J. Nucl. Med. Mol. Imaging* **2018**, *45*, 2139–2146. [CrossRef]

30. Dessole, M.; Petrillo, M.; Lucidi, A.; Naldini, A.; Rossi, M.; De Iaco, P.; Marnitz, S.; Sehouli, J.; Scambia, G.; Chiantera, V. Quality of Life in Women After Pelvic Exenteration for Gynecological Malignancies. *Int. J. Gynecol. Cancer* **2018**, *28*, 267–273. [CrossRef]

31. Perrone, A.M.; Livi, A.; Fini, M.; Bondioli, E.; Concetti, S.; Morganti, A.; Contedini, F.; De Iaco, P. A surgical multi-layer technique for pelvic reconstruction after total exenteration using a combination of pedicled omental flap, human acellular dermal matrix and autologous adipose derived cells. *Gynecol. Oncol. Rep.* **2016**, *18*, 36–39. [CrossRef]

32. Chiantera, V.; Rossi, M.; De Iaco, P.; Koehler, C.; Marnitz, S.; Ferrandina, G.; Legge, F.; Parazzini, F.; Scambia, G.; Schneider, A.; et al. Survival After Curative Pelvic Exenteration for Primary or Recurrent Cervical Cancer: A Retrospective Multicentric Study of 167 Patients. *Int. J. Gynecol. Cancer* **2014**, *24*, 916–922. [CrossRef]

33. Galuppi, A.; Perrone, A.M.; La Macchia, M.; Santini, N.; Medoro, S.; Maccarini, L.R.; Strada, I.; Pozzati, F.; Rossi, M.; De Iaco, P. Local α-Tocopherol for Acute and Short-Term Vaginal Toxicity Prevention in Patients Treated with Radiotherapy for Gynecologic Tumors. *Int. J. Gynecol. Cancer* **2011**, *21*, 1708–1711. [CrossRef]

34. Jeong, Y.Y.; Kang, H.K.; Chung, T.W.; Seo, J.J.; Park, J.G. Uterine Cervical Carcinoma after Therapy: CT and MR Imaging Findings. *Radiographics* **2003**, *23*, 969–981. [CrossRef]

35. Schwarz, J.K.; Siegel, B.A.; Dehdashti, F.; Rader, J.; Zoberi, I. Posttherapy [18F] Fluorodeoxyglucose Positron Emission Tomography in Carcinoma of the Cervix: Response and Outcome. *J. Clin. Oncol.* **2004**, *22*, 2167–2171.

36. Wang, J.; Boerma, M.; Fu, Q.; Hauer-Jensen, M. Radiation responses in skin and connective tissues: Effect on wound healing and surgical outcome. *Hernia* **2006**, *10*, 502–506. [CrossRef] [PubMed]

37. Vincens, E.; Balleyguier, C.; Rey, A.; Uzan, C.; Zareski, E.; Gouy, S.; Pautier, P.; Duvillard, P.; Haie-Meder, C.; Morice, P. Accuracy of magnetic resonance imaging in predicting residual disease in patients treated for stage IB2/II cervical carcinoma with chemoradiation therapy. *Cancer* **2008**, *113*, 2158–2165. [CrossRef] [PubMed]

38. Viswanathan, C.; Faria, S.; Devine, C.; Patnana, M.; Sagebiel, T.; Iyer, R.B.; Bhosale, P. [18F]-2-Fluoro-2-Deoxy-D-glucose–PET Assessment of Cervical Cancer. *PET Clin.* **2018**, *13*, 165–177. [CrossRef]

39. Otero-García, M.M.; Mesa-Álvarez, A.; Nikolic, O.; Blanco-Lobato, P.; Basta-Nikolic, M.; De Llano-Ortega, R.M.; Paredes-Velázquez, L.; Nikolic, N.; Szewczyk-Bieda, M. Role of MRI in staging and follow-up of endometrial and cervical cancer: Pitfalls and mimickers. *Insights Imaging* **2019**, *10*, 19. [CrossRef]

40. Waldenström, A.-C.; Bergmark, K.; Michanek, A.; Hashimi, F.; Norrlund, R.R.; Olsson, C.E.; Gjertsson, P.; Leonhardt, H. A comparison of two imaging modalities for detecting lymphatic nodal spread in radiochemotherapy of locally advanced cervical cancer. *Phys. Imaging Radiat. Oncol.* **2018**, *8*, 33–37. [CrossRef]

41. Meads, C.; Davenport, C.; Małysiak-Szpond, S.; Kowalska, M.; Zapalska, A.; Guest, P.; Martin-Hirsch, P.; Borowiack, E.; Auguste, P.; Barton, P.; et al. Evaluating PET-CT in the detection and management of recurrent cervical cancer: Systematic reviews of diagnostic accuracy and subjective elicitation. *BJOG: Int. J. Obstet. Gynaecol.* **2013**, *121*, 398–407. [CrossRef]

42. Son, S.H.; Jeong, S.Y.; Chong, G.O.; Lee, Y.H.; Park, S.-H.; Lee, C.-H.; Jeong, J.H.; Lee, S.-W.; Ahn, B.-C.; Lee, J.; et al. Prognostic Value of Pretreatment Metabolic PET Parameters in Cervical Cancer Patients with Metabolic Complete Response After Concurrent Chemoradiotherapy. *Clin. Nucl. Med.* **2018**, *43*, e296–e303. [CrossRef]

43. Ryu, S.-Y.; Kim, M.-H.; Choi, S.-C.; Choi, C.-W.; Lee, K.H. Detection of early recurrence with 18F-FDG PET in patients with cervical cancer. *J. Nucl. Med.* **2003**, *44*.

44.   Park, J.J.; Kim, C.K.; Park, S.Y.; Park, B.K. Parametrial Invasion in Cervical Cancer: Fused T2-weighted Imaging and High-b-Value Diffusion-weighted Imaging with Background Body Signal Suppression at 3 T. *Radiology* **2015**, *274*, 734–741. [CrossRef]

45.   Grisaru, D.; Almog, B.; Levine, C.; Metser, U.; Fishman, A.; Lerman, H.; Lessing, J.B.; Even-Sapir, E. The diagnostic accuracy of 18F-Fluorodeoxyglucose PET/CT in patients with gynecological malignancies. *Gynecol. Oncol.* **2004**, *94*, 680–684. [CrossRef] [PubMed]

13

Ten Important Considerations for Ovarian Cancer Screening

Edward J. Pavlik

Division of Gynecologic Oncology, Department of Obstetrics and Gynecology, The University of Kentucky Chandler Medical Center and the Markey Cancer Center, Lexington, KY 40536-0293, USA; epaul1@uky.edu

Academic Editor: Andreas Kjaer

Abstract: The unique intricacies of ovarian cancer screening and perspectives of different screening methods are presented as ten considerations that are examined. Included in these considerations are: *(1) Deciding on the number of individuals to be screened; (2) Anticipating screening group reductions due to death; (3) Deciding on the duration and frequency of screening; (4) Deciding on an appropriate follow-up period after screening; (5) Deciding on time to surgery when malignancy is suspected; (6) Deciding on how screen-detected ovarian cancers are treated and by whom; (7) Deciding on how to treat the data of enrolled participants; (8) Deciding on the most appropriate way to assign disease-specific death; (9) Deciding how to avoid biases caused by enrollments that attract participants with late-stage disease who are either symptomatic or disposed by factors that are genetic, environmental or social; and (10) Deciding whether the screening tool or a screening process is being tested.* These considerations are presented in depth along with illustrations of how they impact the outcomes of ovarian cancer screening. The considerations presented provide alternative explanations of effects that have an important bearing on interpreting ovarian screening outcomes.

Keywords: ovarian; cancer; screening; considerations

1. Introduction

Screening for different cancers, can appear similar; however, closer inspection reveals that there are considerable differences in approaches to cancer screening. This report focuses on the factors, issues and characteristics that uniquely distinguish ovarian cancer screening.

2. The Bare-Bones Basics of Screening

Cancer screening can be over-simplified so that it is conceived as the application of a test that discriminates malignancy. In general, the test for malignancy can be image-based or reagent-based. Image-based screening utilizes the identification of peculiar visual features not unlike correctly finding Waldo in an illustration that contains Waldo and other characters that may resemble Waldo to some degree [1]. Identification skills and sufficient time to complete the visual assignments are central to an image-based approach. Biomarker-based screening utilizes a chemical outcome which gives a result that discriminates malignancy, usually through a cut-off value above which malignancy becomes more likely. This approach can be thought of as asking the test for a "yes" vs. "no" answer about malignancy. This is best illustrated by the cut-off value of CA-125 (*cancer antigen 125*) for recurrent malignancy. However, one should be mindful that CA-125 becomes elevated by a variety of benign conditions [2]. Overlap in the outcome values of both malignant and non-malignant tests on both sides of the cut-off can occur with biomarker-based screening tests.

The key concept described above is "discrimination of malignancy". In simple terms this implies finding malignancy at a high rate, missing malignancy at a low rate, and testing non-malignancy as malignancy at a low rate. To do this, protocols that test screening discrimination must be designed to assess screening effectiveness.

3. Collecting Evidence to Examine Screening Effectiveness—Perspective Analysis for a Prospective Screening Trial

3.1. Consideration 1

Deciding on the Number of Individuals to Be Screened

After the screening tool has been selected, the first step is to make decisions about the size of the screening group framed against a time period needed to accumulate that number of screens. This time frame must be long enough to include a sufficient number of incident cases to give the incident portion of the study power because it is the screening detection of incident cases that can be expected to be at an early stage and demonstrate the clearest benefit from screening. In the Kentucky Ovarian Screening trial, approximately half the malignancies detected by screening were incident [3], and this suggests that the sample size predicted apriori by power analysis probably should be twice as large as a power prediction based on both prevalent and incident cases. For simplicity, incident cases can be defined as those detections that occur after receiving at least one normal screen. This sample enlarged for incidence should be able to distinguish screening effectiveness in prevalent vs. incident cases. A key issue is utilization of a standard of significance to determine power and test results in order to guarantee reproducibility. By comparing Bayesian hypothesis testing with classical hypothesis tests, it has been reported that thresholds for a significance finding should be changed to $p < 0.005$ [4], however, doing such would increase sample size, duration of the trial and ultimately costs [5]. Others favor less stringency and including assessments of actual costs, benefits and probabilities [6]. A potential solution is possible by balancing a weighted sum of type I (false positive) and type II (false negative) errors [7,8]. Bearing in mind that the present status of the UK Collaborative Trial of Ovarian Cancer Screening (UKCTOCS) [9] is an inability to detect a significant statistical difference in survival between screened and unscreened women, the chance of not detecting a difference between groups must be respected [10] by the doubling of sample size as outlined above. Although other factors have been enumerated that are responsible for research findings that are false [11], they do not mitigate the mistake of insufficient power based on choosing too low a level of significance.

3.2. Consideration 2

Anticipating Screening Group Reductions due to Death

Based on family reports and the Social Security Death Index (SSDI), 7.7% of 42,000+ participants in the Kentucky Ovarian Cancer Screening trial died after they began participating, with women over age 75 accounting for 70% of these deaths (Figure 1). Because of participants providing incorrect identifying information and due to the 3-year lag in listing on the SSDI, it is reasonable to expect an overall reduction in the screened population due to death of ~10%. Importantly, as the follow-up window extends to older age groups, a reduction in the screened population due to death of participants that can be followed for disease-specific survival will occur. This increase should be anticipated and used to adjust the group size predicted by power analysis.

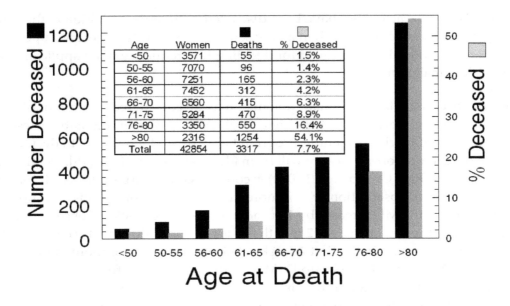

Age	Women	Deaths	% Deceased
<50	3571	55	1.5%
50-55	7070	96	1.4%
56-60	7251	165	2.3%
61-65	7452	312	4.2%
66-70	6560	415	6.3%
71-75	5284	470	8.9%
76-80	3350	550	16.4%
>80	2316	1254	54.1%
Total	42854	3317	7.7%

Figure 1. Age at death of screening participants.

3.3. Consideration 3

Deciding on the Duration and Frequency of Screening

The four major ovarian screening trials [3,9,12,13] used a periodic annual screening approach that accrued participants for 4.6–28.1 years and continued screening after enrollment for 7.7–28.1 years [14]. Two trials have employed a serial evaluation of abnormal screens [9,15]. Duration of the screening portion of the trial is a function of the sample needed and the resources made available to screen. A more difficult question regards frequency of screening. Screening high-risk women every six months has been practiced in the Kentucky trial without prior demonstration of benefit. The repeat screening interval after an abnormal screening exam is more subjective and has been performed at 3–6-month intervals on ovarian abnormalities that appear to be of low risk (cysts and cysts with septations) and at 4-week intervals for 3 months on ovarian tumors of uncertain malignant potential [16]. Annual follow-up for five years has been recommended for ovarian abnormalities that remain stable on several surveillance intervals of < 6 months [16].

A simplified picture of screening frequency is that women with a normal result be scheduled for annual screening, women with a result that is low risk for malignancy are screened more frequently and those with high risk for malignancy or with an abnormality of uncertain malignant potential are screened even more frequently. However, by what method can a result be assigned to one of these categories that minimizes subjectivity? Several characteristics are associated with an expected low risk grouping: (unilocular or septate morphology, morphology index (MI) = 4 or less, ΔMI less than 1.0/month, low-risk Assessment of Different NEoplasias in the adneXa or ADNEX score, absence of Doppler flow, CA125 (Cancer Antigen 125 <200 units/mL premenopausal or < 35 postmenopausal), CA125 stable/month, OVA1 (<5.0 premenopausal or <4.4 postmenopausal, OVA1 is the first multivariate index assay with FDA clearance), low-risk Risk of MAlignancy (ROMA) test, [17], absence of pelvic fluid), while others are associated with considering a high risk grouping (complex or solid morphology, MI >4, ΔMI (1.0/month or greater), high-risk ADNEX score, central Doppler flow, CA125 ($\geq$200 units/mL premenopausal or $\geq$35 postmenopausal), CA125 (doubling within a month), OVA1 ($\geq$5 premenopausal or $\geq$4.4 postmenopausal), high risk ROMA [17], pelvic ascites >60 cm^3). These characteristics have been discussed with more definition in the context of low- and high-risk groups elsewhere [16]. When a new screening modality is decided upon, one or more of these characteristics should be employed for deciding the frequency of its application based upon a potential for risk of malignancy.

An abnormality of uncertain malignant potential may be considered as a tumor of indeterminate status. Following these abnormalities for either resolution or worsening status presents a logical rationale. The Kentucky Ovarian screening Program has activated a protocol to decide if continuing surveillance or a decision-favoring surgery will be made based on findings [18]. In this protocol, four risk groups are defined. Risk Group A (MI$_0$ 0–2) is considered for surgery if the MI increases by 2 or more in the first 4 weeks of observation or 3 or more in the next 12 months. Risk Group B (MI$_0$ 3–4) is considered for surgery if the MI increases by 1 or more in the first 4 weeks of observation or 2 or more in the next 12 months (observation at 3 & 12 months). Risk Group C (MI$_0$ 5–6) is considered for surgery if the MI increases by 1 or more in the first 4 weeks of observation or 1 or more in the next 12 months (observation at 3, 6, 12 months). Risk Group D (MI$_0$ 7–10) is considered for surgery if the MI increases by 1 or more or remains unchanged in the first 4 weeks of observation. Thus, this protocol utilizes variable periods of observation that are determined by the level of risk determined initially (MI$_0$).

3.4. Consideration 4

Deciding on an Appropriate Follow-Up Period after Screening

An overly simple view of follow-up after screening is that it should extend long enough after the last participant in the screening trial has been screened to adequately assess the effect of screening on survival. However, a lesson learned from the UKCTOCS trial is that incident cancers occur after the first screen so that the follow-up for survival can be expected to be extended by one or more years. In the UKCTOCS trial, 4.6 years of screening accrual was coupled to 6.1 years of periodic screening and a final 3.1 years of follow-up. Secondly, over the course of a trial that occupies a decade of time, new treatments can be expected to be introduced that extend survival. Taken together, a longer follow-up extended to 10 years might be more appropriate for the UKCTOCS screening model to adequately assess the effect of screening on survival.

3.5. Consideration 5

Deciding on Time to Surgery When Malignancy Is Suspected

A 40-day tumor doubling time for ovarian malignancy has been estimated using the doubling of CA-125 [19]. While tumor doubling time may vary in different tumors, a 40-day doubling estimate is a good mid-range value [20]. Using this doubling time (Figure 2), comparative increases in size indicate that if the interval between a screen-detected abnormality and surgery is prolonged, tumor size will advance considerably. The mean volume of early stage ovarian malignancies (Stage I & II) detected by the Kentucky Ovarian Cancer Screening Program is 115 cm^3 (±26.7 (SEM)). This represents enlargement to about 75% the size of an orange (Figure 2 black dashed line) and upon removal is associated with significantly extended survival. After 90 days, malignant tumors with an initial volume of up to twice the size of the ovary will approach or exceed the size of an orange and this indicates that the time to surgery should be limited to well under 90 days after a screening is decided to be indicative of malignancy. Efforts in the Kentucky Ovarian Cancer Screening Program limit the time to surgery to less than 30 days to minimize the opportunity for an early stage screening detection to develop into advanced disease diagnosed at surgery. In contrast, the Prostate, Lung, Colorectal and Ovarian Cancer (PLCO) Screening Trial [13] allowed the time to surgery to extend for up to 9 months, a duration that would allow very considerable increases in tumor burden and the opportunity for the development of disease diagnosed at an advanced stage.

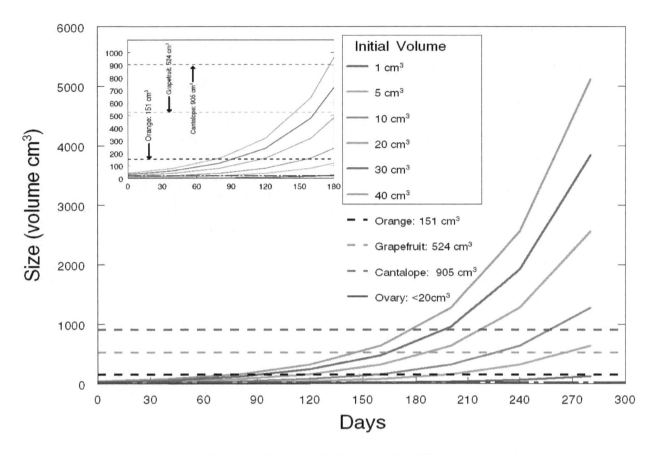

Figure 2. Ovarian Malignancy Doubling.

3.6. Consideration 6

Deciding on How Screen-Detected Ovarian Cancers Are Treated and by Whom

It has recently been recognized that better outcomes are achieved when ovarian cancer is treated by specialists at high volume hospitals [21–29]. No provision for treatment by specialists in high volume hospitals was included in the PLCO trial [13]. Consequently, it is likely that the treatment component of this trial under-performed the detection component and accounted for less than optimal survivals. In order to reduce confounding factors due to treatment that could be deleterious for survival, an ovarian screening trial should limit treatment to high-volume centers by a gynecologic oncologist adhering to National Comprehensive Cancer Network guidelines so that optimal therapy based on staging will be provided. Doing so may be particularly appropriate for early stage ovarian cancer in order that chemotherapy can be utilized in high grade tumors [29,30].

3.7. Consideration 7

Deciding on How to Treat the Data of Enrolled Participants

In the PLCO trial [13], the UKCTOCS trial [9,31] and the Shizuoka Cohort Study of Ovarian Cancer Screening (SCSOCS) trial [12], enrollment in the screening arm was subject to intention to treat (ITT) analysis so that participants were analyzed in the group to which they were originally randomized: "once randomized an individual was always analyzed", even if they were assigned to the screening arm, but never were screened or never received treatment. In this model anything that occurs after randomization is ignored, including non-compliance, protocol deviations, and withdrawal [32]. In contrast, in the Kentucky Ovarian Screening Program [3], only participants that completed the screening and treatment phases of the protocol were analyzed as a per protocol population. ITT analysis strongly favors preserving sample size so that originating power estimates continue to apply. The null hypothesis in a screening trial is that screening does not work. In the simplest sense, this null hypothesis is true if screening is falsely claimed to have a positive effect on disease, but positive screens cannot have a positive effect on disease if treatment is absent or sub-optimal. Individuals in the screening arm that do not receive screening and treatment will make the screening arm less distinguishable from the control arm, while individuals in the non-screening control arm that do receive screening and treatment will make the control arm less distinguishable from the screening arm. ITT analysis gives equal weight to each of these alternatives without testing for balance. Individuals who will seek out, schedule, attend and pay for screening are likely to occur less frequently than those who are assigned to the screening group but become non-compliant for receiving screens and treatment. This imbalance of never-screened individuals in the screening group is more likely to be greater than individuals who cross over to screening in the control group and will dilute the effectiveness of screening. This imbalance will not occur in a protocol-driven trial where unscreened/untreated individuals in the screening arm are censored, as well as individuals, screened independent of the protocol, in the unscreened control arm. In the PLCO trial, this imbalance consisted of 24 never-screened cases within the screening group, 21 untreated screen-positive cases in the screening group, and 8 cases in the screening group that were sub-optimally treated because they did not receive chemotherapy and accounted for 25% of the 212 malignancies reported in the screening group [13]. For the unscreened control arm, 25 untreated cases and 5 sub-optimally treated cases were reported or 17% of the 176 malignancies reported in the control arm [13]. No information was reported on how many cases in the control arm obtained treatment based on seeking access to the screening method. In summary, to test the question "Does screening work?" only cases of positive screens in the intervention group should be included that received treatment adhering to National Comprehensive Cancer Network guidelines, while the control group should identify and censor cross-over cases that obtained out-of-protocol screening.

The PLCO investigators decided to interpret the interval of protection conferred by screening to extend considerably beyond one year. Re-examination of the PLCO data by other investigators that limited the analysis to cancers detected within one year of screening showed that the survival in the screening group was significantly better than in the control group ($p = 0.0017$) and contained fewer Stage IV cases [33]. Thus, it is important to realize that malignancies that appear several years after screening should not be included in the intervention group, and should be censored as an "out-of-screening cycle" event.

3.8. Consideration 8

Deciding on the Most Appropriate Way to Assign Disease-Specific Death

Facile assignment of mortality due to disease is death that occurs with evidence of disease while under treatment for ovarian cancer, meeting the requirement used in both the PLCO and UKCTOS trials that *the disease process and/or associated treatments initiated or sustained a chain of events causally responsible for death.* Conversely, a sudden death with no evidence of disease is a death clearly due to other causes. Conditions for assigning disease-specific death are complicated when disease is evident and a sudden death occurs. Accidents, suicide, diabetic death, stroke and cardiac failure may be responsible for these complications. Difficult assignments of cause of death occur when reporting is incomplete. Both the PLCO trial and the UKCTOCS trial adjudicate disease-specific death differently [34,35]. The PLCO trial incorporated efforts to determine the underlying cause of death through periodic updates of questionnaires, cancer registries, and attempted contacts with next-of-kin and personal physicians (Table 1). Different procedures were used after the first two years of the PLCO trial to ascertain the underlying cause of death. The global resource available to the PLCO trial was the National Death Index which restricts the release of information until three years after any death has occurred. Admittedly, more information was available to the PLCO trial for screened cancers than for unscreened cancers and the control group [35]. The UKCTOCS trial had much greater global access to cancer and death registrations using the National Health Service (NHS) number of participants to access information from the Health & Social Care Information Center, the National Cancer Intelligence Network, Hospital Episodes Statistics, Central Services Agency, the Northern Ireland Cancer Registry, and the Hospital Episodes Statistical records (Table 2). To resolve the underlying cause of death, two pathologists and two gynecologic oncologists relied upon an algorithm involving disease progression (new lesions or increase in size of original lesions by imaging), clinical worsening, or rising biomarkers. Clearly the UKCTOCS had a more comprehensive access to death and factors related to cause of death through information arising in national health services.

Table 1. Mortality review in the Prostate, Lung, Colorectal and Ovarian Cancer Screening (PLCO) trial.

PLCO	PLCO	PLCO
Death due to ovarian cancer	The disease process and/or associated treatments initiated or sustained a chain of events causally responsible for death	Identify other underlying cause of death
Annual update questionnaire	Periodic	
Population-based cancer registries	Whenever possible	
Linkage to National Death Index	Periodic	
Obtained diagnostic medical records: Abstracted by registrars: stage, histology , grade, and treatment	Reviewers blinded to participation in screened vs. unscreened arm	Identify next of kin and personal physician
Underlying cause of death: first 2 years	Death certificate & relevant determinations underlying cause of death	Potential, ovarian cancer deaths, deaths of unknown or uncertain deaths were reviewed by at least 1 member of a panel of expertise (2 reviewers with discrepancies decided by a third)
Underlying cause of death: after year 2	Primary reviewer considered records without access to death certificate	If primary review disagreed with death certificate, a second expert reviewed record & death certificate. Disagreement triggered another independent review which led to a resolution by meeting or teleconference
Attempt to collect identical death information from both screen-detected and non-screen detected cancers	Screen-detected cancers will have more extensive information collected	Less information for both unscreened group participants & screened false positives

Table 2. Mortality review in the UK Collaborative Trial of Ovarian Cancer Screening (UKCTOCS) trial.

UKCTOCS	UKCTOCS	UKCTOCS
Direct communication with participants		
Postal follow-up questionnaires	3–5 years after randomization	
Diagnosis: England & Wales	Linked by NHS number to the Health & Social Care Information Center, the National Cancer Intelligence Network, Hospital Episodes Statistics	Cancer & death registrations
Diagnosis: Northern Ireland	Central Services Agency and the Northern Ireland Cancer Registry	Cancer & death registrations
Surgery outside the trial	Hospital Episodes Statistical records	
Underlying cause of death	Outcomes review committee (2 pathologists & 2 gynecological oncologists)	Final diagnosis based on algorithm: disease progression, (new lesions or increase in size of original lesions by imaging, clinical worsening, or rising biomarkers)

3.9. Consideration 9

Deciding How to Avoid Biases Caused by Enrollments that Attract Participants with Late-Stage Disease Who Are either Symptomatic or Disposed by Factors that Are Genetic, Environmental or Social

It may be possible to explain the failure to detect early stage disease in the PLCO trial in terms of promotions that attracted symptomatic women or women already with late-stage disease. If recruitment inadvertently allowed a biased enrollment of women who already were demonstrating clinical disease, it would certainly explain why early stage disease was not detected. Such a bias could also be contributed to by attracting nulliparous women or women with a family history of ovarian cancer. In contrast to the PLCO trial, the UKCTOCS ran a separate protocol specialized for women at elevated risk for ovarian cancer. Since screening is intended for detecting sub-clinical disease, post-hoc analysis should be performed that censors participants with clinical manifestations of disease when the screening tool is not needed.

3.10. Consideration 10

Deciding Whether the Screening Tool or a Screening Process Is Being Tested

Differences in the screening process between the PLCO and UKCTOCS trials have already been outlined here and in print [14,36] and are likely to have greater impact on outcomes than differences in the screening tools in these two trials. As an aside, completion of full human papillomavirus (HPV) vaccination is subject to age, rural vs. urban location, parental hesitancy/refusal and cultural factors [37,38]. In this example, which utilizes a very effective agent, effectiveness at the population level is limited by these barriers to utilization so that the role of the process assumes great importance even with a very effective vaccination tool. In summary, in a screening trial both the screening tool and the screening process contribute to the overall evaluation so that it is possible for a quite effective screening tool to be utilized in a flawed screening process with the result that overall outcomes are unimpressive. As part of this consideration, the control group is also process driven. If the control group is supposed to receive "usual care", such care could involve no visits to a care-giver as well as timed annual visits that are matched to the frequency of screening visits. In this latter case, the scheduled visits may provide a superior level of care that, based on information related by the subject, leads to imaging with CT or MRI and the potential to identify malignancy. Against this background it is not surprising that individuals in the control arm of clinical trials do better than the overall population.

4. Conclusions

Ten considerations are presented here that can impact the outcomes of ovarian cancer screening. Each should be considered for implementing screening processes and re-considered in post-hoc analyses as alternative explanations of effects that influence screening outcomes.

In addition, the consideration of ovarian cancer risk is appropriate and has been coupled to ovarian cancer screening. The United Kingdom Familial Ovarian Cancer Screening Study (UKFOCS) was begun in 2007 and included 4348 women that received annual screening for five years and follow-up for an additional 4.8 years [39]. The participants met the familial criteria for risk by having had a family member that had been diagnosed with ovarian cancer and would be considered to have a life-time risk $\geq$10%. A shift to early-stage ovarian cancer discovery was observed to result from this screening; however, it is too early to tell if an improved survival will be demonstrated in this screened group of high-risk women. Improved assessments of risk have now been defined based on mutations in $BRCA_1$ (Breast Cancer susceptibility gene 1: 39%–65% life-time risk), and $BRCA_2$ (Breast Cancer susceptibility gene 2: 11%–37% life-time risk) [40,41]. Additional germline mutations in $BRIP_1$, $BARD_1$, $PALB_2$, NBN, $RAD51B$, $RAD51C$, $RAD51D$ [42,43] as well as MLH_1, MSH_2, MSH_6, PMS_2, $EPCAM$, (all associated with Lynch syndrome [44]), TP_{53} (associated with Li-Fraumeni syndrome [45]) and

STK_{11}/LKB_1 (associated with Peutz-Jeghers syndrome [46]) are related to moderately increased risk of ovarian cancer. With the number of germline mutations expanding, there has been support for population-based screening for all women before ovarian cancer develops [47]. Such a position would allow surveillance screening, surgical prophylaxis, or chemoprevention through oral contraceptives. However, utilization of these strategies must be weighed against potential problems (false negative screening, surgical complications, stroke, pre-mature menopause and increasing the risk of other cancers). Thus, with the list of associated gene mutations evolving, more women can be expected to carry some mutation pre-disposing them to ovarian cancer and overall will exceed the 15% of all ovarian cancers attributed to $BRCA_1$ and $BRCA_2$ [46]. In this context, some form of ovarian cancer screening/surveillance will have a role.

References

1. Handford, M. *Where's Waldo?* Candlewick Press: Somerville, MA, USA, 2012.
2. Daoud, E.; Bodor, G. CA-125 concentrations in malignant and nonmalignant disease. *Clin. Chem.* **1991**, *37*, 1968–1974. [PubMed]
3. Nagell, J.R., Jr.; Miller, R.W.; Desimone, C.P.; Ueland, F.R.; Podzielinski, I.; Goodrich, S.T.; Elder, J.W.; Huang, B.; Kryscio, R.J.; Pavlik, E.J. Long-term survival of women with epithelial ovarian cancer detected by ultrasonographic screening. *Obstet. Gynecol.* **2011**, *118*, 1212–1221. [CrossRef] [PubMed]
4. Johnson, V.E. Revised standards for statistical evidence. *Proc. Natl. Acad. Sci. USA* **2013**, *110*, 19313–19317. [CrossRef] [PubMed]
5. Gaudart, J.; Huiart, L.; Milligan, P.J.; Thiebaut, R.; Giorgi, R. Reproducibility issues in science, is *p* value really the only answer? *Proc. Natl. Acad. Sci. USA* **2014**, *111*, E1934. [CrossRef] [PubMed]
6. Gelmana, A.; Rober, C.P. Revised evidence for statistical standards. *Proc. Natl. Acad. Sci. USA* **2014**, *111*, E1933. [CrossRef] [PubMed]
7. Jeffreys, H. *Theory of Probability*; Oxford University Press Inc.: New York, NY, USA, 1961.
8. Pericchi, L.; Pereira, C.A.; Pérez, M.E. Adaptive revised standards for statistical evidence. *Proc. Natl. Acad. Sci. USA* **2014**, *111*, E1935. [CrossRef] [PubMed]
9. Jacobs, I.J.; Menon, U.; Ryan, A.; Gentry-Maharaj, A.; Burnell, M.; Kalsi, J.K.; Amso, N.N.; Apostolidou, S.; Benjamin, E.; Cruickshank, D.; et al. Ovarian cancer screening and mortality in the UK Collaborative Trial of Ovarian Cancer Screening (UKCTOCS): A randomised controlled trial. *Lancet* **2016**, *387*, 945–956. [CrossRef]
10. Stokes, L. Sample size calculation for a hypothesis test. *JAMA* **2014**, *312*, 180–181. [CrossRef] [PubMed]
11. Ioannidis, J.P.A. Why Most Published Research Findings Are False. *PLoS Med.* **2005**, *2*, e124. [CrossRef] [PubMed]
12. Kobayashi, H.; Yamada, Y.; Sado, T.; Sakata, M.; Yoshida, S.; Kawaguchi, R.; Kanayama, S.; Shigetomi, H.; Haruta, S.; Tsuji, Y.; et al. A randomized study of screening for ovarian cancer: A multicenter study in Japan. *Int. J. Gynecol. Cancer* **2008**, *18*, 414–420. [CrossRef] [PubMed]
13. Buys, S.S.; Partridge, E.; Black, A.; Johnson, C.C.; Lamerato, L.; Isaacs, C.; Reding, D.J.; Greenlee, R.T.; Yokochi, L.A.; Kessel, B.; et al. Effect of screening on ovarian cancer mortality—The Prostate, Lung, Colorectal and Ovarian (PLCO) Cancer Screening Randomized Controlled Trial. *JAMA* **2011**, *305*, 2295–2303. [CrossRef] [PubMed]
14. Pavlik, E.J. Ovarian cancer screening effectiveness: A realization from the UK Collaborative Trial of Ovarian Cancer Screening. *Women Health* **2016**, *12*, 5–475. [CrossRef] [PubMed]
15. Pavlik, E.J.; Ueland, F.R.; Miller, R.W.; Ubellacker, J.M.; Desimone, C.P.; Elder, J.; Hoff, J.; Baldwin, L.; Kryscio, R.J.; Nagell, J.R., Jr. Frequency and disposition of ovarian abnormalities followed with serial transvaginal ultrasonography. *Obstet. Gynecol.* **2013**, *122 Pt 1*, 210–217. [CrossRef] [PubMed]
16. Nagell, J.R., Jr.; Miller, R.W. Evaluation and Management of Ultrasonographically Detected Ovarian Tumors in Asymptomatic Women. *Obstet. Gynecol.* **2016**, *127*, 848–858. [CrossRef] [PubMed]
17. Moore, R.G.; Miller, M.C.; Disilvestro, P.; Landrum, L.M.; Gajewski, W.; Ball, J.J.; Skates, S.J. Evaluation of the diagnostic accuracy of the risk of ovarian malignancy algorithm in women with a pelvic mass. *Obstet. Gynecol.* **2011**, *118*, 280–288. [CrossRef] [PubMed]
18. Elder, J.W.; Pavlik, E.J.; Long, A.; Miller, R.W.; DeSimone, C.P.; Hoff, J.T.; Ueland, W.R.; Kryscio, R.J.; van Nagell, J.R., Jr.; Ueland, F.R. Serial ultrasonographic evaluation of ovarian abnormalities with a morphology index. *Gynecol. Oncol.* **2014**, *135*, 8–12. [CrossRef] [PubMed]

19. Han, L.Y.; Karavasilis, V.; Hagen, T.V.; Nicum, S.; Thomas, K.; Harrison, M.; Papadopoulos, P.; Blake, P.; Barton, D.P.; Gore, M.; et al. Doubling time of serum CA125 is an independent prognostic factor for survival in patients with ovarian cancer relapsing after first-line chemotherapy. *Eur. J. Cancer* **2010**, *46*, 1359–1364. [CrossRef] [PubMed]

20. Willemse, P.H.; Aalders, J.G.; de Bruyn, H.W.; Mulder, N.H.; Sleijfer, D.T.; de Vries, E.G. CA-125 in ovarian cancer: Relation between half-life, doubling time and survival. *Eur. J. Cancer* **1991**, *27*, 993–995. [CrossRef]

21. Engelen, M.J.; Kos, H.E.; Willemse, P.H.; Aalders, J.G.; de Vries, E.G.; Schaapveld, M.; Otter, R.; van der Zee, A.G. Surgery by consultant gynecologic oncologists improves survival in patients with ovarian carcinoma. *Cancer* **2006**, *106*, 589–598. [CrossRef] [PubMed]

22. Earle, C.C.; Schrag, D.; Neville, B.A.; Yabroff, K.R.; Topor, M.; Fahey, A.; Trimble, E.L.; Bodurka, D.C.; Bristow, R.E.; Carney, M.; et al. Effect of surgeon specialty on processes of care and outcomes for ovarian cancer patients. *J. Natl. Cancer Inst.* **2006**, *98*, 172–180. [CrossRef] [PubMed]

23. Bristow, R.E.; Zahurak, M.L.; Diaz-Montes, T.P.; Giuntoli, R.L.; Armstrong, D.K. Impact of surgeon and hospital ovarian cancer surgical case volume on in-hospital mortality and related short-term outcomes. *Gynecol. Oncol.* **2009**, *115*, 334–338. [CrossRef] [PubMed]

24. Bristow, R.E.; Palis, B.E.; Chi, D.S.; Cliby, W.A. The National Cancer Database report on advanced-stage epithelial ovarian cancer: Impact of hospital surgical case volume on overall survival and surgical treatment paradigm. *Gynecol. Oncol.* **2010**, *118*, 262–267. [CrossRef] [PubMed]

25. Bristow, R.E.; Chang, J.; Ziogas, A.; Anton-Culver, H. Adherence to treatment guidelines for ovarian cancer as a measure of quality care. *Obstet. Gynecol.* **2013**, *121*, 1226–1234. [CrossRef] [PubMed]

26. Bristow, R.E.; Chang, J.; Ziogas, A.; Randall, L.M.; Anton-Culver, H. High-volume ovarian cancer care: Survival impact and disparities in access for advanced-stage disease. *Gynecol. Oncol.* **2014**, *132*, 403–410. [CrossRef] [PubMed]

27. Cliby, W.A.; Powell, M.A.; Al-Hammadi, N.; Chen, L.; Philip, M.J.; Roland, P.Y.; Mutch, D.G.; Bristow, R.E. Ovarian cancer in the United States: Contemporary patterns of care associated with improved survival. *Gynecol. Oncol.* **2015**, *136*, 11–17. [CrossRef] [PubMed]

28. Bristow, R.E.; Chang, J.; Ziogas, A.; Campos, B.; Chavez, L.R.; Anton-Culver, H. Impact of National Cancer Institute Comprehensive Cancer Centers on ovarian cancer treatment and survival. *J. Am. Coll. Surg.* **2015**, *220*, 940–950. [CrossRef] [PubMed]

29. Lee, J.Y.; Kim, T.H.; Suh, D.H.; Kim, J.W.; Kim, H.S.; Chung, H.H.; Park, N.H.; Song, Y.S.; Kang, S.B. Impact of guideline adherence on patient outcomes in early-stage epithelial ovarian cancer. *Eur. J. Surg. Oncol.* **2015**, *41*, 585–591. [CrossRef] [PubMed]

30. Vernooij, F.; Heintz, A.P.; Witteveen, P.O.; van der Heiden-van der Loo, M.; Coebergh, J.W.; van der Graaf, Y. Specialized care and survival of ovarian cancer patients in The Netherlands: Nationwide cohort study. *J. Natl. Cancer. Inst.* **2008**, *100*, 399–406. [CrossRef] [PubMed]

31. UK Collaborative Trial of Ovarian Cancer Screening. Available online: http://www.isrctn.com/ ISRCTN22488978 (accessed on 11 April 2017).

32. Gupta, S.K. Intention-to-treat concept: A review. *Perspect. Clin. Res.* **2011**, *2*, 109–112. [CrossRef] [PubMed]

33. Koshiyama, M.; Matsumura, N.; Konishi, I. Clinical fficacy of Ovarian Cancer Screening. *J. Cancer* **2016**, *7*, 1311–1316. [CrossRef] [PubMed]

34. Supplimentary Appenidix to Reference 9: Collaborative Trial of Ovarian Cancer Screening (UKCTOCS): A Randomised Controlled Trial. Available online: http://www.thelancet.com/cms/attachment/ 2049825434/2058773146/mmc1.pdf (accessed on 11 April 2017).

35. Miller, A.B.; Yurgalevitch, S.; Weissfeld, J.L. Prostate, Lung, Colorectal and Ovarian Cancer Screening Trial Project Team. Death review process in the Prostate, Lung, Colorectal and Ovarian (PLCO) Cancer Screening Trial. *Control Clin. Trials* **2000**, *231* (Suppl. 6), 400S–406S. [CrossRef]

36. Pavlik, E.J.; Nagell, J.R., Jr. Early detection of ovarian tumors using ultrasound. *Women Health* **2013**, *9*, 39–55. [CrossRef] [PubMed]

37. Sadaf, A.; Richards, J.L.; Glanz, J.; Salmon, D.A.; Omer, S.B. A systematic review of interventions for reducing parental vaccine refusal and vaccine hesitancy. *Vaccine* **2013**, *31*, 4293–4304. [CrossRef] [PubMed]

38. Wilson, R.M.; Brown, D.R.; Carmody, D.P.; Fogarty, S. HPV Vaccination Completion and Compliance with Recommended Dosing Intervals Among Female and Male Adolescents in an Inner-City Community Health Center. *J. Community Health* **2015**, *40*, 395–403. [CrossRef] [PubMed]

39. Rosenthal, A.N.; Lindsay, F.S.M.; Philpott, S.; Manchanda, R.; Burnell, M.; Badman, P.; Hadwin, R.; Rizzuto, I.;

Benjamin, E.; Singh, N.; et al. Evidence of Stage Shift in Women Diagnosed with Ovarian Cancer During Phase II of the United Kingdom Familial Ovarian Cancer Screening Study. *J. Clinl. Oncol.* **2017**. [CrossRef] [PubMed]

40. Antoniou, A.; Pharoah, P.D.; Narod, S.; Risch, H.A.; Eyfjord, J.E.; Hopper, J.L.; Loman, N.; Olsson, H.; Johannsson, O.; Borg, Å.; et al. Average risks of breast and ovarian cancer associated with *BRCA1* or *BRCA2* mutations detected in case series unselected for family history: A combined analysis of 22 studies. *Am. J. Hum. Genet.* **2003**, *72*, 1117–1130. [CrossRef] [PubMed]

41. Evans, D.G.; Shenton, A.; Woodward, E.; Lalloo, F.; Howell, A.; Maher, E.R. Penetrance estimates for BRCA1 and BRCA2 based on genetic testing in a clinical cancer genetics service setting: Risks of breast/ovarian cancer quoted should reflect the cancer burden in the family. *BMC Cancer* **2008**, *8*, 155. [CrossRef] [PubMed]

42. Ramus, S.J.; Song, H.; Dicks, E.; Tyrer, J.P.; Rosenthal, A.N.; Intermaggio, M.P.; Fraser, L.; Gentry-Maharaj, A.; Hayward, J.; Philpott, S.; et al. Germline mutations in the *BRIP1*, *BARD1*, *PALB2*, and *NBN* genes in women with ovarian cancer. *J. Natl. Cancer Inst.* **2015**, *107*, djv214. [CrossRef] [PubMed]

43. Song, H.; Dicks, E.; Ramus, S.J.; Tyrer, J.P.; Intermaggio, M.P.; Hayward, J.; Edlund, C.K.; Conti, D.; Harrington, P.; Fraser, L.; et al. Contribution of germline mutations in the *RAD51B*, *RAD51C*, and *RAD51D* genes to ovarian cancer in the population. *J. Clin. Oncol.* **2015**, *33*, 2901–2907. [CrossRef] [PubMed]

44. Lu, K.H.; Daniels, M. Endometrial and ovarian cancer in women with Lynch syndrome: Update in screening and prevention. *Fam. Cancer* **2013**, *12*, 273–277. [CrossRef] [PubMed]

45. Shulman, L.P. Hereditary breast and ovarian cancer (HBOC): Clinical features and counseling for *BRCA1* and *BRCA2*, Lynch syndrome, Cowden syndrome, and Li-Fraumeni syndrome. *Obstet. Gynecol. Clin. N. Am.* **2010**, *37*, 109–133. [CrossRef] [PubMed]

46. Committee on the State of the Science in Ovarian Cancer Research; Board on Health Care Services; Institute of Medicine; National Academies of Sciences, Engineering, and Medicine. *Ovarian Cancers: Evolving Paradigms in Research and Care*; National Academies Press (US): Washington, DC, USA, 2016.

47. King, M.C.; Levy-Lahad, E.; Lahad, A. Population-based screening for *BRCA1* and *BRCA2*: 2014 Lasker Award. *JAMA* **2014**, *312*, 1091–1092. [CrossRef] [PubMed]

14

Automated Definition of Skeletal Disease Burden in Metastatic Prostate Carcinoma: A 3D Analysis of SPECT/CT Images

Francesco Fiz [1,*], Helmut Dittmann [1], Cristina Campi [2], Matthias Weissinger [1], Samine Sahbai [3], Matthias Reimold [1], Arnulf Stenzl [4], Michele Piana [5], Gianmario Sambuceti [6] and Christian la Fougère [1,7]

[1]   Department of Nuclear Medicine and Clinical Molecular Imaging, University Hospital Tübingen, 72076 Tübingen, Germany; helmut.dittmann@med.uni-tuebingen.de (H.D.); matthias.weissinger@med.uni-tuebingen.de (M.W.); Matthias.Reimold@med.uni-tuebingen.de (M.R.); christian.lafougere@med.uni-tuebingen.de (C.l.F.)

[2]   Department of Medicine-DIMED, Nuclear Medicine Unit, University Hospital of Padua, 35128 Padua, Italy; cristina.campi@gmail.com

[3]   Nuclear Medicine Unit, Hospital Universitaire Henri Mondor, 94010 Créteil, France; sam.sahbai@gmail.com

[4]   Department of Urology, University Hospital Tübingen, 72076 Tübingen, Germany; urologie@med.uni-tuebingen.de

[5]   Department of Mathematics, University of Genoa, 16146 Genoa, Italy; piana@dima.unige.it

[6]   Department of Health Sciences, Nuclear Medicine Unit, University of Genoa, 16146 Genoa, Italy; sambuceti@unige.it

[7]   iFIT Cluster of Excellence, University of Tübingen, 72076 Tübingen, Germany

*   Correspondence: Francesco.Fiz@med.uni-tuebingen.de

Abstract: To meet the current need for skeletal tumor-load estimation in castration-resistant prostate cancer (CRPC), we developed a novel approach based on adaptive bone segmentation. In this study, we compared the program output with existing estimates and with the radiological outcome. Seventy-six whole-body single-photon emission computed tomographies/x-ray computed tomography with 3,3-diphosphono-1,2-propanedicarboxylic acid from mCRPC patients were analyzed. The software identified the whole skeletal volume (S_{Vol}) and classified the voxels metastases (M_{Vol}) or normal bone (B_{Vol}). S_{Vol} was compared with the estimation of a commercial software. M_{Vol} was compared with manual assessment and with prostate specific antigen (PSA) levels. Counts/voxel were extracted from M_{Vol} and B_{Vol}. After six cycles of $^{223}RaCl2$-therapy every patient was re-evaluated as having progressive disease (PD), stable disease (SD), or a partial response (PR). S_{Vol} correlated with that of the commercial software ($R = 0.99$, $p < 0.001$). M_{Vol} correlated with the manually-counted lesions ($R = 0.61$, $p < 0.001$) and PSA ($R = 0.46$, $p < 0.01$). PD had a lower counts/voxel in M_{Vol} than PR/SD (715 ± 190 vs. 975 ± 215 and 1058 ± 255, $p < 0.05$ and $p < 0.01$) and B_{Vol} (PD 275 ± 60, PR 515 ± 188 and SD 528 ± 162 counts/voxel, $p < 0.001$). Segmentation-based tumor load correlated with radiological/laboratory indices. Uptake was linked with the clinical outcome, suggesting that metastases in PD patients have a lower affinity for bone-seeking radionuclides and might benefit less from bone-targeted radioisotope therapies.

Keywords: mCRPC; SPECT/CT; Computer-assisted diagnosis; XOFIGO; Therapy response assessment

1. Introduction

Castration-resistant prostate cancer (CRPC) is defined by rising prostate specific antigen (PSA) levels under androgen blockade and by the eventual diffuse metastatic spread [1–3]. In these patients, skeletal metastases can represent the most relevant prognostic factor, by impairing the static function of the skeleton and by reducing the available space for hematopoiesis [4–6].

Diffuse skeletal CRPC metastatization, once considered a terminal diagnosis, can today be managed by many different approaches, including new-generations of taxanes, second-line hormonal therapy, and radioisotope treatments [7–12]. As these medications might have varying effectiveness and cause different side effects, the choice of therapy sequence usually requires multidisciplinary disease-management. Nevertheless, the most effective sequence of systemic treatments is still a matter of discussion and patient-specific components are likely to play a relevant role [13–15].

Being able to assess treatment response reliably is a pre-requisite for therapy selection and sequencing. Response evaluation may be performed either by analyzing tumor marker blood levels or by serial imaging. Serum PSA level is the most used marker, but alkaline phosphatase might also be helpful in assessing metastasis-dependent bone turnover [16,17].

Circulating markers are, however, dependent on the degree of tumor differentiation and can be altered by concomitant therapies [18–20]. On the other hand, evaluating medical imaging, whether morphological or radioisotope-based, can be challenging in the presence of a high number of metastases or in case of therapy-related changes, such as the "flare" phenomenon [21].

Obtaining an automated evaluation of the skeletal tumor burden is one of the greatest current unmet clinical needs; in recent years, an increasing number of software applications have been developed for this purpose [22]. Existing applications are mostly based on automated thresholding, using standardized uptake value on positron emission tomography (PET) or count values on bone scans; in this setting, telling apart metastases-related uptake from other non-malignant sources of increased bone turnover can be challenging.

To improve the reliability of metastases detection and to obtain a reliable estimation of tumor load, we developed a specific computational tool based on segmentation analysis. This algorithm uses the computed tomography (CT) information to identify and segment all hyperdense localizations within the skeletal system automatically to define the overall metastatic bone compartment. In a second step, information from the co-registered single-photon emission computed tomography (SPECT) or PET images can be extracted for this volume. In this study, we tested this approach on a series of CRPC patients and validated the analysis against different clinical parameters.

2. Results

2.1. Volumetric Assessment and Comparison between Systems

The estimate of total osseous tissue (skeletal volume S_{Vol}, sum of metastases volume M_{Vol}, trabecular volume B_{Vol}, and cortical volume C_{Vol}) showed a tight concordance between our software (EXCALIBUR, University of Genoa, Genoa, Italy) and the commercial application. Mean global skeletal volume was in fact 3875 ± 1513 mL and 3881 ± 1499 mL as measured by the commercial software application and by our computational program, respectively ($R = 0.99$, $p < 0.001$). Mean counts/voxel were 439 ± 71 and 435 ± 61, respectively, with an R correlation index of 0.92 ($p < 0.001$, data not shown). Mean M_{Vol} was 362 ± 249 mL (range 85–1194 mL), corresponding to 27 ± 20% of the total trabecular bone.

The majority of tumor burden was located within the axial skeleton and in the hipbones (M_{Vol} 335 ± 140 mL); 61 patients (81%) had skeletal localizations within the appendicular long bones (M_{Vol} 32 ± 19 mL).

2.2. Volume Characteristics

Mean Hounsfield density was comparable for M_{Vol} (590 ± 136) and C_{Vol} (531 ± 92) but was significantly lower for B_{Vol} (251 ± 78, $p < 0.001$). Higher tracer activity was measured within M_{Vol} (939 ± 279 mean counts/voxel), as compared to B_{Vol} (462 ± 196 mean counts/voxel, $p < 0.001$). Activity concentration within C_{Vol} was even lower (271 ± 106 mean counts/voxel), see Table 1. Mean counts/voxel were directly correlated to mean Hounsfielf Units (HU) for both M_{Vol} (R = 0.52, p < 0.01) and B_{Vol} (R = 0.74, p < 0.001, Figure 1).

Table 1. Radiological and laboratory parameters in patients with or without superscan.

Parameter	All Patients	Superscan	Non-Superscan	p-Value
Mean M_{Vol} (mL)	357 ± 257	527 ± 304	245 ± 187	<0.001
Number of counted lesions	74 ± 30	106 ± 22	61 ± 23	<0.001
INV%	27 ± 20%	40 ± 23%	21 ± 16%	<0.01
PSA (ng/mL)	539 ± 754	1235 ± 959	257 ± 407	<0.001
B_{Vol} mean counts/voxel	466 ± 198	565 ± 243	428 ± 164	NS
M_{Vol} mean counts/voxel	947 ± 277	1104 ± 291	886 ± 251	<0.05
B_{Vol} mean HU	251 ± 78	319 ± 78	223 ± 59	<0.01
M_{Vol} mean HU	590 ± 136	693 ± 132	549 ± 115	<0.001

M_{Vol}: Metastases Volume; INV%: Invasion% or M_{Vol}/B_{Vol} ratio PSA: Prostate-specific antigen; B_{Vol}: Trabecular bone volume; HU: Hounsfield Unit.

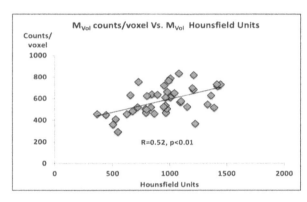
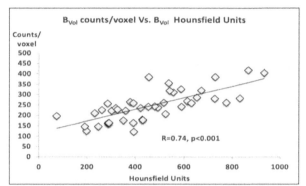
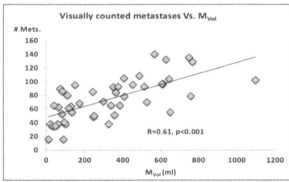
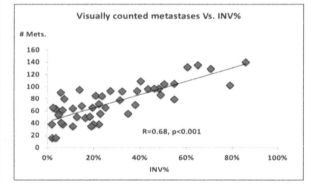

Figure 1. Correlation between counts/voxel and Hounsfield density as well as between volumes and number of metastases. A higher density corresponded to higher mean counts/voxel (top panels). Furthermore, a close correlation was observed between the volumetric estimates and the manual count of metastatic lesions (bottom panels). M_{Vol} = voxels metastases; B_{Vol} = normal bone; INV% = percent of bone invaded by metastases (M_{Vol}/B_{Vol}).

2.3. Tumor Volume, Number of Lesions, and PSA Level

The software based semi-automatic lesion identification (M_{Vol}) and the manual lesion count showed a tight correlation, for the whole skeletal system (R = 0.61, p < 0.001, Figure 1) and the axial segments (R = 0.64, p < 0.001), but not for the appendicular ones (R = 0.07, p = 0.52). Likewise, the number of manually counted lesions correlated with the percent of invasion of the trabecular bone by metastases (INV%) within the whole (R = 0.68) as well as axial (R = 0.69) skeleton, p < 0.001, Figure 1.

Remarkably, PSA level as a marker of tumor load correlated with our measures of bone involvement (M_{Vol} R = 0.46, p < 0.01; number of manually counted lesions R = 0.67, p < 0.001; mean HU of M_{Vol} R = 0.42, p < 0.01; mean HU B_{Vol} R = 0.52, p < 0.001; and M_{Vol}/B_{Vol} ratio R = 0.75, p < 0.001).

2.4. Impact of Superscan Status

Twelve patients (16%) were classified as superscan. CRPC patients with a superscan had a higher mean HU than non-superscan patients in B_{Vol} ($p < 0.001$ Figure 2) as well as in M_{Vol} ($p < 0.01$, Figure 2).

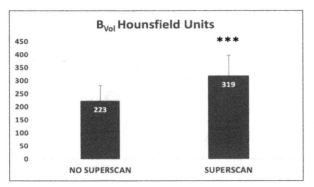
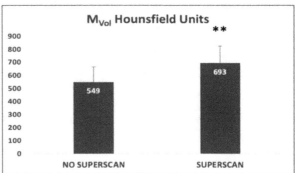
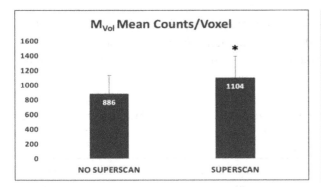
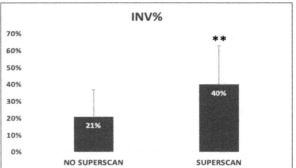

Figure 2. Comparison between superscan and non-superscan patients. Superscan subjects showed a higher density in trabecular bone volume (B_{Vol}) as well as in metastases volume (M_{Vol}) (upper panels). A higher counting rate was observed in the M_{Vol} of superscan patients (bottom left). Finally, percent of trabecular bone space invaded by metastatic lesions was higher in the superscan subjects (bottom right). * $p < 0.05$, ** $p < 0.01$, *** $p < 0.001$. INV% Percent of bone invaded by metastases (M_{Vol}/ B_{Vol}).

Mean counts/voxel in M_{Vol} were higher in superscan subjects than in non-superscan (1104 ± 291 vs. 886 ± 251, $p < 0.05$, Figure 2); conversely, mean counts/voxel in B_{Vol} were not significantly different between the two subpopulations.

Finally, superscan was associated with a higher INV% of trabecular bone by osteoblastic lesions (M_{Vol}/B_{Vol} ratio: 40 ± 23% vs. 21 ± 16%, $p < 0.01$, Figure 5), which was reflected, at qualitative analysis, by a higher number of visually observable metastases (Number of metastases = 106 ± 22 vs. 61 ± 23, $p < 0.001$). See Table 1 for a detailed analysis.

2.5. Therapy Response Assessment

According to the response assessment criteria, which are further detailed in the Material and Methods, 21 patients (28%) were classified with progressive disease (PD), while 35 subjects (46%) were classified with stable disease (SD), and 20 patients (26%) with a partial response (PR).

Patients who presented a PD status after the therapy completion exhibited a markedly lower activity in the M_{Vol} (715 ± 190 counts) in the pre-therapy scan, when compared to those with PR (N = 20, 975 ± 215 counts, $p < 0.05$) or SD (N = 35, 1058 ± 255 counts, $p < 0.01$). Of note, similar findings were found within B_{Vol}, where patients with PD displayed the lowest activity (PD 275 ± 60, PR 515 ± 188 and SD 528 ± 162 counts, $p < 0.001$). See Figure 3.

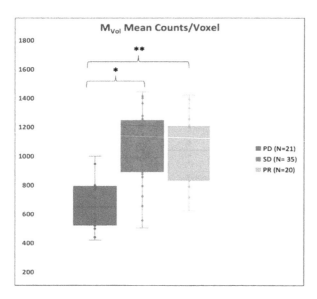
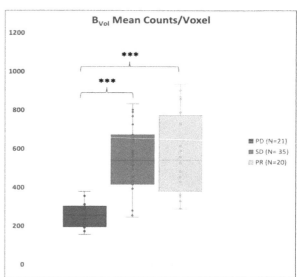

Figure 3. Radioactivity concentration according to response. Patients with progressive disease (PD) after the radioisotope therapy displayed a significantly lower radioactivity concentration at the baseline imaging in metastases volume (M_{Vol}) as well as in trabecular bone volume (B_{Vol}). * $p < 0.05$, ** $p < 0.01$, *** $p < 0.001$. SD = stable disease; PR = partial response.

At receiver operating characteristics (ROC) analysis, both M_{Vol} and B_{Vol} mean counts/voxel were predictive of therapy effectiveness (M_{Vol} 0.895 and B_{Vol} 0.943 for, $p < 0.001$). The best threshold value of mean counts/voxel for discriminating patients with progressive disease was in fact 805 in the M_{Vol} (sensitivity 84%, specificity 81%) and 385 in the B_{Vol} (sensitivity 84%, specificity 100%). No differences were observed in absolute volume of metastases (M_{Vol}) across the therapy outcome groups. See Figure 4.

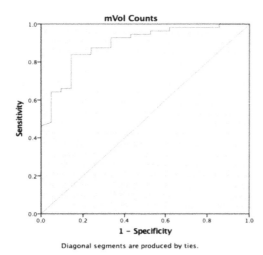
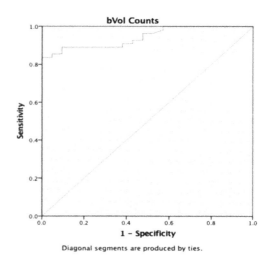

Figure 4. Receiver operating characteristics (ROC) curve of metastases volume (M_{Vol}) and trabecular bone volume (B_{Vol}) counts/voxel values according to progression. Radioactivity concentration was able to discriminate patients with a progressive disease in M_{Vol} as well as in B_{Vol}.

Patients presenting a superscan pattern of radioactivity distribution were evenly distributed among the three groups (PD: 3/21 or 14%, SD 6/35 or 17%, and PR 3/20 15%, p = non significant.

PSA levels showed considerable variations during the therapy. On average, starting from staging to the end of the therapy, it increased by 135 ± 99% in PD patients and by 27 ± 81% in PR subjects. Conversely, PSA decreased by 40 ± 16% in SD patients. However, due to the marked spread of the

PSA-level course among patients, no statistically significant difference could be demonstrated among these groups.

See Table 2 for a detailed analysis.

Table 2. Radiological and laboratory parameters according to response.

Parameter	PD	SD	PR	PD vs. PR	PD vs. SD	PR vs. SD
Mean M_{Vol} (mL)	245 ± 312	342 ± 203	373 ± 254	NS	NS	NS
Number of counted lesions	56 ± 25	80 ± 33	79 ± 26	NS	NS	NS
M_{Vol}/B_{Vol}	19 ± 8%	29 ± 17%	31 ± 23	NS	NS	NS
PSA (ng/mL)	353 ± 540	446 ± 539	746 ± 1004	NS	NS	NS
B_{Vol} mean counts/voxel	275 ± 60	528 ± 162	515 ± 188	<0.001	<0.001	NS
M_{Vol} mean counts/voxel	715 ± 190	1058 ± 255	975 ± 219	<0.05	<0.01	NS
B_{Vol} mean HU	232 ± 81	253 ± 68	264 ± 82	NS	NS	NS
M_{Vol} mean HU	545 ± 157	605 ± 120	610 ± 127	NS	NS	NS

PD: Progressive disease; SD: Stable disease; PR: Partial response; M_{Vol}: Metastases volume; INV%: Invasion% or M_{Vol}/B_{Vol}; PSA: Prostate-specific antigen; B_{Vol}: trabecular bone volume; HU: Hounsfield Units.

3. Discussion

The present paper describes a computational approach to the problem of skeletal tumor burden quantification by means of SPECT/CT data. The robustness of the bone recognition was testified by the tight correlation between the total bone volume as detected by our approach and by a commercial application. The automated identification of bone tumor volume could not be compared with a reference standard, as, to the best of our knowledge, a commercially available CT-based tumor burden estimator does not yet exist. However, the estimates provided by this software tool show a tight concordance with the traditional measures of tumor burden performed with imaging and blood tests.

In our analysis, we considered both the raw figure of tumor volume as well as the percent of invasion, in other words, the ratio between tumor and trabecular volume. Both estimators strongly correlated with the number of manually counted lesions as well as with the PSA values.

As expected, patients with a superscan status at planar bone scans presented a higher tumor volume as well as a higher percent of trabecular bone invaded by bone metastases. These patients presented also a higher bone metastases density and counting rate; however, mean counts in trabecular bone did not significantly differ from those in the trabecular bone of non-superscan patients.

However, the distribution of radioactivity into the metastases, as well as into the trabecular bone, appears to play an important role in the therapeutic effectiveness of $^{223}RaCl_2$. Previous studies have in fact shown that the distribution of the bone scan tracers mirrors that of $^{223}RaCl_2$ [23,24]. In our population, patients who were found to have a disease progression at the end of the therapy presented a lower counting rate at the baseline SPECT/CT not only within the known tumor lesions, but also in the trabecular bone. It might be hypothesized that a lower counting rate at SPECT/CT could correspond to a lesser $^{223}RaCl_2$ avidity and thus to a reduced absorbed dose. Thus, one might hypothesize that micrometastases (if present) in trabecular bone exhibiting only a low counting rate will receive an insufficient therapeutic dose. It is worth noting that tumor volume was conversely and not significantly different across patients with partial response, stable, or progressive disease. As a consequence, semi-quantitative evaluation of bone tracer uptake at baseline might be useful for $^{223}RaCl_2$ therapy stratification.

Patients presenting with a superscan finding were equally distributed in the three response groups, in other words, the presence of a superscan was not per se associated with imaging-based therapy response in our population. Actually, the role of this imaging feature in predicting therapy response in patients treated with $^{223}RaCl_2$ has not been extensively studied. A previous report demonstrated a trend for shorter survival in those patients when compared to those with less than six metastases [25]; however, the relatively low frequency of this condition does not allow us to reach definite conclusions, unless large-scale studies are planned. Nonetheless, our data might suggest that some superscan patients might indeed benefit from a ^{223}RaCl$_2$ treatment.

The robustness of the generated volumetric data and the clinical relevance of the information that has been derived from this analysis suggest a relevant potential for the computer-enhanced evaluation of tumor burden. The relevance of such approaches is testified to by the growing number of computer-assisted techniques, which have been developed in the last few decades to estimate the tumor burden [22]. Different approaches have been presented, for example, the bone-scan index, which is designed to be applied to planar bone scintigraphy [26], but was subject to false-positive findings in the event of a flare phenomenon [27]. Moreover, new 3D-segmentation algorithms have been introduced for PET/CT, one based on a ^{18}F-NaF PET-threshold and requiring specific threshold determination for each individual scanner [28], the other using the tracer uptake of ^{68}Ga-PSMA (prostate-specific membrane antigen) [29], that might be of special interest for upcoming, but currently not approved, PSMA radio-ligand therapies. The main difference of our approach lies on the use of CT-density contrast instead of the PET information for defining tumor volume as well as the applicability to any CT-based hybrid imaging, PET/CT and SPECT/CT, the latter being more widely available and less cost intensive, which is a major advantage of our current approach with SPECT/CT. Finally, the use of bone seeking tracers might better reflect the uptake of ^{223}RaCl$_2$ and thus predict the radiation to the metastases. One algorithm included a segmentation.

Some limitations have to be mentioned. A possible source of error could be a misclassification of non-tumor-related bone thickening [30]. The application automatically excludes non-bone hyperdensity (e.g., vascular calcification) from the edge detection. Likewise, voxel belonging to the spinal canal and hypodense areas (such as bone cysts) are also sorted out. Our approach was shown to be congruent with the estimation of bone volume as provided by a standard commercial software. However, a comparison to an independent imaging-based reference standard provided by means of magnetic resonance or PSMA-PET/CT was not available. Moreover, comparison with other approved methods of tumor load determination, based on planar data, such as the bone scan index [31], was not possible because of their intrinsic difference.

Another significant limitation is that in the SPECT/CT analysis, the limited resolution of the single-photon technique could underestimate the counts in smaller volumes. Finally, we evaluated the therapy response only in subjects who completed the entire ^{223}RaCl$_2$ therapy. This decision was made in order to have a homogenous population and to be able to perform a therapy effectiveness evaluation at the same time point after baseline staging. However, this choice excluded patients who interrupted the therapy due to tumor-progress or because of toxicity; therefore, the information presented in this manuscript applies only to the patient population with a relatively better prognosis [32]. Further studies could shed light on the correlation among tumor load, tracer distribution, and overall survival in patients with in-therapy progression.

4. Materials and Methods

4.1. Patient Population

Seventy-six consecutive patients suffering from CRPC, who underwent whole-body ^{99m}Tc-bisphosphonate-SPECT/CT (mean age 69.5 ± 7, age range 55.5–80.8), were retrospectively analyzed. All examinations were performed for staging in patients with multiple bone lesions, before radionuclide therapy using ^{223}RaCl2. Inclusion criteria comprised histologically confirmed prostate cancer, evidence of prostate specific antigen (PSA) increase under maximal androgen blockade, and presence of clinically symptomatic as well as radiologically confirmed osteoblastic skeletal metastases. Exclusion criteria were the presence of metal implants impeding the analysis of either the axial or the appendicular skeleton (e.g., bilateral total hip replacement, extensive spondylosyndesis, etc.), absence of a signed informed consent, and inability to complete the planned six cycles of ^{223}RaCl$_2$-therapy.

Any previous therapy or combination of treatments was admitted. The PSA level at the time of the scan was recorded.

All patients gave written informed consent for the retrospective analysis of the pseudonymized clinical SPECT/CT data. The investigations were conducted in accordance with the Helsinki Declaration and with national regulations, after approval by the ethics committee of the University of Tübingen. All patients signed a specific consent form, detailing the use of imaging as well as of laboratory data for research purposes.

4.2. Patients' Follow Up

Patients were followed up with throughout the execution of the radionuclide therapy, which included six ^{223}RaCl$_2$ administrations (one per month). A whole-body SPECT/CT scan was carried out at the end of therapy. This scan was re-evaluated by an experienced viewer who was blinded to the results of the computational analysis and who stratified the patients according to therapy response as follows: if new lesions were detected (whether on CT or in the SPECT images), the case was classified as progressive disease (PD). On the contrary, if no new lesions were observed, the patient was considered having a stable disease (SD). Finally, if no new lesions were observed and the uptake intensity was visibly diminished, the case was judged as partial response (PR). This study was approved by the Local Ethics Committee of the University of Tübinngen (No. 747/2017BO1) on 9 March 2015.

4.3. Scan Protocol

Patients were scanned on a hybrid SPECT/CT device (Discovery 670 Pro, GE Healthcare, Chicago, IL, USA), three hours after injection of 8–10 MBq/Kg of ^{99m}Tc-3,3-diphosphono-1,2-propanedicarboxylic acid (CIS bio, Berlin, Germany). To minimize artifacts caused by the presence of radioactive urine in the excretory system, patients were asked to drink at least 1000 mL of water during the uptake time and to void immediately before the scan. No urinary bladder catheterization was used.

The acquisition protocol comprised a whole-body planar scan. This part was followed by a whole-body SPECT/CT scan, from vertex up to mid-distal femur, which was obtained by reconstructing and fusing three sequential fields-of-view on a dedicated workstation (Xeleris 3®, GE Healthcare, Chicago, IL, USA). SPECT acquisition was carried out with the two camera heads in H-Mode; parameters for each field-of-view were as follows: energy window 140.5 ± 1 0%, angular step 6°, time per step 15″. The transaxial field-of-view and pixel size of the reconstructed SPECT images were 54 cm and 5 × 5 mm, respectively, with a matrix size of 128 × 128. SPECT raw data were reconstructed using ordered-subset expectation maximization iterative protocol (2 iterations, 10 subsets).

The technical parameters of the 16-detector row, helical CT scanner included a gantry rotation speed of 0.8 s and a table speed of 20 mm per gantry rotation. The scan was performed at 120 kV voltage and 10–80 mA current. A dose modulation system (OptiDose®, GE Healthcare, Chicago, IL, USA) was applied to optimize total exposure according to the patient's body size. No contrast medium was injected.

4.4. Image Analysis

Segmentation of bone volumes was performed on the CT data according to the previously validated method [33–35]. Briefly, the algorithm identified the skeleton on CT images by assuming that compact bone is the structure with the highest X-ray attenuation coefficient in the human body. This assumption implies a stark HU value difference between soft tissue and cortical bone. The program functions by reading the HU values of every voxel in any given slice horizontally; when it encounters a sharp variation of HU density, it assumes that it had reached the bone outer border. From that point, it samples a 2-pixel ring, which corresponds to the cortical bone. It then samples the average density of this cortical bone volume. Thereafter, it categorizes every voxel on the inside of this volume as trabecular bone (bone volume, B_{Vol}) or as osteoblastic metastases volume (M_{Vol}). This is done by using the mean density of the cortical volume as the cutoff value, assuming the osteoblastic metastases will have an average density at least equal to that of cortical bone. Therefore, the final output of this process consists of the following volumes:

- Cortical Volume (C_{Vol}): the bone surface
- Trabecular Volume (B_{Vol}): the normal trabecular bone
- Metastases Volume (M_{Vol}): osteoblastic metastases (tumor burden)
- Skeletal Volume (S_{Vol}): entire skeletal volume (sum of C_{Vol}, B_{Vol}, and M_{Vol})
- %INV: percent of invasion (M_{Vol}/B_{Vol} ratio)

A graphical overview of the segmentation process and an example of the program's work on the original slices are shown in Figures 5 and 6.

For details on the mathematical rationale underlying the bone recognition algorithm, please see the original work from Sambuceti et al. [33]. For an overview on the principle of tumor burden estimation, we refer to our previous work [6].

After an initial automatic segmentation, the program displayed the resulting images to the operator, who could manually exclude all benign hyperdensities (e.g., osteochondrosis, osteophytes, metal implants). Purely lytic areas, having a HU inferior to 30, were automatically removed.

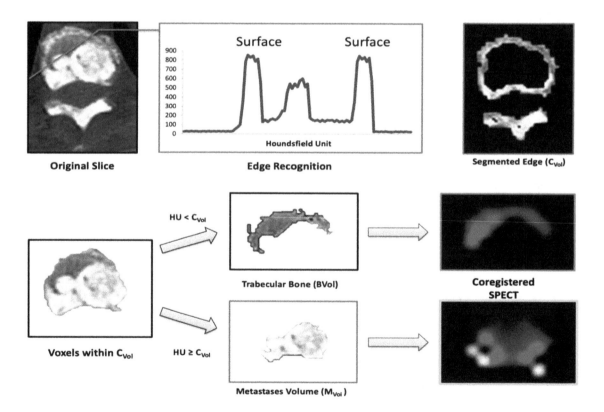

Figure 5. Functioning of the segmentation process. The software analyzes sequentially the Hounsfield Unit (HU) density of voxel within a single slice (top left). The bone border is identified as an increase of HU values (top center). After definition of the cortical volume (C_{Vol}, top right), its mean HU density is calculated. This value is used to classify all voxels located on the inside of C_{Vol} as pertinent to bone metastases (M_{Vol}) or to normal trabecular bone (B_{Vol}, middle and left bottom panels). Afterwards, mean counts/voxel are extracted from the co-registered images (bottom right).

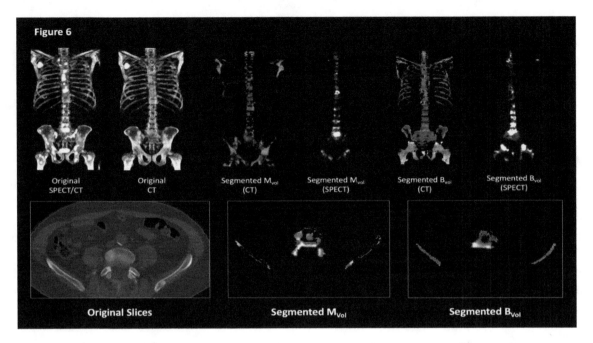

Figure 6. Examples of the segmentation output. Three-dimensional maximum intensity projections representations (top panels) and transaxial views (bottom panels) of the original images (left) and of the processed imaging outputs (center and right).

In the next step, masks corresponding to the M_{Vol} and the B_{Vol} were generated and exported onto the co-registered SPECT images; here, mean radioactivity concentration (counts/voxel) was calculated. The program's output included the volume (in mL), the mean HU density, and the mean counts of both volumes M_{Vol} and B_{Vol}. For the purpose of the present study, the skull was excluded from the analysis. Separate computations were then conducted for the whole-body skeleton (the whole skeleton from atlas until the distal femurs), the axial skeleton (vertebrae and sternum), and the appendicular bones (humeral and femoral shafts).

4.5. Validation of the Computational Technique and Comparison with Controls

In order to correlate the information obtained by the new program with known indices, we compared the magnitude of volumes, density values, and tracer distribution with approved radiological, clinical, and laboratory standards of reference. In the first step, we aimed to verify the correctness of the bone identification by our program. To do so, we compared the total S_{Vol} with a volumetric estimate of the whole skeleton obtained by a licensed commercial application (QMetrix®, General Electric, Boston, MA, USA). This comparison was done to ensure that our method could correctly recognize the bone volume on the CT images.

In the second step, we compared the M_{Vol} (as an estimate of the tumor burden) with the absolute number of metastatic lesions, which were manually counted on the SPECT/CT images by an expert reader. Finally, M_{Vol}, mean M_{Vol} HU, average M_{Vol} counts, and ratio between M_{Vol} and B_{Vol} were correlated to PSA levels.

To further stratify disease aggressiveness, both HU values and counts of M_{Vol} were compared between patients with or without a superscan finding at planar imaging. Superscan was defined as the presence of uniformly increased activity within the skeleton, with very faint or absent visualization of the renal system [36].

4.6. Statistical Analysis

Data are presented as mean ±standard deviation. The t-test for unpaired data was used to compare values between patients' subgroups. To verify the probability of therapy response as a function of the measured counts within the segmented volumes, ROC analyses were performed, and areas-under-curve (AUC) calculated. Correlations between indices were assessed with bivariate analyses, using Pearson's R index. Prevalence of superscan patients among groups was tested using the Chi-squared test.

A p-value of <0.05 was considered significant. The SPSS statistical program (SPSS®, v. 21.0, IBM, Armonk NY, USA) was employed.

5. Conclusions

This study aimed to contribute to the transition to tailored treatments in the field of metastasized castration-resistant prostate cancer. The availability of reliable indices of disease burden and the capability to measure therapy response accurately, as well to predict its clinical course, are key in ensuring the best possible treatment to every single patient. The present paper presents a method by which disease-specific indices, mirroring the corresponding parameters of disease status, can be obtained. The capability to extract this data can potentially be used, pending further studies, to ameliorate the imaging-based disease stratification and to improve the therapeutic schedule, therefore improving treatment effectiveness in these patients.

Author Contributions: Individual contribution are as follows: Conceptualization: F.F., C.l.F and G.S.; methodology: M.R., H.D., C.C. and A.S.; Software: C.C. and M.P.; Formal analysis: M.W. ans S.S.; Visualization: M.W. and S.S.; Writing (draft preparation): F.F., M.W. and H.D.; Writing (review and editing): F.F., C.l.F., H.D., A.S., M.P. and G.S.; Supervision: C.l.F.

References

1. Seruga, B.; Ocana, A.; Tannock, I.F. Drug resistance in metastatic castration-resistant prostate cancer. *Nat. Rev. Clin. Oncol.* **2011**, *8*, 12–23. [CrossRef] [PubMed]
2. Cookson, M.S.; Roth, B.J.; Dahm, P.; Engstrom, C.; Freedland, S.J.; Hussain, M.; Lin, D.W.; Lowrance, W.T.; Murad, M.H.; Oh, W.K.; et al. Castration-resistant prostate cancer: AUA Guideline. *J. Urol.* **2013**, *190*, 429–438. [CrossRef] [PubMed]
3. Bubendorf, L.; Schopfer, A.; Wagner, U.; Sauter, G.; Moch, H.; Willi, N.; Gasser, T.C.; Mihatsch, M.J. Metastatic patterns of prostate cancer: An autopsy study of 1589 patients. *Hum. Pathol.* **2000**, *31*, 578–583. [CrossRef] [PubMed]
4. Huang, X.; Chau, C.H.; Figg, W.D. Challenges to improved therapeutics for metastatic castrate resistant prostate cancer: From recent successes and failures. *J. Hematol. Oncol.* **2012**, *5*, 35. [CrossRef] [PubMed]
5. Benjamin, R. Neurologic complications of prostate cancer. *Am. Fam. Physician* **2002**, *65*, 1834–1840. [PubMed]
6. Fiz, F.; Sahbai, S.; Campi, C.; Weissinger, M.; Dittmann, H.; Marini, C.; Piana, M.; Sambuceti, G.; la Fougere, C. Tumor Burden and Intraosseous Metabolic Activity as Predictors of Bone Marrow Failure during Radioisotope Therapy in Metastasized Prostate Cancer Patients. *Biomed. Res. Int.* **2017**, *2017*, 3905216. [CrossRef] [PubMed]
7. Kantoff, P.W.; Higano, C.S.; Shore, N.D.; Berger, E.R.; Small, E.J.; Penson, D.F.; Redfern, C.H.; Ferrari, A.C.; Dreicer, R.; Sims, R.B.; et al. Sipuleucel-T immunotherapy for castration-resistant prostate cancer. *N. Engl. J. Med.* **2010**, *363*, 411–422. [CrossRef] [PubMed]
8. Kwon, E.D.; Drake, C.G.; Scher, H.I.; Fizazi, K.; Bossi, A.; van den Eertwegh, A.J.; Krainer, M.; Houede, N.; Santos, R.; Mahammedi, H.; et al. Ipilimumab versus placebo after radiotherapy in patients with metastatic castration-resistant prostate cancer that had progressed after docetaxel chemotherapy (CA184-043): A multicentre, randomised, double-blind, phase 3 trial. *Lancet Oncol.* **2014**, *15*, 700–712. [CrossRef]
9. Pezaro, C.J.; Omlin, A.G.; Altavilla, A.; Lorente, D.; Ferraldeschi, R.; Bianchini, D.; Dearnaley, D.; Parker, C.; de Bono, J.S.; Attard, G. Activity of cabazitaxel in castration-resistant prostate cancer progressing after docetaxel and next-generation endocrine agents. *Eur. Urol.* **2014**, *66*, 459–465. [CrossRef] [PubMed]
10. Hoskin, P.; Sartor, O.; O'Sullivan, J.M.; Johannessen, D.C.; Helle, S.I.; Logue, J.; Bottomley, D.; Nilsson, S.; Vogelzang, N.J.; Fang, F.; et al. Efficacy and safety of radium-223 dichloride in patients with castration-resistant prostate cancer and symptomatic bone metastases, with or without previous docetaxel use: A prespecified subgroup analysis from the randomised, double-blind, phase 3 ALSYMPCA trial. *Lancet Oncol.* **2014**, *15*, 1397–1406. [CrossRef]

11. Kratochwil, C.; Giesel, F.L.; Stefanova, M.; Benesova, M.; Bronzel, M.; Afshar-Oromieh, A.; Mier, W.; Eder, M.; Kopka, K.; Haberkorn, U. PSMA-Targeted Radionuclide Therapy of Metastatic Castration-Resistant Prostate Cancer with 177Lu-Labeled PSMA-617. *J. Nucl. Med.* **2016**, *57*, 1170–1176. [CrossRef] [PubMed]

12. Kratochwil, C.; Bruchertseifer, F.; Giesel, F.L.; Weis, M.; Verburg, F.A.; Mottaghy, F.; Kopka, K.; Apostolidis, C.; Haberkorn, U.; Morgenstern, A. 225Ac-PSMA-617 for PSMA-Targeted alpha-Radiation Therapy of Metastatic Castration-Resistant Prostate Cancer. *J. Nucl. Med.* **2016**, *57*, 1941–1944. [CrossRef] [PubMed]

13. Sartor, A.O.; Fitzpatrick, J.M. Urologists and oncologists: Adapting to a new treatment paradigm in castration-resistant prostate cancer (CRPC). *BJU Int.* **2012**, *110*, 328–335. [CrossRef] [PubMed]

14. Sartor, O. State-of-the-Art Management for the Patient with Castration-Resistant Prostate Cancer in 2012. *Am. Soc. Clin. Oncol. Educ. Book* **2012**, 289–291. [CrossRef]

15. Chung, P.H.; Gayed, B.A.; Thoreson, G.R.; Raj, G.V. Emerging drugs for prostate cancer. *Expert Opin. Emerg. Drugs* **2013**, *18*, 533–550. [CrossRef]

16. Yu, E.Y.; Gulati, R.; Telesca, D.; Jiang, P.; Tam, S.; Russell, K.J.; Nelson, P.S.; Etzioni, R.D.; Higano, C.S. Duration of first off-treatment interval is prognostic for time to castration resistance and death in men with biochemical relapse of prostate cancer treated on a prospective trial of intermittent androgen deprivation. *J. Clin. Oncol.* **2010**, *28*, 2668–2673. [CrossRef]

17. Bahl, A.K.; Bertelli, G.; Lewis, P.D.; Jenkins, P.; Aziz, A.; Davies, P.J.; Persad, R.; Smith, C.G.; Hurley, K.; Mason, M.D. Correlation of elevated alkaline phosphatase (ALP) and survival in metastatic castration-resistant prostate cancer (CRPC) treated with docetaxel chemotherapy: Results of SWSW Uro-oncology Group study from three U.K. centers. *J. Clin. Oncol.* **2011**, *29*, 206. [CrossRef]

18. Piper, C.; van Erps, T.; Pfister, D.J.; Epplen, R.; Porres, D.; Heidenreich, A. Frequency and prognostic significance of the PSA flare-up phenomenon in men with castration-resistant prostate cancer (CRPC) who undergo docetaxel-based chemotherapy. *J. Clin. Oncol.* **2012**, *30*, 92. [CrossRef]

19. Schroder, F.H.; Tombal, B.; Miller, K.; Boccon-Gibod, L.; Shore, N.D.; Crawford, E.D.; Moul, J.; Olesen, T.K.; Persson, B.E. Changes in alkaline phosphatase levels in patients with prostate cancer receiving degarelix or leuprolide: Results from a 12-month, comparative, phase III study. *BJU Int.* **2010**, *106*, 182–187. [CrossRef]

20. Qin, J.; Liu, X.; Laffin, B.; Chen, X.; Choy, G.; Jeter, C.R.; Calhoun-Davis, T.; Li, H.; Palapattu, G.S.; Pang, S.; et al. The PSA(-/lo) prostate cancer cell population harbors self-renewing long-term tumor-propagating cells that resist castration. *Cell Stem Cell* **2012**, *10*, 556–569. [CrossRef]

21. Pollen, J.J.; Witztum, K.F.; Ashburn, W.L. The flare phenomenon on radionuclide bone scan in metastatic prostate cancer. *AJR Am. J. Roentgenol.* **1984**, *142*, 773–776. [CrossRef] [PubMed]

22. Fiz, F.; Dittman, H.; Campi, C.; Morbelli, S.; Marini, C.; Brignone, M.; Bauckneht, M.; Piva, R.; Massone, A.M.; Piana, M.; et al. Assessment of Skeletal Tumor Load in Metastasized Castration-Resistant Prostate Cancer Patients: A Review of Available Methods and an Overview on Future Perspectives. *Bioengineering* **2018**, *5*, 58. [CrossRef] [PubMed]

23. Carrasquillo, J.A.; O'Donoghue, J.A.; Pandit-Taskar, N.; Humm, J.L.; Rathkopf, D.E.; Slovin, S.F.; Williamson, M.J.; Lacuna, K.; Aksnes, A.K.; Larson, S.M.; et al. Phase I pharmacokinetic and biodistribution study with escalating doses of (2)(2)(3)Ra-dichloride in men with castration-resistant metastatic prostate cancer. *Eur. J. Nucl. Med. Mol. Imaging* **2013**, *40*, 1384–1393. [CrossRef] [PubMed]

24. Pacilio, M.; Ventroni, G.; De Vincentis, G.; Cassano, B.; Pellegrini, R.; Di Castro, E.; Frantellizzi, V.; Follacchio, G.A.; Garkavaya, T.; Lorenzon, L.; et al. Dosimetry of bone metastases in targeted radionuclide therapy with alpha-emitting (223)Ra-dichloride. *Eur. J. Nucl. Med. Mol. Imaging* **2016**, *43*, 21–33. [CrossRef] [PubMed]

25. Fosbol, M.O.; Petersen, P.M.; Kjaer, A.; Mortensen, J. (223)Ra Therapy of Advanced Metastatic Castration-Resistant Prostate Cancer: Quantitative Assessment of Skeletal Tumor Burden for Prognostication of Clinical Outcome and Hematologic Toxicity. *J. Nucl. Med.* **2018**, *59*, 596–602. [CrossRef] [PubMed]

26. Petersen, L.J.; Mortensen, J.C.; Bertelsen, H.; Zacho, H.D. Computer-assisted interpretation of planar whole-body bone scintigraphy in patients with newly diagnosed prostate cancer. *Nucl. Med. Commun* **2015**, *36*, 679–685. [CrossRef]

27. Ryan, C.J.; Shah, S.; Efstathiou, E.; Smith, M.R.; Taplin, M.E.; Bubley, G.J.; Logothetis, C.J.; Kheoh, T.; Kilian, C.; Haqq, C.M.; et al. Phase II study of abiraterone acetate in chemotherapy-naive metastatic castration-resistant prostate cancer displaying bone flare discordant with serologic response. *Clin. Cancer Res.* **2011**, *17*, 4854–4861. [CrossRef] [PubMed]

28. Rohren, E.M.; Etchebehere, E.C.; Araujo, J.C.; Hobbs, B.P.; Swanston, N.M.; Everding, M.; Moody, T.; Macapinlac, H.A. Determination of Skeletal Tumor Burden on 18F-Fluoride PET/CT. *J. Nucl. Med.* **2015**, *56*, 1507–1512. [CrossRef]

29. Bieth, M.; Kronke, M.; Tauber, R.; Dahlbender, M.; Retz, M.; Nekolla, S.G.; Menze, B.; Maurer, T.; Eiber, M.; Schwaiger, M. Exploring New Multimodal Quantitative Imaging Indices for the Assessment of Osseous Tumor Burden in Prostate Cancer Using 68Ga-PSMA PET/CT. *J. Nucl. Med.* **2017**, *58*, 1632–1637. [CrossRef]

30. Horger, M.; Bares, R. The role of single-photon emission computed tomography/computed tomography in benign and malignant bone disease. *Semin. Nucl. Med.* **2006**, *36*, 286–294. [CrossRef]

31. Nakajima, K.; Edenbrandt, L.; Mizokami, A. Bone scan index: A new biomarker of bone metastasis in patients with prostate cancer. *Int. J. Urol.* **2017**, *24*, 668–673. [CrossRef] [PubMed]

32. Dadhania, S.; Alonzi, R.; Douglas, S.; Gogbashian, A.; Hughes, R.; Dalili, D.; Vasdev, N.; Adshead, J.; Lane, T.; Westbury, C.; et al. Single-centre Experience of Use of Radium 223 with Clinical Outcomes Based on Number of Cycles and Bone Marrow Toxicity. *Anticancer Res.* **2018**, *38*, 5423–5427. [CrossRef] [PubMed]

33. Sambuceti, G.; Brignone, M.; Marini, C.; Massollo, M.; Fiz, F.; Morbelli, S.; Buschiazzo, A.; Campi, C.; Piva, R.; Massone, A.M.; et al. Estimating the whole bone-marrow asset in humans by a computational approach to integrated PET/CT imaging. *Eur. J. Nucl. Med. Mol. Imaging* **2012**, *39*, 1326–1338. [CrossRef] [PubMed]

34. Fiz, F.; Marini, C.; Piva, R.; Miglino, M.; Massollo, M.; Bongioanni, F.; Morbelli, S.; Bottoni, G.; Campi, C.; Bacigalupo, A.; et al. Adult advanced chronic lymphocytic leukemia: Computational analysis of whole-body CT documents a bone structure alteration. *Radiology* **2014**, *271*, 805–813. [CrossRef] [PubMed]

35. Fiz, F.; Marini, C.; Campi, C.; Massone, A.M.; Podesta, M.; Bottoni, G.; Piva, R.; Bongioanni, F.; Bacigalupo, A.; Piana, M.; et al. Allogeneic cell transplant expands bone marrow distribution by colonizing previously abandoned areas: An FDG PET/CT analysis. *Blood* **2015**, *125*, 4095–4102. [CrossRef] [PubMed]

36. Constable, A.R.; Cranage, R.W. Recognition of the superscan in prostatic bone scintigraphy. *Br. J. Radiol.* **1981**, *54*, 122–125. [CrossRef] [PubMed]

15

Ultrasound Monitoring of Extant Adnexal Masses in the Era of Type 1 and Type 2 Ovarian Cancers: Lessons Learned from Ovarian Cancer Screening Trials

Eleanor L. Ormsby [1,2,*], Edward J. Pavlik [3] and John P. McGahan [1]

[1]   Department of Radiology, University of California Davis Medical Center, 4860 Y Street, Suite 3100, Sacramento, CA 95817, USA; jpmcgahan@ucdavis.edu

[2]   Department of Radiology, Kaiser Permanente Sacramento, 2025 Morse Ave, CA 95825, USA

[3]   Division of Gynecologic Oncology, Department of Obstetrics and Gynecology, University of Kentucky Chandler Medical Center-Markey Cancer Center, Lexington, KY 40536, USA; Epaul1@uky.edu

*   Correspondence: eormsby@gmail.com

Academic Editor: Andreas Kjaer

Abstract: Women that are positive for an ovarian abnormality in a clinical setting can have either a malignancy or a benign tumor with probability favoring the benign alternative. Accelerating the abnormality to surgery will result in a high number of unnecessary procedures that will place cost burdens on the individual and the health delivery system. Surveillance using serial ultrasonography is a reasonable alternative that can be used to discover if changes in the ovarian abnormality will occur that favor either a malignant or benign interpretation. Several ovarian cancer screening trials have had extensive experiences with changes in subclinical ovarian abnormalities in normal women that can define growth, stability or resolution and give some idea of the time frame over which changes occur. The present report examines these experiences and relates them to the current understanding of ovarian cancer ontology, presenting arguments related to the benefits of surveillance.

Keywords: ovary; cancer; screening; monitoring; surveillance; serial ultrasonography

---

1. Introduction

Ovarian cancer is the deadliest cancer that women face, causing more deaths than any other cancer of the female reproductive system [1]. However, the prevalence of ovarian cancer is low, responsible for only about 3% of all cancers in women [2] and accounting for a lifetime risk of 1.3% (1 in 75) [3]. Transvaginal ultrasound (TVS) has been widely recognized as the first line for evaluating adnexal masses presenting both low risk and low cost. Prospective ovarian cancer screening trials have utilized TVS to detect early stage malignancies. The five-year survival rate for women diagnosed with stage I ovarian cancer has been reported to be as high as 95% [4,5] in contrast to only 30% for women with stage III disease [6]. While large prospective screening trials have focused on how best to identify malignancies in asymptomatic women in the general population, adnexal masses are commonly identified by ultrasound ordered for a wide variety of indications in routine clinical practice even when a patient does not present with relevant symptoms. While the US Preventive Services Task Force (USPSTF) has recommended against population screening for ovarian cancer [7], many women undergo ultrasound for various symptoms. This paper reviews recent prospective ovarian cancer screening trial findings for clinical application on how women with adnexal masses, found by ultrasound, for various reasons other than for screening purposes, should be managed and followed.

Ovarian cysts are often observed sonographically even in post-menopausal women with a reported incidence rate of up to 21% [8]. The question of how best to manage these masses has been the subject of much interest and debate among clinicians including obstetric gynecologists, primary care physicians, radiologists and gynecology oncologists. Several reports have asserted that resected ovarian cysts do not contain malignancy [9–11], but that if left unmonitored, ovarian cysts can progress to ovarian cancers [12,13]. Therefore, all ovarian cysts may present some source of concern. Historically, this concern has led to a conundrum among radiologists and clinicians. Should these cysts be monitored (how frequently and for how long) or should ovarian cysts be managed operatively at the risk of potential harm from surgical complications and medical expenses?

In 2010, a consensus panel of the Society of Radiologists in Ultrasound (SRU) that was composed of 19 experts in radiology, obstetric gynecology, and gynecology oncology, as well as pathology released a recommendation regarding the management of adnexal masses found sonographically in asymptomatic women [14]. The panel analyzed literature available at the time of the conference (October 2009) and strategies in clinical practice with the goal of reaching a consensus on: (1) which masses might not require follow-up, (2) which masses would need imaging follow-up, as well as when follow-up evaluation should occur, and (3) which masses should warrant referral to a gynecologic oncologist for surgical evaluation. The consensus agreed that it is reasonable to perform annual ultrasound follow-up of cysts larger than 5 cm in premenopausal women and those larger than 1 cm in postmenopausal women, although such cysts are unlikely to be malignant [14]. A recent expert review suggested that low risk abnormalities can undergo an initial three-month follow-up with those that remain stable or decreasing in size being examined every 12 months for five years [15].

Since the SRU guidelines from 2010 [14], differences over how best to manage adnexal masses persisted and were recently addressed by the first international consensus conference on adnexal masses [15]. This panel included representatives of societies in the fields of gynecology, gynecologic oncology, radiology and pathology and clinicians from Europe, Canada and the United States. While many of the adnexal masses are benign appearing (i.e., simple cysts or hemorrhagic cysts), for many more, it is not clear whether the mass may contain foci of malignancy and consequently are classified as *indeterminate*. As a clarification of terminology, "simple cysts" and "unilocular cysts" are the same and are characterized as being anechoic structures that are absent papillae, solid areas and septa (complete or incomplete). The low prevalence of ovarian cancer (3%) [2] establishes the likelihood that most ovarian cysts are benign yet cysts cannot be dismissed because they occur with a high incidence rate (21–35%) [8]. Some cysts are not simple and include morphologic elements that can demonstrate multiseptations or small solid nodules. No specific guideline had been established for indeterminate masses by the SRU consensus due to the fact that data analyzing long-term follow up of adnexal masses at the time was insufficient. The SRU stated that "as research continues, the recommendations regarding management of adnexal cysts may vary". The present review examines the evidence from recent research in histopathology of ovarian cancer types, ovarian cancer screening trials and ultrasound morphology of adnexal masses to establish a framework for surveillance of these masses.

2. Type 1 and Type 2 Ovarian Cancers Found in Ultrasound Imaging

Currently, ovarian cancers now include two distinct types of malignancy: Type 1 or 2 based on histologic pathogenesis, molecular alterations and clinical progression (Table 1). Type 1 ovarian cancers include low grade serous carcinoma, endometrioid carcinoma, and clear cell carcinoma. Type 1 ovarian cancers demonstrate a step-wise progression originating from a benign precursor or borderline tumor or endometriosis [16–18]. For example, low grade serous carcinomas may arise via transformation of benign and borderline serous tumors that are thought to be derived from inclusion cysts originating from the ovarian surface or tubal epithelium. This progression is analogous to the adenoma-to-carcinoma sequence seen in colorectal carcinoma pathogenesis or the hyperplasia-to-carcinoma sequence in endometrioid carcinoma of the endometrium [19].

In contrast, Type 2 ovarian cancers are highly aggressive and include high grade serous, high grade endometrioid and undifferentiated carcinomas, as well as malignant mixed mesodermal carcinomas, usually presenting at an advanced stage [17,19,20]. Type 2 ovarian cancers often have TP53 mutations but rarely have mutations that are associated with Type 1 ovarian malignancies [17,20]. Some Type 2 ovarian cancers (in particular, high grade serous carcinoma) are associated with *BRCA* (BReast CAncer susceptibility gene) inactivation [21]. Compelling evidence indicates that these malignancies may originate from the epithelium of the fimbrial portion of the fallopian tube as serous tubal intraepithelial carcinomas (STIC) [22–32]. Finally, some high grade serous carcinomas have been reported to develop from transformation of serous borderline tumors or low grade Type 1 serous carcinomas [17–20]. While pathogenesis may differ, the morphology of the high-grade serous carcinomas that develop in the Type 2 pathway is similar to high-grade serous carcinomas that are transformed from Type 1 tumors with shared clinical behaviors [17]. Using this paradigm, a stratified treatment plan can be devised. However, currently there is no prospective means that differentiates between the subtypes of ovarian cancer based on ultrasound imaging. Based on recent ovarian cancer screening results, abnormalities with lesser degrees of morphologic complexity may harbor micro foci of ovarian cancer indicating that a wide spectrum of abnormal morphology should be considered for ultrasound follow up and active surveillance.

Table 1. Summary of Type 1 and Type 2 ovarian carcinomas.

Tumor Type	Type 1 Tumors	Type 2 Tumors
Behavior	Indolent	Aggressive
Diagnosis at	Early Stage	Advanced Stage
Survival Rate at 5 years	About 55%	About 30%
Type/Precursor	-Endometrioid carcinoma/Endometriosis -Clear cell carcinoma/Endometriosis Mucinous carcinoma/Mucinous Cystadenoma, Endometriosis, Teratoma, -Brenner Tumor, and Mucinous borderline tumor -Low grade serous carcinoma/Serous cystadenoma, Adenofibroma, Atypical proliferative serous tumor, Mullerian epithelial cyst -Transitional cell carcinoma or Malignant Brenner tumor/Brenner tumor	-High grade serous carcinoma/Probably de novo starting at the tubo, ovarian surface epithelium, serous tubal intraepithelial carcinomas (STIC) or ovarian hilum stem cell -Undifferentiated carcinoma? -Malignant mixed carcinoma?

2.1. Summary of Information from Recent Prospective Ovarian Cancer Screening Trials

There have been four large prospective ovarian cancer screening trials utilizing ultrasound in asymptomatic women [5,33–35]. The first randomized control trial in the US was the Prostate, Lung, Colorectal and Ovarian Cancer Screening (PLCO) Trial, a randomized controlled trial (RCT) of 68,616 women aged 55 to 74 of whom 30,630 underwent screening between 1993 and 2007 [34]. Women were screened using serum CA-125 (cancer antigen 125) at a cut-off of ≥35 kU/L and transvaginal ultrasound (TVS) for four years followed by CA-125 alone for an additional two years. Endpoint analysis showed that screening with the combination of CA-125 and transvaginal ultrasound had no mortality benefit compared to the unscreened control group [34]. Importantly, in the PLCO study, surgical decisions were made on the basis of a single ultrasound exam and an absolute CA-125 level of 35 units/mL. More importantly, the PLCO trial had no uniform evaluation and treatment algorithm for patients with screen-detected adnexal masses so that women identified in the screening arm could be treated up to nine months after ultrasound detection, allowing their disease to progress to later stages during this time.

In the multicenter prospective randomized Shizuoka Cohort Study of Ovarian Cancer Screening (SCSOCS) trial in Japan [33], conducted between 1985 and 1999, asymptomatic postmenopausal women were assigned either to a screening arm ($n = 41,688$) or to a control arm ($n = 40,799$). Furthermore,

63% of ovarian cancers detected by screening were stage I disease versus 38% in the control arm. Importantly, optimal tumor debulking was achieved more often in women whose ovarian cancer was detected by screening [33]. Assessment of ovarian cancer specific survival was not completed in the SCSOCS trial.

More recent studies have been published with a screening strategy that improves on using a single ultrasound exam or a single CA-125 value at 35 units/mL, an approach that did not achieve an acceptable positive predictive value (PPV) in the PLCO trial [34]. These strategies include the use of serial ultrasound instead of a single ultrasound exam dictating the surgical decision and the utilization of multimodalities keying on changes in serial CA 125 determinations. The University of Kentucky Ovarian Cancer Screening Trial utilized a prospective single arm that focused on annual ultrasound screening study of 25,327 women from 1987 to 2012 [36]. In the Kentucky study, serial ultrasound follow up of the 6807 women with ovarian abnormalities displaying varying ultrasonographic morphologic features resulted in a 304% improved PPV from 8.1% to 25% and reduced unnecessary surgery on benign tumors [36]. Importantly, this study found that women in the screening group had a higher rate of earlier stage cancer discovery (68% stage I or II disease) than the unscreened comparison group (27% stage I or II, $p < 0.01$) [36–38]. Overall five-year survival of women who had epithelial ovarian cancer (EOC) found during the serial ultrasound follow up including false negative cancers was 74.8% ± 6.6% compared to 53.7% ± 2.3% for women who were clinically detected ($p < 0.01$) [37,38]. Using the serial ultrasound approach, differentiating benign from malignant tumors was based on the regression of benign masses [36]. Extending serial ultrasound to include a quantitative index showed that malignant tumors demonstrated increasing morphology index scores over time [37,39].

Others have evaluated serial CA-125 level or other biomarkers such as human epididymis protein 4 (HE4) to improve the detection of ovarian cancer [40–42]. The Risk of Ovarian Cancer Algorithm (ROCA) is a multivariate linear model based on longitudinal data from women with ovarian cancer and estimates intermediate and high risk for malignancy based on changes in CA-125 levels relative to an individual's previous levels. ROCA with multiple CA-125 determinations has performed better in detecting ovarian cancer than a single level since CA-125 levels vary greatly depending on the menopausal status, fertility drug use, current cigarette use, race, pelvic inflammation and irregular menstruation [43]. Using an absolute CA-125 cut off value of 35 units/mL may result in a high false negative rate because only 50–60% of women with stage 1 EOC will have CA-125 elevated above this level and borderline, and Type 1 or low grade tumors are known to express low levels of CA-125 [44].

In the United Kingdom Collaborative Trial of Ovarian Cancer Screening (UKCTOC), the largest randomized control screening trial to date, performed between 2001–2005, 202,638 women from the general population were assigned to a control group (no intervention) or to annual screening using either transvaginal ultrasound (USS) or serum CA-125 interpreted by ROCA with transvaginal ultrasound as a second line test (multimodal screening, MMS) [12,35,44]. The stage distribution of the screen-detected primary invasive cancers was similar in both the multimodality group and the group that received only ultrasonography [35]. In addition, 50% of primary invasive ovarian and tubal malignancies detected by serial ultrasound screening alone had stage I or II disease versus 26% in the control cases detected clinically (i.e., without screening) [35]. Screening produced a significant increase in the detection of early stage ovarian malignancy. A report on the survival benefit from the UKCTOCS has been published, which showed that, when prevalent cases were excluded, a significant mortality reduction was noted after 7–14 years within the multimodality arm [35]. Similar but lesser mortality reduction was seen with ultrasound alone. The trial is currently undergoing additional follow up to further examine mortality reduction. Based on these data, it was concluded that 641 screens are needed to prevent one ovarian cancer death [35].

Recently, it has been reported that ovarian cancer screening detects more indolent and less aggressive Type 1 cancers [45] and that the frequency of Type 2 cancer is ~75% is higher than Type 1 with higher mortality rate for Type 2 cancer due to its faster rate of growth and metastasis. This result is in contrast to findings from the Kentucky Ovarian Cancer Screening trial where 83.3% of early stage malignancies were aggressive Type 2 cancers [5,35,36,38]. In the UKCTOC ultrasound arm trial, both Type 1 and Type 2 cancers were detected albeit more Type 1 than Type 2 [35]. Of the 23 Type 2 cancers diagnosed in the UKCTOC ultrasound arm, 15 were associated with adnexal abnormalities, while eight had normal ultrasound with subsequent diagnosis of ovarian cancer within 16 months (ranging 6–13 months with median of 10) [12]. No women with persisting normal ultrasound results were found to have Type 1 ovarian cancers of the 32 women with Type 1 cancer who were detected by ultrasound in the ultrasound arm of the UKCTOC [12]. Based on these observations, it may be concluded that many Type 2 cancers are found in women brought to clinical practice by symptoms and that Type 2 cancers have been shown to be quite possible to find through ovarian cancer screening using ultrasonography. Therefore, serial ultrasound follow up of persistent masses may benefit women in clinical practice by discriminating lethal Type 2 ovarian cancers as well as by reducing unnecessary surgery in cases where complexity moderates or abnormalities resolve.

2.2. Can Type 2 Ovarian Cancers Be Detected by Ultrasound?

Using a growth model of serous cystadenocarcinoma (Type 2) based on retrospective analysis of $BRCA_1$ carriers who had undergone prophylactic bilateral salpingo-oophorectomies (PBSOs), it was noted that high grade serous carcinoma likely spends approximately 4.3 years as histopathologically detectable but clinically occult early stage tumors [46]. This analysis also stated that more than 50% of serous carcinomas advanced to stage III/IV by the time they reached 3 cm in diameter. Assuming spherical shape, this would be a volume of 14 cm^3 (note that the normal ovary is 10–20 cm^3 and a walnut is 22 cm^3). The report postulated that the tumor would double in volume every two and a half months so that, at best, ultrasound follow up may only lead to the detection of low volume high grade Type 2 cancers rather than early stage cases. However, early stage disease detected in the Kentucky Ovarian Screening Program was larger than postulated by this model (Stage I Type 2: 65.4 cm^3 $\pm$ 27.6, 27, 4.1, 366, $n = 13$; Stage II Type 2: 131.1 cm^3 $\pm$ 33.4, 95.8, 10, 351.4, $n = 14$ (mean $\pm$ SEM, median, min, max)) [5,37]. Thus, the prediction made by the model [46] that to achieve 50% sensitivity in detecting tumors before they advance to Stage III, an annual screen would need to detect tumors of 1.3 cm in diameter is inaccurate and not supported by empirical screening data. Other investigators modeling the levels of CA-125 associated with the smallest progressing ovarian cancers reported that these cancers could develop unnoticed for 10.1 years and presented the view that the largest tumor below the resolution of ultrasound (0.5 cm diameter) could progress to a detectable size (1.2–2.5 cm) in 1–2 years [47]. Based on this estimation [47] and the Kentucky findings summarized above, early stage Type 2 ovarian malignancies are well within the range of discovery by ultrasound. In the context of surveillance monitoring, it would seem that arbitrary cessation as suggested by one retrospective study [48] of ultrasound follow up of small complex adnexal masses, which are less than 6 cm at seven months would miss both small volume high grade Type 2 cancers and the indolent Type 1 tumors that can potentially progress to higher grade invasive cancer.

3. Risk of Ovarian Cancer When There Is an Adnexal Mass

Adapting the information from these prospective ovarian cancer screening trials to non-screening applications in day-to-day clinical practice needs consideration. The USPSTF has recommended against ultrasound exams for ovarian cancer screen in asymptomatic women [7] based on prior randomized prospective ovarian cancer trials that failed to show mortality benefits while focusing on the risk of unnecessary surgery with a small immediate complication rate or more long-term effects of premature menopause from oophorectomy such as bone density loss. However, women present clinically with a wide variety of indications including nonspecific symptoms, as well as more gynecologic symptoms such as vaginal bleeding, pelvic fullness or pain. Sometimes, women may be referred for follow up ultrasound on incidental abnormal findings from other diagnostic radiology exams such as CT that have been obtained for unrelated reasons. Women who had any adnexal mass had a much higher relative risk of developing ovarian cancer as observed in the UKCTOC trial, compared to women who had no adnexal mass [12]. The relative risk ratio for all EOC (Types 1 and 2) was 49.2 for women with a multilocular solid cyst and 38.4 for women with a solid mass when compared to women with normal ultrasound exams [12]. For the most deadly and aggressive ovarian cancers (Type 2), the relative risk was 31.3 for women with a multilocular cysts with solid components and 38.4 for women with a solid mass [12].

Even benign appearing unilocular and multilocular cysts without any solid elements have been reported to be associated with epithelial ovarian cancer. In the UKCTOC report, unilocular and multilocular cysts without any solid components had a relative risk for EOC within three years of 5.3 (95% CI (confidence interval) 1.9–15.2) and 6.8 (95% CI 1.9–22.9), respectively, compared to normal ultrasound exams [12]. Among the primary EOC detected in the UKCTOC ultrasound screening trial, 16% (nine out of 55) developed from unilocular cysts while 9% (five out of 55) developed from multilocular cysts within three years of an initial scan. Among the borderline tumor and Type 1 epithelial cancers, 16% (five out of 32) developed from unilocular cysts while 13% (four out of 32) developed from multilocular cysts [12]. In another series by a separate research group, 11% (4/35) of borderline tumors and 4% (1/24) of epithelial ovarian cancers were classified as unilocular cysts at ultrasound examination performed by an ultrasound expert in a tertiary referral center for gynecological ultrasound [49].

Valentin et al. noted in their cohort that the overall malignancy rate for unilocular cysts was 1% and was higher among postmenopausal women (2.76%) then premenopausal women (0.54%) [50]. While the rates were very low, the difference was statistically significant between the two age groups. The authors of the study noted that, upon pathologic inspection, seven of the 11 malignant cysts described as unilocular on ultrasounds were found to contain small papillary projections or solid components, which were not observed sonographically [50]. Careful scrutiny of ultrasound images was advocated because subjective error or ultrasound resolution may provide explanations for the failure to observe the papillary projections. While there are limitations to ultrasound, the degree to which these limitations contribute to ultrasound results is small as shown by high sensitivities ($\geq$80%) and high negative predictive values (>99%) [5,37,38].

3.1. The Risk Profile for Abnormal Ultrasound Findings

Among postmenopausal women in the general US population, the overall risk of ovarian cancer rises with age to a 9–13% lifetime risk [51]. Relative risk increases when symptoms are present for which a pelvic ultrasound is often performed in clinical practice, mostly because of pelvic pain. The great majority of women with symptoms alone do not have an ovarian malignancy. The majority of women with both symptoms and an ovarian abnormality on ultrasound also do not have a malignancy due to the low prevalence of ovarian cancer; however, women with symptoms have been found to have a higher prevalence of ovarian cancer than that reported for asymptomatic women in screening trials using ultrasonography [52–54]. Differences between screening trial pelvic ultrasound outcomes and those in clinical settings result because symptoms predominate in clinical settings.

3.2. Benefit of Serial Ultrasound Follow-Up

Serial ultrasound and a subsequent increase in morphologic complexity of an adnexal mass have been used as the basis for surgical decisions in the single arm trial at the University of Kentucky [37] and in the UKCTOC [35]. In the University of Kentucky trial, the majority of ovarian abnormalities resolved within a year with serial ultrasound, including indeterminate masses. More than half of women (63%) with ovarian cystic abnormalities had resolution in the subsequent follow-up with near exponential resolution of ovarian abnormalities so that, by 1–2 years, only a fraction of the ovarian abnormalities persisted (Figure 1, from [36]).

Ovarian abnormalities that continue to persist comprise only a fraction of the ovarian abnormalities that are identified and are candidates for ongoing serial observation until their indeterminate status changes due to an increase in morphologic complexity. Therefore, serial ultrasound surveillance can mitigate the potential risk from surgical complications due to prematurely resecting indeterminate adnexal masses, especially if an adnexal mass demonstrates signs of resolving. Ultrasound follow-up is advantageous because it is cost effective and low risk. The cost of ultrasound follow-up is nominal compared to the cost of surgical treatment for women [55] and provides a greater margin of safety than dismissing an extant adnexal mass without follow-up based on presuming benign status due to an initial indeterminate ultrasound morphology.

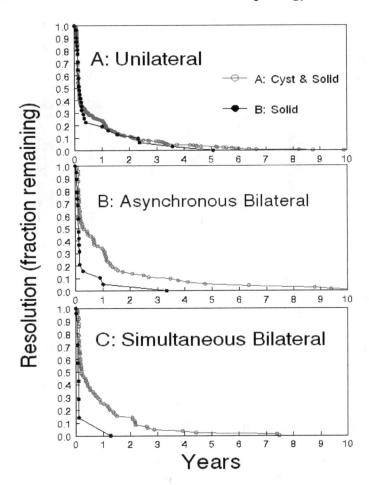

Figure 1. Resolution of complex ovarian abnormalities. (**A**) unilateral abnormalities, never simultaneously on both sides; (**B**) intermittent unilateral abnormalities consisting of ovarian abnormality on one side or the other at different times; (**C**) bilateral abnormalities occurring simultaneously on both sides. Cysts with solid components: red open circles. Solid components: black solid circles. Intrapanel comparisons, (**A**): not statistically different. (**B**) $p < 0.001$, (**C**) $p < 0.001$. Interpanel comparisons: **A** vs. **C** $p < 0.01$, **A** vs. **B** and **B** vs. **C**, not significantly different.

4. Subjectivity

4.1. Does Stability Over Time Argue Against Malignancy?

To address this question, work that focused on the ultrasound discovery of adnexal masses was reviewed [13]. Malignancy has been found in stable masses, which enlarged and increased in morphologic complexity in up to three years after initial detection in the UKCTOCS [12]. To put the risk of prematurely terminating ultrasound surveillance in perspective, the definition of the acceptable risk level (ARL) from environmental studies [56] of no more than 1 extra death/100,000 was used to normalize the UKCTOCS trial data. Using this approach, the absolute risks for the appearance of malignancy in up to three years after an initial ultrasound exam as calculated from the UKCTOCS data [12] are considerably elevated (Figure 2). The risk of malignancy is higher after finding any of the ovarian ultrasound abnormalities as judged by the 95% CI (Figure 2). Even allowing the 0.001% ARL to be relaxed 10 fold would still lead to the expectation of a considerable number of extra malignancies within three years of the first scan. If prematurely stopping surveillance caused 50% or more of these malignancies to be diagnosed at an advanced stage, likely destined to be fatal, then extra deaths due to curtailing surveillance can be expected to be high and emphasizes the peril of limiting ultrasound surveillance [13].

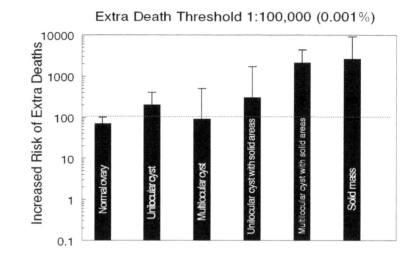

Figure 2. Estimation of risk in terms of extra deaths in women diagnosed with Type 2 primary epithelial ovarian cancer within three years after an ultrasound exam. Data were collected in the United Kingdom Collaborative Trial of Ovarian Cancer Screening Protocols as published [12] and normalized by the acceptable level of risk of no more than one extra death per 100,000 in environmental studies. Absolute risk of subsequent malignancy is shown by the bar labeled with each type of finding on the first ultrasound exam. The 95% confidence interval extends upward from each bar. The dashed line indicates the 95% confidence interval of the normal ovary extended across all types of findings.

4.2. The Conundrum of Ultrasound: Subjectivity and Technical Considerations

Subjectivity and operator-dependent errors are intrinsic to ultrasound imaging even when the images are acquired and interpreted by expert radiologists or gynecologists and contain subtle features that can go unreported or be missed. While the term *expert sonographer* is in wide use, there is no definition that provides an understanding of this status or terminology. Ultrasounds are very often performed by technologists whose varying skills and expertise are acquired and honed in the practice in which they are employed. For experts and technologists alike, small lesions can be missed due to various technical factors such as subject motion, lack of patient cooperation, large body habitus with poor acoustic penetration, bowel gas shadowing which obscures pelvic organs, positioning of the ovarian structure behind the uterus, etc. For some large masses, complete visualization of the wall and internal morphology cannot be obtained because the signal from the transvaginal probe cannot adequately reach the entire mass. When this is the case, the SRU recommendations advocate pelvic magnetic resonance images (MRIs) for better characterization and full visualization of large masses [14]. Small papillary projections within unilocular cysts can be absent on ultrasound, but later confirmed by surgical pathology. Thus, there can be situations where information from ultrasound can be inadequate.

Although ultrasound is highly sensitive, subjectivity inherent to the interpretation of ultrasound images accounts for variation in ultrasound reports especially for indeterminate adnexal masses. Recently, the International Ovarian Tumor Analysis (IOTA) study showed that there is considerable uncertainly and inter-observer disagreement when solid components and papillary projection were present [57]. Most disagreement was on the definition of a papillary projection, but there was also uncertainty leading to disagreement about whether a certain structure should be classified as a solid component or as a collection of septa, a collection of small cysts or as ovarian stroma. Including Doppler imaging can introduce variability because some septa can only be visualized with Doppler and, therefore it can change the type of morphology that is reported.

In addition to physiological cysts, serous and mucinous cystadenomas, transitional and germ cell tumors, struma ovarii, stromal cell tumors, fibromas, endometriomas, low malignant potential (borderline) tumors, and malignancies, and other structures that are expected to have the potential to be reported as having solid components in ultrasound exams of the adnexa include: inflammations, infections and abscesses. Only after surgery has been performed is it possible to establish the histopathologic identity of an ovarian abnormality seen on ultrasound. Histopathological identification is not a possibility in serial ultrasound surveillance when solid structures resolve as has been reported in the Kentucky study [36]. In brief, this study reported that while cysts with solid components had the highest risk for epithelial ovarian cancer, many complex abnormalities (cysts with apparent solid areas) and apparent solid masses were more likely to resolve within a year of surveillance (76.5–80.6%) than unilocular cysts and cysts with septations (32.8–43.9%, $p < 0.001$) [36]. Complex abnormalities and solid masses had a median time to resolution of 7.8–8.7 weeks, while unilocular cysts and cysts with septations had a median time to resolution of 53–55.6 weeks. The expectation is that if these were truly solid masses that are highly suspicious for cancer, they should not resolve. There are several possibilities to explain this observation. First, something other than the ovary was measured in the ultrasound report (i.e., overlapping adjacent tissue like a bowel loop). Second, the plane through which a partially solid ovarian structure was sonographically examined exaggerated the extent to which the structure appeared to be solid. Third, unverified factors like inflammation, infection or abscess were responsible for reporting solid areas in the ultrasound report, providing pseudo-findings. Serial ultrasonography provides a protection against a pseudo-finding of solid structure whenever there is evidence of a resolving process or resolution. Few would argue that uncertainty can be eliminated in ultrasound exams, especially with subjective interpretation providing the foundation for what is reported. The degree to which subjective interpretation can account for the identification of apparently "solid components" that subsequently resolve is not presently known, but can be corrected by a serial ultrasound imaging approach in diagnostic imaging. Moreover, the utilization of complementary Doppler imaging could contribute to differentiating a truly solid mass as distinct from a mass of clotted blood. However, even with Doppler imaging, not all solid masses will be able to demonstrate Doppler flow if there is too much tissue for the ultrasound beam to penetrate or if certain tumors are not sufficiently vascularized for detection by Doppler imaging. Thus, in the absence of definitive Doppler identification, the best solution for distinguishing apparently solid components is serial ultrasonography.

5. Ovarian Mass Ultrasound Morphology

There is considerable overlap between the ultrasonographic morphology of ovarian masses. In the UKCTOCS study, 25 (78.1%) of the borderline/Type 1 cancers had adnexal abnormalities with solid elements (unilocular solid/multilocular solid cysts or solid masses) on the initial ($n = 23$) or subsequent ($n = 2$) scans [12]. Of the 23 women diagnosed with Type 2 EOC, 15 had sonographic adnexal abnormalities where eleven (47.8%) had solid elements or ascites on the initial scan [12]. While in the UKCTOCS study, the strongest association between ovarian morphology and epithelial ovarian cancer was the presence of "solid component(s)", borderline, and Type 1 and Type 2 cancers were found across all sonographic morphologies including unilocular and multilocular cysts without solid components. In contrast, benign pathology was the norm for all morphologies including cysts with solid components [36]. The challenge for radiologists and gynecologic oncologists is correctly diagnosing epithelial ovarian cancers associated with indeterminate masses having multiple thick septations and or solid components that can be seen across borderline, indolent Type 1 tumors, aggressive Type 2 tumors and benign masses. This challenge is complicated by the low prevalence of ovarian cancer. Clear expressions of ovarian abnormalities seen ultrasonographically are presented in Figure 3. Tumors of low malignant potential (i.e., borderline tumors) account for 15% of all epithelial ovarian cancers (Figure 3A). Nearly 75% of these tumors are stage I at the time of diagnosis. They represent a heterogeneous group and occur in younger women with favorable prognosis. However, symptomatic recurrence and death may be found as long as 20 years after therapy in some patients. While low grade serous tumors (Type 1) occur less frequently, pernicious high-grade serous carcinomas (Type 2) predominate, accounting for over half of ovarian malignancies, Figure 3B. Undifferentiated carcinomas (Figure 3C, 2%), malignant mixed mesodermal tumors (Figure 3D, 3%) and high grade transitional cell carcinomas (Figure 3E, 2%) (all Type 2) each carry a serious prognosis, but together account for less than 10% of ovarian malignancies. Endometriod carcinomas comprise ~20% of ovarian malignancies with low and high grade endometriod carcinomas appearing ultrasonographically similar (Figure 3F,G). Together with clear cell carcinomas (Figure 3H, 3%), malignant Brenner's tumor (Figure 3I, <1%) and mucinous carcinomas (Figure 3J,K, 5%) are recognized as being responsive to treatment. Overlapping morphological components characterize all of these tumors. To discriminate malignant from benign abnormalities, a Morphology Index (MI) has been developed at the University of Kentucky [58]. The MI grades an abnormality on the basis of both size and structure (morphology) as shown in Figure 4. Increasing MI scores correlate well with the risk of an abnormality being malignant [39].

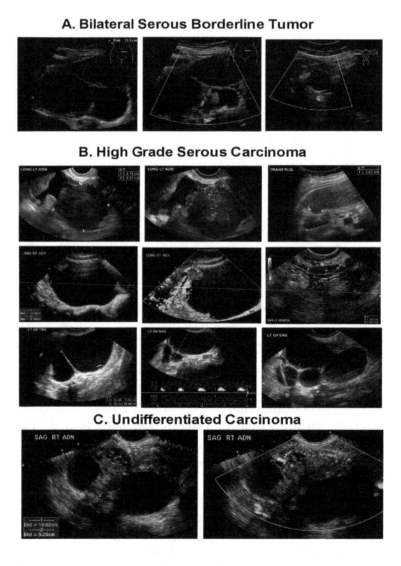

Figure 3. *Cont.*

D. Malignant Mixed Mesodermal Tumor

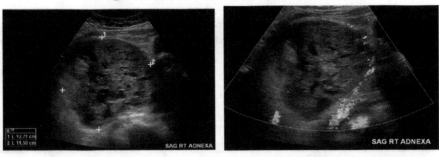

E. High Grade Transitional Cell Carcinoma

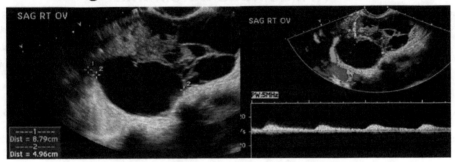

F. Low Grade Endometriod Carcinoma

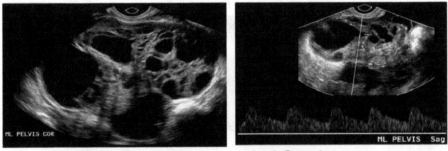

G. High Grade Endometriod Carcinoma

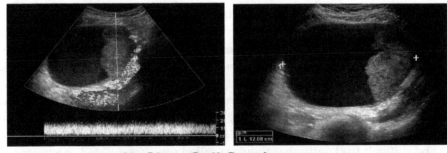

H. Clear Cell Carcinoma

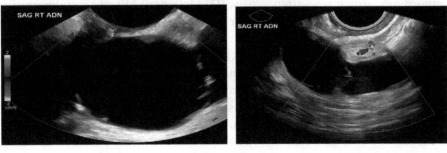

Figure 3. *Cont.*

J. Mucinous Borderline Tumor

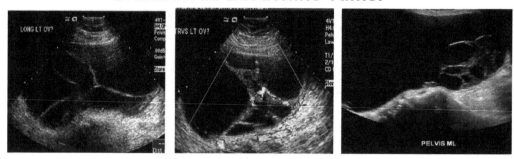

K. Mucinous Carcinoma

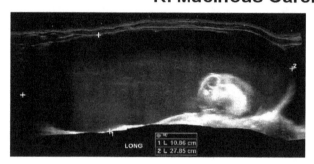 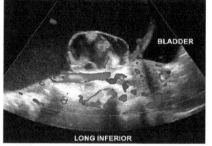

I. Malignant Brenner Tumor

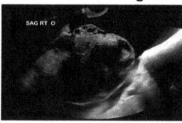 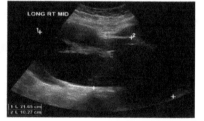

Figure 3. Ultrasonographic appearance of borderline, Type 1 and Type 2 ovarian cancers. (**A**) Bilateral Serous Borderline Tumor: tumors of low malignant potential (i.e., borderline tumors) account for 15% of all epithelial ovarian cancers. Nearly 75% of these tumors are stage I at the time of diagnosis. They represent a heterogeneous group and occur in younger women with favorable prognosis. However, symptomatic recurrence and death may be found as long as 20 years after therapy in some patients. (**B**) High Grade Serous Carcinoma (Type 2): serous carcinomas comprise the majority of ovarian carcinomas. Unlike low-grade serous carcinoma, *TP53* mutation occurs in up to 80% of high-grade tumors [17,20]. (**C**) Undifferentiated Carcinoma (Type 2): about 5% of ovarian cancers are so poorly differentiated and difficult to classify that they are called undifferentiated carcinomas and occur as large, solid hemorrhagic structures with necrosis. (**D**) Malignant Mixed Mesodermal Tumor (Type 2): occur almost exclusively in postmenopausal women. (**E**) High grade transitional cell carcinoma (Type 2) is probably not a distinct entity but a poorly differentiated form of serous or endometrioid carcinoma. (**F**) Low Grade Endometrioid Carcinoma (Type 1): endometriosis a likely precursor of endometrioid carcinoma. (**G**) High grade Endometriod carcinoma (Type 2) is morphologically indistinguishable from high grade serous carcinoma. (**H**) Clear Cell Carcinoma (Type 1): as with endometrioid carcinomas, there is a close association between endometriosis and clear cell carcinoma. (**I**) Malignant Brenner Tumor (Type 1): relatively uncommon neoplasm. Most Brenner tumors are benign, only 2–5% being malignant. (**J**) Mucinous Borderline Tumor (Type 1): 53.3% of borderline tumors are serous tumors and 42.5% are mucinous tumors (42.5%). (**K**) Mucinous Carcinoma (Type 1): frequently has a heterogeneous composition with coexisting elements of cystadenoma, stromal microinvasion, noninvasive carcinoma, and invasive carcinoma.

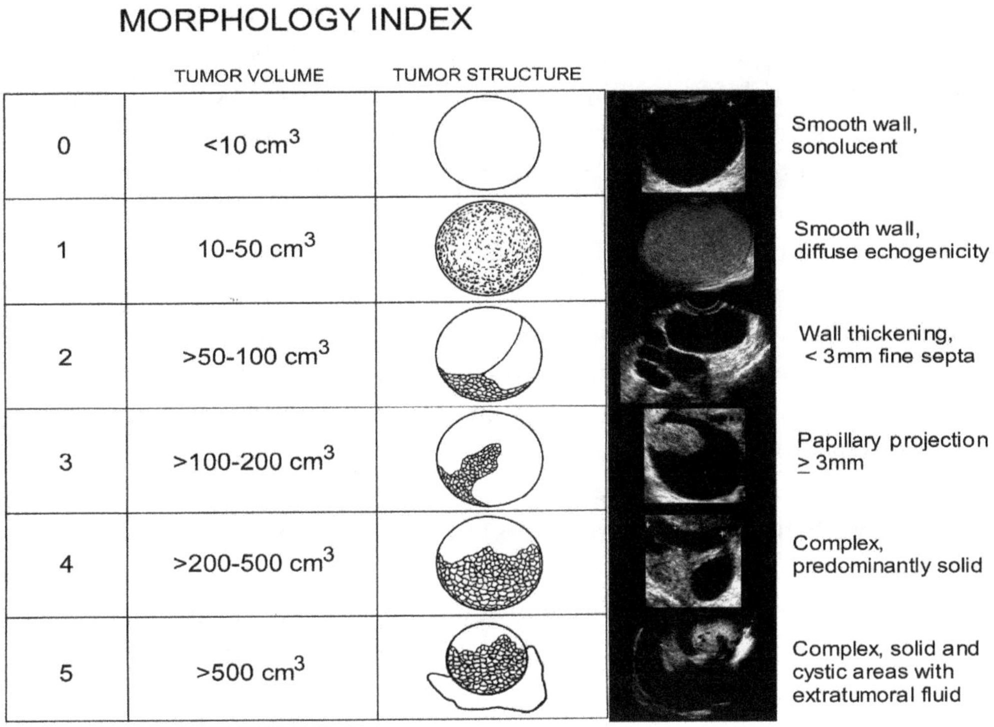

MORPHOLOGY INDEX

	TUMOR VOLUME	TUMOR STRUCTURE		
0	<10 cm^3			Smooth wall, sonolucent
1	10-50 cm^3			Smooth wall, diffuse echogenicity
2	>50-100 cm^3			Wall thickening, < 3mm fine septa
3	>100-200 cm^3			Papillary projection ≥ 3mm
4	>200-500 cm^3			Complex, predominantly solid
5	>500 cm^3			Complex, solid and cystic areas with extratumoral fluid

Figure 4. Morphology Index evaluation of ovarian abnormalities. Part of the figure is reprinted from [39,58].

5.1. Malignant Degeneration of Benign Masses

It is well known that epithelial ovarian carcinomas can develop from ovarian endometriosis [59–63]. The strongest association is seen with endometrioid and clear cell carcinomas [64–66], which have been reported to be associated with ovarian endometriosis in 30–40% and 40–70% of cases, respectively [66,67]. Endometrioid cancer is considered as a Type 1 tumor while clear cell carcinoma is a more intermediate type [16]. Twenty-eight per cent of benign and 38% of borderline endometrioid tumors were reported to be associated with endometriosis in one series [68,69]. Thus, there are benign entities that can become malignant.

5.2. Psychosocial Elements in Prospective Ovarian Cancer Screening Trials

In an age when patients can freely review their medical charts, including their entire radiology report, and access the Internet for information, we enter uncharted territory in how to communicate our findings with patients. The cost in following an ovarian mass by ultrasound is nominal compared to surgery or extensive chemo-radiation treatment when ovarian cancer is detected at a later stage. When women were polled about screening for ovarian cancer by the University of Kentucky Ovarian Cancer trial team, 97% of the women surveyed reported that they wanted to be screened and that they would even pay for screening themselves because ovarian cancer has a mortality ratio that is four times greater than breast cancer, despite an incidence rate that is low [70] even with potential complications that range from long-term physiological changes such as bone density loss to surgical mortality.

It is legitimate to consider if serial ultrasound and surveillance impacts psychosocial well-being. Non-physical or psychological harm to women has been examined in the Kentucky Ovarian Screening trial. When compared to an age and education matched group with no history of ovarian screening, women in the Kentucky trial had more ovarian cancer-specific distress/anxiety, less optimism, and less knowledge about risk factors upon entry [71]. Thus, some distress or anxiety relative to ovarian cancer appears to play a motivating role for entering the Kentucky screening trial. As part of these efforts, the validity of self-reporting by women in the Kentucky trial was evaluated and found to be very high [72]. In a study with baseline, two-week and four-month measurement, recipients of a normal ovarian screening exam showed decreased ovarian cancer-related distress, increased positive effects and increased knowledge of risk factors [73], indicating, for the vast majority of women screened, that there are beneficial effects on ovarian cancer-specific anxiety, attitude and knowledge. Women who received an abnormal TVS screening result were found to have an elevated ovarian cancer-specific distress (but not general distress) at a two-week follow-up that returned to baseline at the four-month follow-up [74]. Results were influenced by a monitoring coping style, low optimism and family history of ovarian cancer. Needs that have been identified in women with an abnormal TVS screening result deal with anticipation, emotional responses, role of the sonographer and impact of prior cancer experiences [75]. In examining social cognitive processing vs. cognitive social health processing after an abnormal TVS screening, analyses found that greater distress was associated with greater social constraint [76]. Thus, psychological conditions that are apparently associated with ovarian screening are governed by different underlying factors in different women and not the screening result per se. Furthermore, recent published findings from the UKCTOCS data showed that screening does not necessarily provoke an unacceptable level of anxiety or psychological morbidity [77]. Taken together, these results support the position that surveillance and serial ultrasonography may not negatively impact perceptions of well-being, particularly if more women were made aware that some tumors may be low grade and slow growing.

6. Executive Summary of What We Already Know

There has been significant advancement in our understanding of ovarian cancer since the first randomized prospective ovarian cancer screen trials were initiated to detect cancers in early stages to reduce the mortality of this disease. We now know that ovarian cancer is a large heterogeneous group consisting of Type 1 (indolent and low grade tumor) and Type 2 (aggressive and high grade tumor) based on molecular, genetic make-up of the cancer and how they progress based on their precursors or genetic predisposition [16–32]. The evidence indicates that surgical treatment based on limited imaging or tumor marker data based on single or short-term exams has led to unnecessary surgery with potential for morbidity or mortality [34]. Ultrasounds in ovarian cancer screening have detected both Type 1 and Type 2 cancers even at early stages [5,12,35–38]. Because benign and malignant ovarian neoplasms share overlapping ultrasound morphologies, accounting for a high ratio of benign to malignant surgical findings and because ovarian cancer prevalence is low while the prevalence of ovarian abnormalities is high, active ultrasonographic surveillance of ovarian abnormalities based on the morphologic index provides the best means for detecting Type 2 ovarian cancers. Theoretical modeling on how Type 2 cancers behave has shown that it may be possible to detect low volume high grade cancer with better outcomes utilizing close follow-up with ultrasounds [46,47]. Ovarian cancer screening with ultrasound has detected a stage shift that finds malignancies at an earlier stage and serial ultrasound has increased the positive predictive value of this approach while decreasing false positive cases [5,36–38]. Medical-legal risk may enter the consideration when an indeterminate mass is not followed, often leading to surgery that proves unnecessary. Unnecessary surgery on false positive cases can have serious immediate complication rates ranging from 2–15% [12,34], but, if serial ultrasound indicates that the abnormality is resolving, then the need for surgery could be circumvented. Based on a comprehensive review of the literature, it can be concluded that:

(1)   there are benefits in ultrasound monitoring of persisting indeterminate masses;
(2)   resolution of sonographic abnormality defines benign status;
(3)   stability over time may not equate with benign status particularly for Type 1 tumors;
(4)   for certain types of tumors benign lesions are precursors of malignant lesions;
(5)   repeated ultrasound monitoring does not negatively impact psychosocial well-being.

7. Conclusions

In conclusion, ultrasounds are inexpensive, associated with low morbidity, widely available, have high sensitivity in detecting abnormalities and are free of risk in image acquisition. Decisions for following ovarian masses detected by ultrasound in day-to-day practice differ from decisions for annual ovarian cancer screening in asymptomatic women with normal risk. The goal of ovarian cancer screening is to detect early stage ovarian cancer with improved mortality benefit. The role of ultrasounds in adnexal mass management should be to increase positive predictive value of detecting ovarian cancer to minimize unnecessary surgeries and to avoid failures to detect ovarian cancers. Findings from ovarian cancer screening trials and advances in our understanding of ovarian cancer pathogenesis can guide the management of adnexal masses found in clinical practice, especially since screening studies have observed that women with ovarian masses found by ultrasounds have a higher risk for ovarian cancer than those women who do not have an ovarian mass. Serial ultrasound surveillance using a morphologic index allows quantitative surveillance and the ability to distinguish benign masses based upon stable index scores (absence of growth, stable morphology) or decreasing index scores (resolution), while increasing index scores are strongly linked to malignancy. Concomitant use of serial CA-125 as in the ROCA model should also increase the positive predictive value of detecting malignancy. All improvements should promote a close working relationship between diagnostic radiology and clinicians using standardized structured reporting models as advocated by the American College of Radiology as seen in the Breast Imaging Reporting Data System (BI-RADS) or the Liver Imaging Reporting Data System (LI-RADS) to reduce ambiguous terminology, decrease variability in interpretation and improve communication.

Author Contributions: Eleanor L. Ormsby Edward J. Pavlik and John P. McGahan contributed equally to the writing, review and editing of this manuscript.

References

1. Siegel, R.L.; Miller, K.D.; Jemal, A. Cancer Statistics, 2015. *CA Cancer J. Clin.* **2015**, *65*, 5–29. [CrossRef] [PubMed]
2. U.S. Cancer Statistics Working Group. United States Cancer Statistics: 1999–2013 Incidence and Mortality Web-based Report. U.S. Department of Health and Human Services, Centers for Disease Control and Prevention and National Cancer Institute: Atlanta, 2016. Available online: www.cdc.gov/uscs (accessed on 25 April 2017).
3. American Cancer Society Surveillance Research 2015. Available online: http://www.cancer.org/acs/groups/content/@editorial/documents/document/acspc-044512.pdf (accessed on 25 April 2017).
4. Jemal, A.; Siegel, R.; Ward, E.; Murray, T.; Xu, J.; Thun, M.J. Cancer Statistics, 2007. *CA Cancer J. Clin.* **2007**, *57*, 43–66. [CrossRef] [PubMed]
5. Van Nagell, J.R., Jr.; Miller, R.W.; DeSimone, C.P.; Ueland, F.R.; Podzielinski, I.; Goodrich, S.T.; Elder, J.W.; Huang, B.; Kryscio, R.J.; Pavlik, E.J. Long-term survival of women with epithelial ovarian cancer detected by ultrasonographic screening. *Obstet. Gynecol.* **2011**, *118*, 1212–1221. [CrossRef]
6. Salani, R.; Bristow, R.E. Surgical management of epithelial ovarian cancer. *Clin. Obstet. Gynecol.* **2013**, *55*, 75–95. [CrossRef] [PubMed]
7. U.S. Preventive Services Task Force. Final Recommendation Statement Ovarian Cancer: Screening. September 2012. Available online: http://www.uspreventiveservicestaskforce.org/Page/Document/RecommendationStatementFinal/ovarian-cancer-screening (accessed on 29 December 2016).
8. Hartge, P.; Hayes, R.; Reding, D.; Sherman, M.E.; Prorok, P.; Schiffman, M.; Buys, S. Complex ovarian cysts in postmenopausal women are not associated with ovarian cancer risk factors: Preliminary data from the prostate, lung, colon, and ovarian cancer screening trial. *Am. J. Obstet. Gynecol.* **2000**, *183*, 1232–1237. [CrossRef] [PubMed]
9. Bailey, C.L.; Ueland, F.R.; Land, G.L.; DePriest, P.D.; Gallion, H.H.; Kryscio, R.J.; van Nagell, J.R., Jr. The malignant potential of small cystic ovarian tumors in women over 50 years of age. *Gynecol. Oncol.* **1998**, *69*, 3–7. [CrossRef] [PubMed]

10. Modesitt, S.C.; Pavlik, E.J.; Ueland, F.R.; DePriest, P.D.; Kryscio, R.J.; Nagell, J.R., Jr. Risk of malignancy in unilocular ovarian cystic tumors less than 10 centimeters in diameter. *Obstet. Gynecol.* **2003**, *102*, 594–599. [CrossRef]

11. Saunders, B.A.; Podzielinski, I.; Ware, R.A.; Goodrich, S.; Desimone, C.P.; Ueland, F.R.; Seamon, L.; Ubellacker, J.; Pavlik, E.J.; Kryscio, R.J.; et al. Risk of malignancy in sonographically confirmed septated cystic ovarian tumors. *Gynecol. Oncol.* **2010**, *118*, 278–282. [CrossRef] [PubMed]

12. Sharma, A.; Apostolidou, S.; Burnell, M.; Campbell, S.; Habib, M.; Gentry-Maharaj, A.; Amso, N.; Seif, M.W.; Fletcher, G.; Singh, N.; et al. Risk of epithelial ovarian cancer in asymptomatic women with ultrasound-detected ovarian masses: A prospective cohort study within the UK collaborative trial of ovarian cancer screening (UKCTOCS). *Ultrasound Obstet. Gynecol.* **2012**, *40*, 338–344. [CrossRef]

13. Ormsby, E.L.; Pavlik, E.J.; Van Nagell, J.R. Ultrasound follow up of an adnexal mass has the potential to save lives. *Am. J. Obstet. Gynecol.* **2015**, *213*, 657–661. [CrossRef] [PubMed]

14. Levine, D.; Brown, D.L.; Andreotti, R.F.; Benacerraf, B.; Benson, C.B.; Brewster, W.R.; Coleman, B.; DePriest, P.; Doubilet, P.M.; Goldstein, S.R.; et al. Society of Radiologists in Ultrasound. Management of asymptomatic ovarian and other adnexal cysts imaged at US Society of Radiologists in Ultrasound Consensus Conference Statement. *Radiology* **2010**, *26*, 121–131.

15. Glanc, P.; Benacerraf, B.; Bourne, T.; Brown, D.; Coleman, B.; Crum, C.; Dodge, J.; Levine, D.; Pavlik, E.; Timmerman, D.; et al. First International Consensus Report on Adnexal Masses: Management Recommendations. *J. Ultrasound Med.* **2017**. [CrossRef] [PubMed]

16. Kurman, R.J.; Shih, I. The origin and pathogenesis of epithelial ovarian cancer: A proposed unifying theory. *Am. J. Surg. Pathol.* **2010**, *34*, 433–443. [CrossRef] [PubMed]

17. Koshiyama, M.; Matsumura, N.; Konishi, I. Recent concepts of ovarian carcinogenesis: Type I and type II. *Biomed. Res. Int.* **2014**. [CrossRef] [PubMed]

18. Lim, D.; Olivia, D.E. Precursors and pathogenesis of ovarian carcinoma. *Pathology* **2013**, *45*, 229–242. [CrossRef] [PubMed]

19. Vang, R.; Shih, I.; Kurman, R.J. Ovarian low-grade and high-grade serous carcinoma: Pathogenesis, clinicopathologic and molecular biologic features, and diagnostic problems. *Adv. Anat. Pathol.* **2009**, *16*, 267–282. [CrossRef] [PubMed]

20. Cho, K.R.; Shih, I. Ovarian cancer. *Ann. Rev. Pathol.* **2009**, *4*, 287–313. [CrossRef] [PubMed]

21. Senturk, E.; Cohen, S.; Dottino, P.R.; Senturk, E.; Cohen, S.; Dottino, P.R.; Martignetti, J.A. A critical re-appraisal of *BRCA₁* methylation studies in ovarian cancer. *Gynecol. Oncol.* **2010**, *119*, 376–383. [CrossRef] [PubMed]

22. Alvarado-Cabrero, I.; Navani, S.S.; Young, R.H.; Scully, R.E. Tumors of the Fimbriated End of the Fallopian Tube: A Clinicopathologic Analysis of 20 Cases, Including Nine Carcinomas. *Int. J. Gynecol. Pathol.* **1997**, *16*, 189–196. [CrossRef] [PubMed]

23. Colgan, T.J.; Murphy, J.; Cole, D.E.; Narod, S.; Rosen, B. Occult carcinoma in prophylactic oophorectomy specimens: Prevalence and association with *BRCA* germline mutation status. *Am. J. Surg. Pathol.* **2001**, *25*, 1283–1289. [CrossRef] [PubMed]

24. Cass, I.; Holschneider, C.; Datta, N.; Barbuto, D.; Walts, A.E.; Karlan, B.Y. *BRCA*-mutation-associated fallopian tube carcinoma: A distinct clinical phenotype? *Obstet. Gynecol.* **2005**, *106*, 1327–1334. [CrossRef] [PubMed]

25. Medeiros, F.; Muto, M.G.; Lee, Y.; Elvin, J.A.; Callahan, M.J.; Feltmate, C.; Garber, J.E.; Cramer, D.W.; Crum, C.P. The tubal fimbria is a preferred site for early adenocarcinoma in women with familial ovarian cancer syndrome. *Am. J. Surg. Pathol.* **2006**, *30*, 230–236. [CrossRef] [PubMed]

26. Kindelberger, D.W.; Lee, Y.; Miron, A.; Hirsch, M.S.; Feltmate, C.; Medeiros, F.; Callahan, M.J.; Garner, E.O.; Gordon, R.W.; Birch, C.; et al. Intraepithelial Carcinoma of the Fimbriae and Pelvic Serous Carcinoma: Evidence for a Causal Relationship. *Am. J. Surg. Pathol.* **2007**, *31*, 161–169. [CrossRef] [PubMed]

27. Crum, C.R.; Drapkin, R.; Miron, A.; Ince, T.A.; Muto, M.; Kindelberger, D.W.; Lee, Y. The distal fallopian tube: A new model for pelvic serous carcinogenesis. *Curr. Opin. Obstet. Gynecol.* **2007**, *19*, 3–9. [CrossRef] [PubMed]

28. Guth, U.; Huang, D.J.; Bauer, G.; Stieger, M.; Wight, E.; Singer, G. Metastatic patterns at autopsy in patients with ovarian carcinoma. *Cancer* **2007**, *110*, 1272–1280. [CrossRef] [PubMed]

29. Landen, C.N.; Birrer, M.J.; Sood, A.K. Early Events in the Pathogenesis of Epithelial Ovarian Cancer. *J. Clin. Oncol.* **2008**, *26*, 995–1005. [CrossRef] [PubMed]

30. Lengyel, E. Ovarian Cancer Development and Metastasis. *Am. J. Pathol.* **2010**, *177*, 1053–1064. [CrossRef] [PubMed]

31. Crum, C.P.; Mckeon, F.D.; Xian, X. The oviduct and ovarian cancer: Causality, clinical implications, and "targeted prevention". *Clin. Obstet. Gynecol.* **2012**, *55*, 24–35. [CrossRef] [PubMed]

32. Malpica, A.; Deavers, M.T.; Lu, K.; Bodurka, D.C.; Atkinson, E.N.; Gershenson, D.M.; Silva, E.G. Grading ovarian serous carcinoma using a two-tier system. *Am. J. Surg. Pathol.* **2004**, *28*, 496–504. [CrossRef] [PubMed]

33. Kobayashi, H.; Yamada, Y.; Sado, T.; Sakata, M.; Yoshida, S.; Kawaguchi, R.; Kanayama, S.; Shigetomi, H.; Haruta, S.; Tsuji, Y.; et al. A randomized study of screening for ovarian cancer: A multicenter study in Japan. *Int. J. Gynecol. Cancer* **2008**, *18*, 414–420. [CrossRef] [PubMed]

34. Buys, S.S.; Partridge, E.; Black, A.; Johnson, C.C.; Lamerato, L.; Isaacs, C.; Reding, D.J.; Greenlee, R.T.; Yokochi, L.A.; Kessel, B.; et al. Effect of screening on ovarian cancer mortality: The Prostate, Lung, Colorectal and Ovarian (PLCO) Cancer Screening Randomized Controlled Trial. *JAMA* **2011**, *305*, 2295–2303. [CrossRef] [PubMed]

35. Jacobs, I.J.; Menon, U.; Ryan, A.; Gentry-Maharaj, A.; Burnell, M.; Kalsi, J.K. Ovarian cancer screening and mortality in the UK Collaborative Trial of Ovarian Cancer Screening (UKCTOCS): A randomised controlled trial. *Lancet* **2016**, *387*, 945–956. [CrossRef]

36. Pavlik, E.J.; Ueland, F.R.; Miller, R.W.; Ubellacker, J.M.; Desimone, C.P.; Elder, J.; Hoff, J.; Baldwin, L.; Kryscio, R.J.; van Nagell, J.R., Jr. Frequency and disposition of ovarian abnormalities followed with serial transvaginal ultrasonography. *Obstet. Gynecol.* **2013**, *122*, 210–217. [CrossRef] [PubMed]

37. Van Nagell, J.R., Jr.; Miller, R.W. Evaluation and Management of Ultrasonographically Detected Ovarian Tumors in Asymptomatic Women. *Obstet. Gynecol.* **2016**, *127*, 848–858. [CrossRef] [PubMed]

38. Van Nagell, J.R., Jr.; Hoff, J.T. Transvaginal ultrasonography in ovarian cancer screening: Current perspectives. *Int. J. Womens Health.* **2014**, *6*, 25–33. [CrossRef] [PubMed]

39. Elder, J.W.; Pavlik, E.J.; Long, A.; Miller, R.W.; Desimone, C.P.; Hoff, J.T.; Ueland, W.R.; Kryscio, R.J.; Nagell, J.R., Jr.; Ueland, F.R. Serial ultrasonographic evaluation of ovarian abnormalities with a morphology index. *Gynecol. Oncol.* **2014**, *135*, 8–12. [CrossRef] [PubMed]

40. Kaijser, J.; van Gorp, T.; van hoorde, k.; van Holsbeke, C.; Sayasneh, A.; Vergote, I.; Bourne, T.; Timmerman, D.; van Calster, B. A comparison between an ultrasound based prediction model (LR2) and the risk of ovarian malignancy algorithm (ROMA) to assess the risk of malignancy in women with an adnexal mass. *Gynecol. Oncol.* **2013**, *129*, 377–383. [CrossRef] [PubMed]

41. Urban, N.; Thorpe, J.D.; Bergan, L.A.; Forrest, R.M.; Kampani, A.V.; Scholler, N.; O'Briant, K.C.; Anderson, G.L.; Cramer, D.W.; Berg, C.D.; et al. Potential role of HE4 in multimodal screening for epithelial ovarian cancer. *J. Natl. Cancer Inst.* **2011**, *103*, 1630–1634. [CrossRef] [PubMed]

42. Moore, R.G.; MacLaughlan, S.; Bast, R.C. Current state of biomarker development for clinical application in epithelial ovarian cancer. *Gynecol. Oncol.* **2010**, *116*, 240–245. [CrossRef] [PubMed]

43. Skates, S.J.; Mai, P.; Horick, N.K.; Piedmonte, M.; Drescher, C.W.; Isaacs, C.; Armstrong, D.K.; Buys, S.S.; Rodriguez, G.C.; Horowitz, I.R.; et al. Large Prospective Study of Ovarian Cancer Screening in High risk Women: CA-125 Cut-point Defined by Menopausal Status. *Cancer Prev. Res. (Phila)* **2011**, *4*, 1401–1408. [CrossRef] [PubMed]

44. Menon, U.; Gentry-Maharaj, A.; Hallett, R.; Ryan, A.; Burnell, M.; Sharma, A.; Lewis, S.; Davies, S.; Philpott, S.; Lopes, A.; et al. Sensitivity and specificity of multimodal and ultrasound screening for ovarian cancer, and stage distribution of detected cancers: Results of the prevalence screen of the UK Collaborative Trial of Ovarian Cancer Screening (UKCTOCS). *Lancet Oncol.* **2009**, *10*, 327–340. [CrossRef]

45. Havrilesky, L.; Sanders, G.; Kulasingam, S.; Chino, J.; Berchuck, A.; Marks, J.; Evan, R.; Myers, E. Development of an ovarian cancer screening decision model that incorporates disease heterogeneity. *Cancer* **2010**, *117*, 545–553. [CrossRef] [PubMed]

46. Brown, P.O.; Palmer, C. The Preclinical Natural History of Serous Ovarian Cancer: Defining the Target for Early Detection. *PLoS Med.* **2009**, *6*. [CrossRef] [PubMed]

47. Hori, S.S.; Gambhir, S.S. Mathematical Model Identifies Blood Biomarker–Based Early Cancer Detection Strategies and Limitations. *Sci. Transl. Med.* **2011**, *3*, 109ra116.

48. Suh-Burgmann, E.; Hung, Y.Y.; Kinney, W. Outcomes from ultrasound follow-up of small complex adnexal masses in women over 50. *Am. J. Obstet. Gynecol.* **2014**, *211*, 623.e1–623.e7. [CrossRef] [PubMed]

49. Yazbek, J.; Raju, K.S.; Ben-Nagi, J.; Holland, T.; Hillaby, K.; Jurkovic, D. Accuracy of ultrasound subjective

"pattern recognition" for the diagnosis of borderline ovarian tumors. *Ultrasound Obstet. Gynecol.* **2007**, *29*, 489–495. [CrossRef] [PubMed]

50. Valentin, L.; Ameye, L.; Franchi, D.; Guerriero, S.; Jurkovic, D.; Savell, L.; Fischerova, D.; Lissoni, A.; van Holsbeke, C.; Fruscio, R.; et al. Risk of malignancy in unilocular cysts: A study of 1148 adnexal masses classified as unilocular cysts at transvaginal ultrasound and review of the literature. *Ultrasound Obstet. Gynecol.* **2013**, *41*, 80–89. [CrossRef] [PubMed]
51. Yancik, R.; Ries, L.G.; Yates, J.W. Ovarian cancer in the elderly: An analysis of surveillance. *Am. J. Obstet. Gynecol.* **1986**, *154*, 639–647. [CrossRef]
52. Pavlik, E.J.; van Nagell, J.R. Early Detection of Ovarian Tumors Using Ultrasound. *Womens Health* **2013**, *9*, 39–55. [CrossRef] [PubMed]
53. Gilbert, L.; Basso, O.; Sampalis, J.; Karp, I.; Martins, C.; Feng, J.; Piedimonte, S.; Quintal, L.; Ramanakumar, A.V.; Takefman, J.; et al. Assessment of symptomatic women for early diagnosis of ovarian cancer: Results from the prospective DOvE pilot project. *Lancet Oncol.* **2012**, 285–291. [CrossRef]
54. Rossing, M.A.; Wicklund, K.G.; Cushing-Haugen, K.L.; Weiss, N.S. Predictive value of symptoms for early detection of ovarian cancer. *J. Natl. Cancer Inst.* **2010**, *102*, 222–229. [CrossRef] [PubMed]
55. Cooper, A.L.; Nelson, D.F.; Doran, S.; Ueland, F.R.; DeSimone, C.P.; DePriest, P.D.; McDonald, J.M.; Saunders, B.A.; Ware, R.A.; Pavlik, E.J.; et al. Long-Term Survival and Cost of Treatment in Patients with Stage IIIC Epithelial Ovarian Cancer. *Curr. Women's Health Rev.* **2009**, *5*, 44–50.
56. McColl, S.; Hicks, J.; Craig, L.; Shortreed, J. *Environmental Health Risk Management: A Primer for Canadians*; Graphic Services University of Waterloo: Waterloo, ON, Canada, 2000.
57. Zannoni, L.; Savelli, L.; Jokubkiene, L.; Di Legge, A.; Condous, G.; Testa, A.C.; Sladkevicius, P.; Valentin, L. Intra-and interobserver agreement with regard to describing adnexal masses using International Ovarian Tumor Analysis terminology: Reproducibility study involving seven observers. *Ultrasound Obstet. Gynecol.* **2014**, *44*, 100–108. [CrossRef] [PubMed]
58. Ueland, F.R.; DePriest, P.D.; Pavlik, E.J.; Kryscio, R.J.; Nagell, J.R., Jr. Preoperative differentiation of malignant from benign ovarian tumors: The efficacy of morphology indexing and Doppler flow sonography. *Gynecol. Oncol.* **2003**, *91*, 46–50. [CrossRef]
59. Testa, A.C.; Timmerman, D.; van Hosbeke, C.; Zannoni, G.F.; Fransis, S.; Moerman, P.; Vellone, V.; Mascilini, F.; Licameli, A.; Ludovisi, M.; et al. Ovarian cancer arising in endometrioid cysts: Ultrasound findings. *Ultrasound Obstet. Gynecol.* **2011**, *38*, 99–106. [CrossRef] [PubMed]
60. Fukunaga, M.; Nomura, K.; Ishikawa, E.; Ushigome, S. Ovarian atypical endometriosis: Its close association with malignant epithelial tumours. *Histopathology* **1997**, *30*, 249–255. [CrossRef] [PubMed]
61. Heaps, J.M.; Nieberg, R.K.; Berek, J.S. Malignant neoplasms arising in endometriosis. *Obstet. Gynecol.* **1990**, *75*, 1023–1028. [CrossRef]
62. Moll, U.M.; Chumas, J.C.; Chalas, E.; Mann, W.J. Ovarian carcinoma arising in atypical endometriosis. *Obstet. Gynecol.* **1990**, *75*, 537–539. [PubMed]
63. Sainz de la Cuesta, R.; Eichhorn, J.H.; Rice, L.W.; Fuller, A.F., Jr.; Nikrui, N.; Goff, B.A. Histologic transformation of benign endometriosis to early epithelial ovarian cancer. *Gynecol. Oncol.* **1996**, *60*, 238–244. [CrossRef] [PubMed]
64. Stern, R.C.; Dash, R.; Bentley, R.C.; Snyder, M.J.; Haney, A.F.; Robboy, S.J. Malignancy in endometriosis: Frequency and comparison of ovarian and extraovarian types. *Int. J. Gynecol. Pathol.* **2001**, *20*, 133–139. [PubMed]
65. Ogawa, S.; Kaku, T.; Amada, S.; Kobayashi, H.; Hirakawa, T.; Ariyoshi, K.; Kamura, T.; Nakano, H. Ovarian endometriosis associated with ovarian carcinoma: A clinicopathological and immunohistochemical study. *Gynecol. Oncol.* **2000**, *77*, 298–304. [CrossRef] [PubMed]
66. Mostoufizadeh, M.; Scully, R.E. Malignant tumors arising in endometriosis. *Clin. Obstet. Gynecol.* **1980**, *23*, 951–963. [CrossRef] [PubMed]
67. Russell, P. The pathological assessment of ovarian neoplasms. I: Introduction to the common "epithelial" tumours and analysis of benign "epithelial" tumours. *Pathology* **1979**, *11*, 5–26. [CrossRef] [PubMed]
68. Bell, D.A.; Scully, R.E. Atypical and borderline endometrioid adenofibromas of the ovary: A report of 27 cases. *Am. J. Surg. Pathol.* **1985**, *9*, 205–214. [CrossRef] [PubMed]
69. Snyder, R.R.; Norris, H.J.; Tavassoli, F. Endometrioid proliferative and low malignant potential tumors of the ovary: A clinicopathologic study of 46 cases. *Am. J. Surg. Pathol.* **1988**, *12*, 661–671. [CrossRef] [PubMed]

70. Pavlik, E.J.; van Nagell, J.R., Jr. Ovarian cancer screening—What women want. *Int. J. Gynecol. Cancer* **2012**, *22*, S21–S23. [CrossRef] [PubMed]

71. Salsman, J.M.; Pavlik, E.; Boerner, L.M.; Andrykowski, M.A. Clinical, demographic, and psychological characteristics of new, asymptomatic partipants in a transvaginal ultrasound screening program for ovarian cancer. *Prev. Med.* **2004**, *39*, 315–322. [CrossRef] [PubMed]

72. Lykins, E.L.; Pavlik, E.; Andrykowski, M.A. Validity of self-reports of return for routine repeat screening in an ovarian screening program. *Cancer Epidemiol. Biomark. Prev.* **2007**, *16*, 490–493. [CrossRef] [PubMed]

73. Gaugler, J.E.; Pavlik, E.; Salsman, J.M.; Andrykowski, M.A. Pyschological and behavioral impact of receipt of a "normal" ovarian cancer screening test. *Prev. Med.* **2006**, *42*, 463–470. [CrossRef] [PubMed]

74. Andrykowski, M.A.; Boerner, L.M.; Salsman, J.M.; Pavlik, E. Psychological response to test results in an ovarian cancer screening program: A prospective, longitudinal study. *Health Psychol.* **2004**, *23*, 622–666. [CrossRef] [PubMed]

75. Ryan, P.Y.; Graves, K.D.; Pavlik, E.J.; Andrykowski, M.A. Abnormal ovarian cancer screening test result: Women's informational, psychological and practical needs. *J. Psychosoc. Oncol.* **2007**, *25*, 1–18. [CrossRef] [PubMed]

76. Andrykowski, M.A.; Pavlik, E. Response to an abnormal ovarian cancer-screening test result: Test of the social cognitive processing and cognitive social health information processing models. *Psychol. Health* **2011**, *26*, 383–397. [CrossRef] [PubMed]

77. Barrett, J.; Jenkins, V.; Farewell, V. BJOG: Psychological morbidity associated with ovarian cancer screening: Results from more than 23,000 women in the randomised trial of ovarian cancer screening (UKCTOCS). *BJOG* **2014**, *121*, 1071–1079. [CrossRef] [PubMed]

16

Gold Nanoparticle Mediated Multi-Modal CT Imaging of Hsp70 Membrane-Positive Tumors

Melanie A. Kimm [1], Maxim Shevtsov [2,3,4], Caroline Werner [2], Wolfgang Sievert [2], Wu Zhiyuan [2], Oliver Schoppe [2,5], Bjoern H. Menze [2,5], Ernst J. Rummeny [1], Roland Proksa [6], Olga Bystrova [4], Marina Martynova [4], Gabriele Multhoff [2] and Stefan Stangl [2,*]

[1] Department of Diagnostic and Interventional Radiology, Klinikum rechts der Isar der Technischen Universität München, 81675 Munich, Germany; Melanie.Kimm@tum.de (M.A.K.); Ernst.Rummeny@tum.de (E.J.R.)

[2] Central Institute for Translational Cancer Research (TranslaTUM), Klinikum rechts der Isar der Technischen Universität München, 81675 Munich, Germany; Maxim.Shevtsov@tum.de (M.S.); c.werner@tum.de (C.W.); Wolfgang.Sievert@tum.de (W.S.); zhiyuan2012.wu@tum.de (W.Z.); Oliver.Schoppe@tum.de (O.S.); Bjoern.Menze@tum.de (B.H.M.); Gabriele.Multhoff@tum.de (G.M.)

[3] Pavlov First Saint Petersburg State Medical University, 197022 St. Petersburg, Russia

[4] Institute of Cytology of the Russian Academy of Sciences (RAS), 194064 St. Petersburg, Russia; o3608338@gmail.com (O.B.); mgmart14@mail.ru (M.M.)

[5] Institute for Advanced Studies, Department of Informatics, Technical University of Munich, 85748 Garching, Germany

[6] Philips GmbH Innovative Technologies, Research Laboratories, 22335 Hamburg, Germany; roland.proksa@philips.com

[*] Correspondence: Stefan.Stangl@tum.de

Abstract: Imaging techniques such as computed tomographies (CT) play a major role in clinical imaging and diagnosis of malignant lesions. In recent years, metal nanoparticle platforms enabled effective payload delivery for several imaging techniques. Due to the possibility of surface modification, metal nanoparticles are predestined to facilitate molecular tumor targeting. In this work, we demonstrate the feasibility of anti-plasma membrane Heat shock protein 70 (Hsp70) antibody functionalized gold nanoparticles (cmHsp70.1-AuNPs) for tumor-specific multimodal imaging. Membrane-associated Hsp70 is exclusively presented on the plasma membrane of malignant cells of multiple tumor entities but not on corresponding normal cells, predestining this target for a tumor-selective in vivo imaging. In vitro microscopic analysis revealed the presence of cmHsp70.1-AuNPs in the cytosol of tumor cell lines after internalization via the endo-lysosomal pathway. In preclinical models, the biodistribution as well as the intratumoral enrichment of AuNPs were examined 24 h after i.v. injection in tumor-bearing mice. In parallel to spectral CT analysis, histological analysis confirmed the presence of AuNPs within tumor cells. In contrast to control AuNPs, a significant enrichment of cmHsp70.1-AuNPs has been detected selectively inside tumor cells in different tumor mouse models. Furthermore, a machine-learning approach was developed to analyze AuNP accumulations in tumor tissues and organs. In summary, utilizing mHsp70 on tumor cells as a target for the guidance of cmHsp70.1-AuNPs facilitates an enrichment and uniform distribution of nanoparticles in mHsp70-expressing tumor cells that enables various microscopic imaging techniques and spectral-CT-based tumor delineation in vivo.

Keywords: gold nanoparticle; heat shock protein 70; molecular imaging; biomarker; spectral-CT

1. Introduction

Detection of all malignant tumor cells in a patients' body is a prerequisite for a successful therapy outcome. In established clinical routine, combined positron emission tomography (PET)/computed tomography (CT) imaging is commonly used for tumors exceeding 0.5–1 cm^3. For standard clinical PET imaging, ^{18}F-glucose is often used as a PET tracer. However, glucose-based PET/CT imaging faces several disadvantages, such as false-positive and/or false-negative signals, e.g., triggered by the fact that only metabolically active but not resting cells can be visualized, the low tumor-to-background contrast, and the relatively low resolution of the technique [1]. With improved settings, a spatial resolution of 2 mm is technically feasible, as demonstrated in patients with prostate cancer [2].

The introduction of gold nanoparticles (AuNP)-based contrast agents added a new value to imaging techniques. Functionalization of novel metal-based nanoparticles with tumor-specific antibodies [3] and their utilization in imaging techniques such as photoacoustic tomography or CT combine the advantages of a molecular, tumor-specific imaging with the unique attributes of AuNP in clinical imaging. For instance, spectral-CT technology employs a photon-counting detector which registers the interactions of individual photons, creating a certain energy spectrum which can subsequently be converted into a color image. At the same time, a nonspectral attenuation image can be acquired. This combination allows a precise spatial information with a high resolution. With the emergence of clinical spectral-CT scanners, the need of tumor-specific contrast agents further increased. In this setting, AuNPs might play a crucial role as the energy-dependent X-ray attenuation properties (K-edge at 80.7 keV) allow an excellent separation from calcium (K-edge at 4 keV) and iodine (K-edge at 33.2 keV) [4].

For in vivo application, it is also essential that the applied nanoparticles are nontoxic, biodegradable or inert, and easily transportable in the blood and/or lymphatic system. Biocompatible camouflage of the NP surface is a prerequisite to avoid immediate uptake by macrophages. Small AuNPs (<100 nm) demonstrated to be beneficial for utilization in clinical applications [5–7]. Apart from the formulation of AuNPs, tumor imaging with nanoparticle-based contrast agents can be further improved and specified by functionalization with antibodies targeting tumor-specific, membrane-bound biomarkers. For an improved signal-to-background ratio and a high tumor specificity, candidate markers should be selectively expressed on tumor cells while being absent on healthy cells. Membrane-bound Heat shock protein 70 (Hsp70, Hsp70-1, HspA1A, #3303) has been found to fulfill these criteria, exhibiting a remarkable tumor-specific targeting capability [8,9]. In addition to the physiological, cytosolic expression in all nucleated cells, Hsp70 is also found on the plasma membrane of malignantly transformed cells. Upon stress, this molecular chaperone has been found to be increased in the cytosol and on the plasma membrane of different murine and human tumor cells. Screening of tumor biopsies of over 1200 patients has shown that the majority of the primarily diagnosed carcinoma samples but none of the tested corresponding normal tissues exhibited a membrane Hsp70-positive phenotype [10–13]. After therapy of tumors with standard regimens, such as radiotherapy or chemotherapy, the membrane expression density of Hsp70 on tumor cells is increased [14], which in turn further improves targeting of membrane Hsp70-positive tumors after standard therapies. Furthermore, an upregulated membrane Hsp70 density could be detected on relapse tumors and metastases compared to primary tumors. In multiple studies, the malignancy of tumors correlates positively with the Hsp70 expression density in the cytoplasm and on the plasma membrane [8,11].

For a specific in vivo tumor targeting which is mediated by membrane-bound Hsp70, we developed the membrane Hsp70-specific antibody cmHsp70.1 [9,15]. To utilize the beneficial features of targeting membrane Hsp70 with the imaging capabilities of gold as a contrast agent, we developed an AuNP formulation, functionalized with cmHsp70.1 monoclonal antibody to target membrane-bound Hsp70 on tumor cells in vitro and in vivo. In previous studies, we could demonstrate a rapid and specific binding, uptake, and internalization of cmHsp70.1-AuNPs into tumor cells in vitro, leading to a high intracellular accumulation. Furthermore, following incubation of viable tumor cells with cmHsp70.1-AuNPs, no severe toxic side effects were observed up to a concentration of 10 µg/mL [16].

2. Results

2.1. Functionalization of AuNPs with cmHsp70.1 Antibody

For the coupling of mouse IgG1 isotype-matched or cmHsp70.1 antibody to AuNPs, we used a standard maleimide coupling reaction (Figure 1A). The size of the mean hydrodynamic diameter of unconjugated AuNPs was determined to be 45 ± 14 nm (Figure 1B, top panel). The sizes of cmHsp70.1 antibody-conjugated cmHsp70-AuNPs were 54 ± 11 nm (Figure 1B, middle panel) and 59 ± 18 nm for IgG1 isotype-matched control antibody-conjugated gold nanoparticles (IgG1-AuNPs) (Figure 1B, bottom panel). No self-aggregation was observed in aliquotes of the conjugated as well as the unconjugated AuNPs in phosphate buffered saline (PBS) at 37 °C during 24 h. After 4 weeks of storage at 4 °C, self-aggregation of the particles was observed. An exemplary size distribution histogram is given in Figure A1. To determine the Hsp70-specific binding capacity of cmHsp70.1-AuNPs, we performed analysis of the interaction of cmHsp70.1-AuNPs as well as IgG-AuNPs with recombinant human Hsp70, using an agglomeration assay, as described by Shevtsov et al. [17]. Following a 4 h incubation period with recombinant Hsp70, the size of the formed clusters, as determined by dynamic light scattering (DLS), was larger after incubation with cmHsp70.1-AuNPs (mean event sizes: 152 nm and 2420 nm) than with IgG1-AuNPs (52.9 nm), indicating the formation of ligand-mediated agglumerates. The hydrodynamic diameter of recombinant Hsp70 was determined to be 9.7 nm (Figure A2).

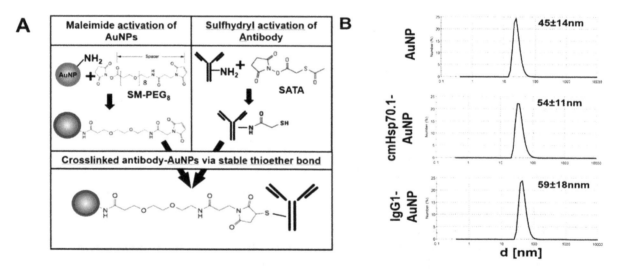

Figure 1. Antibody conjugation of gold nanoparticles (AuNPs) and characterization: (**A**) Coupling reaction of maleimide-activated AuNPs and sulfhydryl-activated monoclonal antibodies. (**B**) Size distribution of the differently functionalized AuNPs, given in size by number histograms.

2.2. Uptake and Internalization of Functionalized AuNPs in Tumor Cells In Vitro

To verify the binding capacities and specific uptake of cmHsp70.1-AuNPs in comparison to control nanoparticles (AuNPs and IgG1-AuNPs) in vitro, we performed binding tests on viable, membrane Hsp70-positive tumor cells. To determine the density of the target antigen, the cell lines 4T1 and CT26 were analyzed for their membrane and cytosolic expression of Hsp70. The Hsp70 high expressing cell line 4T1 showed a membrane Hsp70-positive phenotype on 67% ± 9% of the cells, whereas CT26 cells showed a positive phenotype on 43% ± 6% of the cells (Figure 2A). For determination of the total Hsp70 density in the cell lines, an in-cell ELISA technique was established for cells grown in chamber slides. The Hsp70 mean signal intensity in 4T1 and CT26 cell lines were $150.11 \times 10^3 \pm 24.92 \times 10^3$ a.u.

and $89.39 \times 10^3 \pm 17.19 \times 10^3$ a.u., respectively (Figure 2C). These data were verified by a sandwich ELISA of cell lysates derived from 10×10^6 cells of each cell line, resulting in Hsp70 contents of 4.28 ± 1.74 ng/mL and 1.17 ± 0.72 ng/mL for 4T1 and CT26 cells, respectively (Figure 2C). Subsequently, both cell lines were incubated with the three different types of AuNPs for 24 h at 37 °C to mimic and $89.39 \times 10^3 \pm 17.19 \times 10^3$ a.u., respectively (Figure 2B). These data were verified by a sandwich ELISA of cell lysates derived from 10×10^6 cells of each cell line, resulting in Hsp70 contents of 4.28 ± 1.74 ng/mL and 1.17 ± 0.72 ng/mL for 4T1 and CT26 cells, respectively (Figure 2C). Subsequently, both cell lines were incubated with the three different types of AuNPs for 24 h at 37 °C to mimic the uptake in living cells. In both cell lines, the content of AuNPs was visualized by brightfield and electron microscopy (Figure 3). Compared to blank AuNPs (Figure 3A, left panel) and IgG1-AuNPs (Figure 3A, middle panel), which showed minor cytosolic uptake, cmHsp70.1-AuNPs displayed the strongest accumulation in both 4T1 and CT26 cells (Figure 3A, right panel). In transmission electron microscopy (TEM), the cmHsp70.1-AuNPs have been found to accumulate in intracellular vesicles of both 4T1 and CT26 cells 24 h after incubation. A representative image of cmHsp70.1-AuNPs in 4T1 cells is shown in Figure 3B.

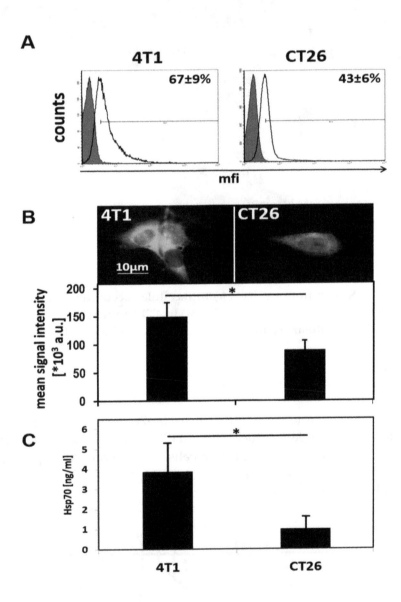

Figure 2. Quantification of Hsp70 in target tumor cell lines: (**A**) Plasma-membrane bound Hsp70 on 4T1 (left) and CT26 (right) cell lines, as determined by flow cytometry. (**B**) Quantitative staining of total Hsp70 in 4T1 and CT26 cells (upper panel) and quantification (lower panel), as determined by an in-cell ELISA technique. (**C**) Quantification of total Hsp70 in whole cell lysates of 4T1 and CT26 cell lines, as determined by an Hsp70 sandwich ELISA. * $p < 0.05$.

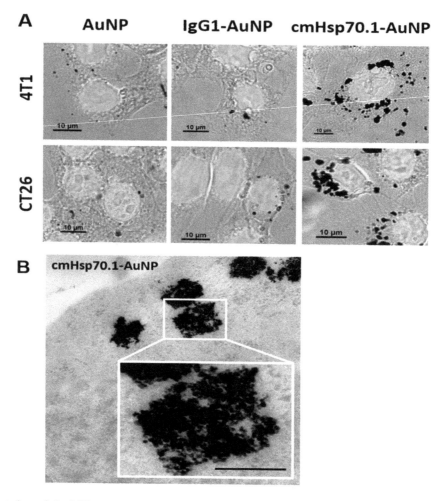

Figure 3. Uptake of AuNPs in tumor cells: (**A**) Intracellular accumulation of blank AuNPs (left), IgG1-AuNPs (middle), and cmHsp70.1-AuNPs (right) in 4T1 (upper panel) and CT26 (lower panel) cells. (**B**) TEM image of intracellular accumulations in 4T1 cells. Magnification is of the indicated area (white box). Scale bar, 1 μm.

2.3. Accumulation of Functionalized AuNPs in Tumors In Vivo

To investigate the specificity and sensitivity of cmHsp70.1-conjugated AuNPs to target tumors in vivo, syngeneic tumor models in Balb/c mice were established. Animals were injected orthotopically (o.t.) with 4T1 and subcutaneously with CT26 tumor cells, respectively. When tumors reached a size of 200 mm^3, two times 2.5 mg of AuNPs of each group (AuNP, IgG1-AuNP, and cmHsp70.1-AuNP) were injected i.v. consecutively at an interval of 24 h (Figure 4).

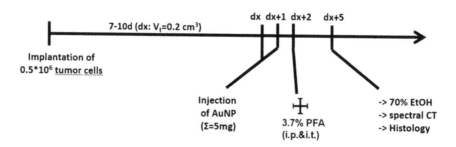

Figure 4. Timeline of the in vivo experiments.

Twenty-four hours after the second injection, mice were euthanized and fixed and subsequently imaged using spectral-CT or tumors and organs were directly applied to histological analysis. In parallel, single cell suspensions of tumors of both models have been analyzed for their plasma membrane Hsp70 status. To characterize the tumor models regarding the main features which determine the accumulation of molecular functionalized contrast agents in vivo, tumors were histologically analyzed for the target antigen content (Hsp70) in the cytosol as well as on the plasma membrane. Their vascularization status (CD31) and the presence of tumor infiltrating macrophages (F4/80) have been investigated as well. Both tumor types, 4T1 (o.t.) and CT26 (s.c.), displayed similar vascularization and infiltration of macrophages, indicating comparable effects on the NP input through these routes. Immunohistological Hsp70 staining revealed a strong expression in both tumor models, featuring cytosolic as well as nuclear Hsp70 expression. However, 4T1 tumors showed a more patterned architecture of the Hsp70 density. To investigate the membrane Hsp70 status of the tumors in vivo, a single cell suspension of freshly dissected tumors was investigated. With 76% ± 7% and 67% ± 13% membrane Hsp70-positive viable tumor cells, 4T1 and CT26 tumors grown in vivo, respectively, showed a slightly higher Hsp70 expression density compared to the in vitro cultured cells. However, the increased width of the cytometric data, as given in histograms, indicates an increased heterogeneity in the membrane Hsp70 expression pattern in in vivo grown tumors (Figure 5).

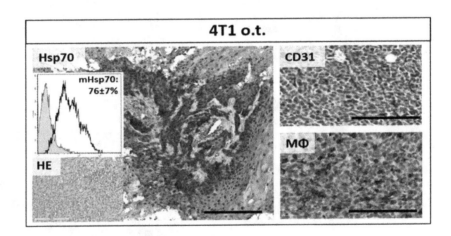

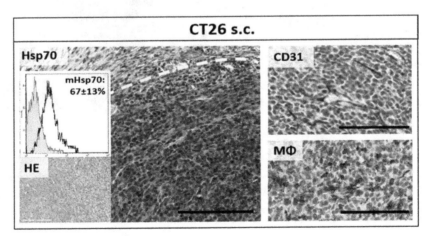

Figure 5. Tumor characterization: Orthotopic (o.t.) 4T1 (upper panel) and subcutaneous (s.c.) CT26 (lower panel) tumors were analyzed with regard to membrane (flow cytometry analysis, upper inlay) and overall (immunohistochemistry, IHC) Hsp70 expression as well as their content of CD31 positive vessels (IHC and CD31) and the infiltration of macrophages (MΦ, IHC, and F4/80). Hematoxylin & Eosin (H&E) was used as an overview stain (lower inlay). Scale bars, 200 μm (Hsp70) and 100 μm (CD31 and MΦ).

In a next step, we investigated the feasibility of cmHsp70.1-AuNPs as a contrast agent in a first cohort of tumor-bearing mice. For this pilot study, three mice with subcutaneous CT26 tumors underwent spectral CT imaging postmortem. Each mouse had received one type of AuNP 24 h before sacrifice. Interestingly, in all animals, we were able to detect AuNPs in the tumors with the highest density of nanoparticles in the tumor periphery. Nevertheless, we also noticed some striking differences. The mouse which was treated with IgG1-AuNPs presented the lowest content of AuNPs inside the tumor (3.3 μg Au/mm^3 tumor) with a very low accumulation of particles within the tumor center (Figure 6C,D). In the mouse which was treated with unconjugated AuNPs, 4.3 μg Au/mm^3 was detected in total but mainly at the periphery of the tumor, with considerably less AuNPs in the tumor center (Figure 6A,B). In case of an injection of cmHsp70.1-AuNPs, 4.4 μg Au/mm^3 was found inside the tumor. Despite similar amounts of different AuNPs in the tumor area, the distribution pattern of the AuNP formulation differed drastically. CmHsp70.1-AuNPs were found to be located in the tumor periphery and highly dispersed in the tumor center (Figure 6E,F).

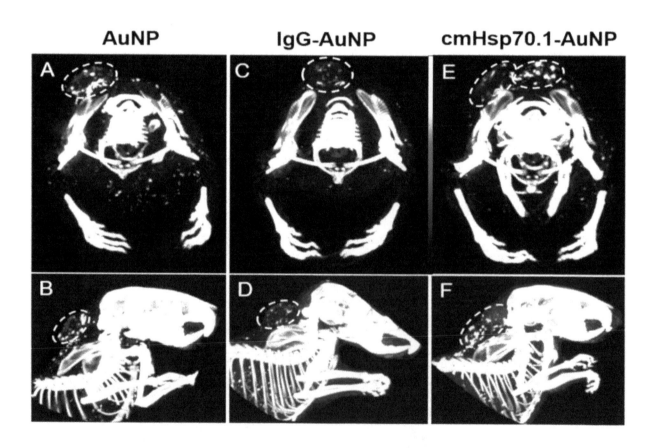

Figure 6. Tumor detection using spectral-CT. Upper Row (**A,C,E**): axial view, bottom row (**B,D,F**): sagital view. AuNP amounts are pseudo-coloured from black (6.5 mg/mL) over red (10 mg/mL) to white (13.5 mg/mL). (**A,B**) spectral CT-views of mice injected with AuNPs; (**C,D**) spectral CT-views of mice injected with IgG-AuNPs; (**E,F**) spectral CT-views of mice injected with cmHsp70.1-AuNPs.

The spectral CT-based biodistribution analysis detected a high accumulation of AuNPs in the spleen, lower amounts in the liver, and very low amounts of AuNPs in the lung. The other organs did not exhibit concentrations which were high enough to generate a signal in the spectral CT measurements. However, to prove data for statistical significance, the number of mice within the study groups have to be increased to relevant numbers in future experiments. The tumors were further analyzed for their gold content by histology (Figure 7).

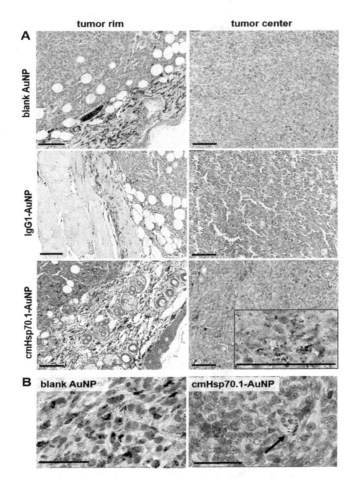

Figure 7. AuNP uptake and distribution in CT26 tumors: (**A**) Silver enhancement of AuNPs. Upper row: blank AuNPs, middle row: IgG1-AuNPs, bottom row: cmHsp70.1-AuNPs. Left: Region of Interest (ROI) at tumor rim area, right: ROI set to tumor center. Scale bars, 100 μm. (**B**) Double staining of Macrophages (F4/80, brown) and silver enhancement of AuNPs (black). Arrow: single-positive cells for AuNPs. Scale bars: 5 μm.

Sections were treated with silver enhancement to visualize AuNPs by light microscopy (Figure 7A). As revealed by spectral-CT, histological analysis confirmed the varying intratumoral distribution of the three groups of AuNPs. In tumors of mice which were treated with cmHsp70.1-AuNPs, a rather homologous distribution of NPs was observed throughout the whole tumor volume compared to the blank AuNPs or IgG1-AuNPs. Notably, the enrichment of AuNPs at the tumor rim following i.v. injection of blank AuNPs was most likely due to F4/80 positive monocyte/macrophage lineages with internalized AuNPs (Figure 7B, left). In contrast, next to the payload introduction via macrophages, cmHsp70.1-AuNPs were also found in large amounts in F4/80-negative tumor cells. Consequently, an extended accumulation of the cmHsp70.1-AuNPs was also detected in the tumor center. In this region, we also identfied less AuNP containing macrophages (Figure 7B, right). IgG1-AuNPs showed the lowest accumulation in all regions of the tumor (Figure 7A, middle). These NPs, besides their lack of targeting ability, exhibited equal biocompatibility to that of cmHsp70.1-AuNPs due to the conjugation of the murine IgG1 antibody. Consequently, these IgG1NPs resulted in the lowest intratumoral accumulation yield.

To obtain the in vivo biodistribution characteristics of cmHsp70.1-AuNPs, 24 h following systemic application, we further analyzed silver enhanced sections of tumors, liver, spleen, kidneys, heart, lungs, and intestines of another group of tumor-bearing Balb/c mice (after subcutaneous and orthotopic injection) (Figure 8).

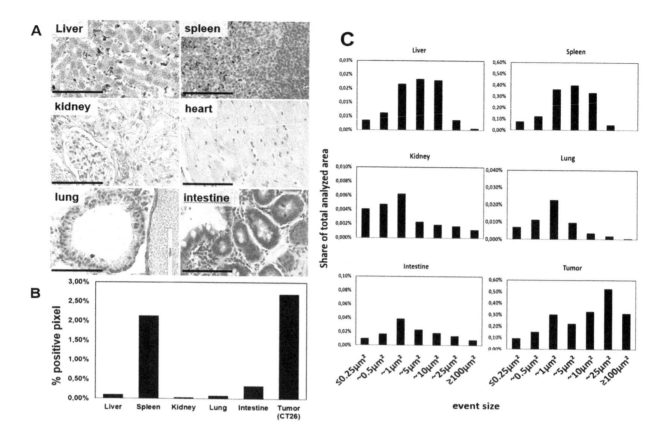

Figure 8. Biodistribution of cmHsp70.1-AuNPs: (**A**) Silver enhancement staining of liver, spleen, kidney, heart, lung, and intestine. Scale bar, 100 μm. (**B**) Pixel analysis of silver enhancement stainings in tumors and organs, given in positive pixel/mm^2 tissue. (**C**) size distribution of silver enhanced cmHsp70.1-AuNP signals in different organs following i.v. injection.

For an improved accuracy of the analysis, we used a machine-learning approach. The algorithm for the analysis of sections was trained on 28 slides in total and was applied for the analysis of 14 slides. In comparison to the organs, the highest accumulation of cmHsp70.1-AuNPs was found in the tumors, with $85.98 \times 10^3 \pm 4.94 \times 10^3$ positive pixel per mm^2, which equals to 2.7% positive pixels per section (Figure 8B). Using the machine-learning approach, we found the majority of the nanoparticles accumulated in spleen ($14.04 \times 10^3 \pm 1.37 \times 10^3$ pixel/mm^2) (2.13% signal/section), liver ($13.34 \times 10^3 \pm 0.7 \times 10^3$ pixel/mm^2) (0.11% signal/section), and intestine ($9.48 \times 10^3 \pm 1.37 \times 10^3$ pixel/mm^2) (0.34% signal/section), followed by lungs ($6.28 \times 10^3 \pm 1.30 \times 10^3$ pixel/mm^2) (0.09% signal/section). In muscle, as represented by heart tissue, the accumulation of AuNPs was below the detection limit. Kidney was rarely affected, indicating an enterohepatic secretion of the AuNPs. In addition to the analysis of the overall entry of AuNPs in the organs and tumors, we utilized the machine-learning approach to analyze the size distribution of the nanoparticle agglumerations within the organs. The majority of positively stained events in liver and spleen resulted in a size range up to 10 μm. Accumulation of events in this size range might be suggested to be due to incorporation of the AuNP by macrophages and Kupffer cells, as indicated also in Figure 7B. The majority of AuNPs in kidney, lung, and intestine yielded in agglumerates of about 1 μm in size. In the tumor, cmHsp70.1-AuNP spots of 25 μm^2 were dominant, followed by spots of 1 μm^2 (Figure 8C). As tumor-associated macrophages exhibit large cytoplasmatic volumes, the accumulation of AuNPs above 10 μm^2 suggest the appearance of this cell type. However, aggregates of 1 μm^2 point to tumor cells with smaller cytoplasmic space as tumor cells. This finding is also supported by microscopical analysis of in vitro grown tumor cells with the majority of NP accumulating in cellular organelles of about 1 μm, following endocytosis (Figure 3).

3. Discussion

The discovery of suitable contrast agents for the visualization of tumors is one of the most important areas in clinical oncology. In tumor imaging, CT imaging is the most commonly used technique featuring fast scanning speed with high spatial resolution of a large portion of the body. Functional molecular imaging can be accomplished with positron-electron-tomography (PET), often used in combination with CT. However, certain limitations affect the quality of tumor visualization. PET imaging using ^{18}F-FDG is highly dependent on a high tumor cell metabolism compared to the surrounding normal tissue. Furthermore, PET tracers need to exert ionizing effects, which in turn increases the patient's risk to accumulate DNA mutations. An approach to overcome the limiting effects of PET/CT led to the development of spectral-CT analyzers [6,18], which use the k-edge discrimination of elements, allowing for their specific identification inside the body [19]. Another advantage of the spectral segmentation is the possibility to utilize multiple contrast agents within one imaging session, which reduces the X-ray expositions of the patient.

One further limitation of PET imaging is the spatial detection limit, leading to a potential miss of small lesions. Therefore, the usage of tumor-specific markers is beneficial.

Herein, the major stress-inducible member of the HSP70 family, Hsp70 (HspA1A), was used as a target for the tumor-specific uptake of functionalized AuNPs in different tumor entities. Hsp70 is expressed on the plasma membrane of a variety of tumor entities, whereas normal cells lack an Hsp70 membrane expression [9]. However, further studies investigate the role of membrane-associated Hsp70 in the context of inflammatory diseases, such as sepsis. It was found that membrane Hsp70 also plays a role in the regulation of inflammatory responses. A study of Hirsch et al. described polymorphonuclear neutrophils (PMNs), expressing mHsp70. These PMNs are recognized and lysed by $\gamma\delta$ T-lymphocytes and therefore protect the host cells from inflammation-induced damage [20].

In previous studies, we observed that tumor cell membrane-associated Hsp70 is rapidly internalized and therefore mediates an efficient uptake of Hsp70-binding probes into the cytoplasm, such as fluorescence-labeled cmHsp70.1 antibody [15] and tumor-penetrating peptide (TPP) [21,22]. Since the binding epitope of cmHsp70.1 antibody is identical in mouse and human tumor cells [9], murine CT26 colon and mammary 4T1 tumor cell lines were used in the present study.

The application of AuNPs for imaging in vivo is a promising new approach in the field of in vivo imaging [7,23,24]. The uptake of antibody-conjugated nanoparticles into tumor cells is dependent on several factors: the expression density of receptors, which are expressed on the target cells; the distribution of the target epitopes throughout the cells [25]; the affinity of the tracer to the membrane epitope; and the speed of internalization [21,26].

In order to monitor the efficiency of functionalized AuNPs in vitro and in vivo, we applied different imaging modalities. Dynamic light scattering is a widely used technique to determine the hydrodynamic diameter of AuNPs in the nm–μm range.

Furthermore, the quantification of AuNPs within tumor cells is of relevance to estimate the concentration of nanoparticles that is necessary for noninvasive in vivo imaging of tumors as well as for their use as therapeutic agent. In our in vivo/ex vivo setup, we were able to detect aggregates of AuNPs in tumors and organs in perinuclear areas of around 1–2 μm in diameter as well as larger aggregates of around 25 μm in diameter. The presented machine-learning approach has proven to be beneficial for the analysis of the distribution of AuNPs. Next to calculating the quantity of gold signal within tumors and organs, we were able to separate the signal into groups, which allows for an easy analysis of AuNPs within different cell types. This is important for a more precise prediction of the biodistribution and possible toxic side effects of AuNPs.

Toxic side effects of AuNPs following i.v. application were investigated in previous studies [27,28]. No negative side effects such as loss in body weight or organic dysfunctions were observed in these experiments up to a concentration of 500 μg/mL [29]. Concordantly, in the in vivo experiments of this study, we did not observe any sign of toxicity at the injected concentration of 5 mg AuNPs per mouse. However, additional pharmacological and toxicological studies are needed to prove safety.

On the basis of the specific and quantitative uptake of cmHsp70.1-AuNPs in Hsp70-positive tumor cells and its imaging properties, our approach hints at a possible beneficial use in radiation therapy. Numerous studies have reported on the radiation-enhancing effect of AuNPs within tumor tissue [30,31].

First, promising findings for radiotherapy enhancement of AuNPs were achieved in preclinical mammary carcinoma studies [32]. The results of Hainfeld et al. showed an 86% 1-year survival for a combinatorial therapy of irradiation in presence of NPs compared to 20% for radiotherapy alone. Probable mechanisms involved in radiosensitization are, besides changes in the cell cycle or an elevated reactive oxygen species, the production and the release of secondary Auger electrons by gold in very close proximity to the nucleus [31]. In previous in vitro studies on the intracellular distribution of Hsp70 targeting AuNPs, we observed an increased accumulation of the NPs in close proximity to the nucleus 24 to 48 h after incubation [16], indicating possible beneficial effects of this approach for radiotherapeutical interventions. In summary, we demonstrate that the functionalization of AuNPs with cmHsp70.1 antibody is a highly promising approach for in vivo tumor targeting. Our preclinical studies show that the accumulation of AuNPs within the investigated tumors was sufficient for visualization by spectral-CT which allows 3D reconstructions and quantifications.

4. Materials and Methods

4.1. Antibody Coupling of AuNPs

Coupling of Hsp70-specific antibody (cmHsp70.1, multimmune, Germany) or an isotype-matched control IgG1 antibody (Sigma Aldrich, St. Luis, Mo, USA) to AuNPs (Nanopartz, Loveland, CO, USA) was done as described before [16]. Briefly, polyethylenglycol (PEG)-amine-coated spherical gold nanoparticles of 30 nm diameter were maleimide activated (Pierce, Thermo Fischer Scientific, Rockford, IL, USA) and incubated over night with sulfhydryl-activated antibodies. Antibody-coupled AuNPs or unconjugated AuNPs were analyzed and used for experiments within 24 h. Nanoparticles were analyzed (size, aggregation) by dynamic light scattering (DLS, Zetasizer NanoS, Malvern Instruments, Malvern, UK). Measurements were done in triplets and mean values were calculated.

4.2. Characterization of AuNPs

Antibody-conjugated AuNPs or unconjugated AuNPs were used for experiments directly after coupling. For AuNP characterization and controlling their aggregation, particle size was analyzed by dynamic light scattering (Zetasizer NanoS; Malvern Instruments, Malvern, UK). Only nanoparticles that produced single peaks were used for experiments. For analysis of the specific interaction of differentially functionalized AuNPs with Hsp70, 150 µg/mL nanoparticles dissolved in PBS were incubated with recombinant Hsp70 protein at a concentration of 0.5 µg/mL. Following a 4-h incubation time, the size of the clusters formed by IgG1-AuNP + Hsp70 and cmHsp70.1-AuNP + Hsp70, respectively, was analyzed by DLS.

4.3. Cell Culture

Murine colon carcinoma cell line CT26 (CT26.WT; American type culture collection (ATCC) #CRL-2638) and the mouse mammary carcinoma cell line 4T1 (ATCC #CRL-2539) were cultured in Roswell Park Memorial Institute 1640 medium supplemented with 10% (v/v) heat-inactivated fetal calf serum, 2 mM L-glutamine, 1 mM sodium pyruvate, and antibiotics (100 IU/mL penicillin and 100 µg/mL streptomycin). Cells were incubated at 37 °C in 95% humidity and 5% (v/v) CO_2 and cultivated twice a week.

4.4. Assessment of Hsp70 Content of the Tumor Cells

The Hsp70 membrane phenotype of the cells was assessed by flow cytometry. Single cell suspensions of tumor cell lines were incubated with fluorescein-isothiocyanate (FITC)-conjugated cmHsp70.1 mAb for 30 min on ice. As controls, conjugation of an IgG1 isotype-matched antibody was done. After washing and adding propidium-iodide (PI) for life and dead discrimination, binding of antibodies was measured using a FACSCalibur instrument (BD Biosciences, Heidelberg, Germany). Data were analyzed using CellQuest Pro 6.0 software. Only PI-negative, viable cells were analyzed. To determine the membrane Hsp70 status of tumors grown in vivo, single cell suspension of freshly dissected tumors was generated by combined chopping and trypsin treatment of the tumors. Here, anti-mouse CD45 APC antibody was added to cmHsp70.1-FITC to distinguish tumor cells from mononuclear blood cells and infiltrated macrophages.

In-cell ELISA was performed, as described previously [21]. Briefly, cells grown in chamber slides were fixed with DAKO Fix & Perm kit (DAKO, Jena, Germany) and cellular membranes were permeabilized and incubated with cmHsp70.1-FITC antibody. Following microscopy with comparable settings, quantification of fluorescence signal was determined on the mean signal intensity values by ImageJ 1.52a image analysis software.

Quantification of the Hsp70 content was confirmed by an Hsp70 sandwich ELISA, as described elsewhere [33]. Shortly, after determination of the cell count, cells were lysed by incubation in Tris-HCl-based buffer containing 1% Triton-X100 and SDS. After centrifugation, the Hsp70 concentration in the supernatant was measured by total Hsp70 ELISA kit (R&D systems, Minneapolis, MN, USA) as described by the manufacturer. Each supernatant sample was measured in duplicates.

4.5. Animals

All animal procedures and their care were conducted in conformity with national and international guidelines (EU 2010/63) with approval from the local authorities of the Government of Upper Bavaria and ethical committee of Pavlov First Saint Petersburg State Medical University (St. Petersburg, Russia) (2015/068) and supervised by respective animal care and use committees. Animals were housed in standard animal rooms in individually ventilated cage systems (IVS Techniplast, Buggugiate, Italy) under specific pathogen-free conditions with free access to water and standard laboratory chow ad libitum. In total, 6 female Balb/c mice (aged 10–14 weeks, Charles River Laboratories, Sulzfeld, Germany) were used. Induction of subcutaneous tumors was done under inhalation anesthesia (1.8% isoflurane with medical O_2) by injection of 5×10^5 CT26 cells subcutaneously in the neck area or of 5×10^5 4T1 cells orthotopically in the 4th mammary fat pad. When tumors reached a size of 200 mm³, AuNPs were intravenously injected using standard procedures. In total, 5 mg unconjugated, IgG1-, or cmHsp70.1-AuNPs, suspended in phosphate buffered saline, were injected in a consecutive pattern of two times 2.5 mg per day within 48 h. Another 24 h after the second application, mice were euthanized under deep anesthesia, fixed in 4% neutral-buffered formalin for 5 days, and stored in 70% ethanol for further analysis.

4.6. Bright Field Microscopy

For light microscopy, cells were grown in 8-well chamber slides (NUNC-Nalgene; Thermo Fisher Scientific, Pittsburgh, PA, USA) at a concentration of 10,000 cells per well. Upon adherence, cells were incubated with AuNPs at a nontoxic concentration of 1 µg/mL. Cellular uptake of AuNPs or quantum dots of the same size were analyzed with a Zeiss Observer Z1 (Zeiss, Germany).

4.7. Transmission Electron Microscopy

Cells were co-incubated with functionalized and non-conjugated AuNPs (at a concentration 100 µg/mL) for 24 h. Following, incubation cells were washed with PBS, fixed for 1 h at 4 °C in 2.5% glutaraldehyde in 0.1 M cacodylate buffer (pH = 7.4), postfixed in 1% aqueous OsO4 (for 1 h), dehydrated, and embedded in Araldite-Epon mixture. Sections were assessed employing Zeiss Libra 120 electron microscope (Carl Zeiss, Germany).

4.8. Histology and Immunohistochemistry

Tumors and organs were either dissected following whole-body fixation of mice or fixed in 3.7% neutral-buffered formaldehyde and embedded in paraffin. Two-μm sections of the organs and tumors were prepared, and the morphology was visualized by standard H&E staining. For immunohistochemistry, the activity of the endogenous peroxidase was blocked with 1% hydrogen peroxide and 0.1% sodium azide. After antigen retrieval in citric acid buffer (pH 6) at 100 °C, sections were incubated with anti-Hsp70 antibody cmHsp70.1, followed by horse radish peroxidas (HRP)-labelled secondary rabbit anti-mouse antibody (Dako, Jena, Germany). Diaminobenzidine (Dako) was used as a chromogen. Sections were counterstained with 1% Mayer's hematoxylin. To visualize the AuNPs by light microscopy, silver-enhancement staining was used according to the manufacturers' protocol (Sigma-Aldrich, Darmstadt, Germany), followed by counterstaining of the nuclei with 0.1% Nuclear Fast Red solution (Morphisto, Frankfurt a.M., Germany). Slides were digitalized with a digital slide scanner (AT2, Leica, Wetzlar, Germany).

4.9. Spectral-CT Imaging and Image Acquisition

Spectral CT images were acquired at a Philips spectral CT scanner, as described before [18]. Briefly, a preclinical spectral photon-counting CT system (Philips Healthcare, Hamburg, Germany) was used to obtain axial scans over 360 ° at a beam voltage of 100 kVp. For optimal discrimination of the signals of AuNPs, a threshold was set at the k-edge energy of gold.

4.10. Spectral CT Image-Based Gold Quantification

Osirix® MD v10.0.5 software (Pixmeo SARL, Bern, Switzerland) was used for analysis. Mean background was measured from several ROIs in the spleen. Gold amounts were calculated over the whole tumor volume (μg gold/mm^3).

4.11. Deep Learning-Based Quantification of AuNP Histology

The biodistribution of silver-stained AuNPs in histological slides was assessed with the help of a deep neural network. Regions of interest in each slide were defined via manual delineation. Slides were subdivided into smaller, slightly overlapping patches of 1000 × 1000 pixels to meet memory constraints. In a first preliminary step, AuNP concentrations were segmented with the help of color-channel-specific dynamic thresholding and morphological operations (opening and closing with fixed kernels). Parameters were manually tuned to optimize results for the majority of slides. In a second step, the best resulting binary masks were manually selected and partially manually corrected. In a third step, a deep neural network was trained to segment AuNP concentrations on this basis. In a final step, the trained network was used to derive segmentations of AuNP concentrations for all slide patches. A k-fold rotation of data splits was applied so that the network yields segmentations on data samples that were not used for training, ensuring that the segmentation represents the result of the learned task rather than replicates the threshold-derived training data. This procedure yielded substantially more accurate and consistent segmentations of AuNP concentrations as compared to the preliminary thresholding procedure. Subsequent re-concatenation of slightly overlapping slide patches ruled out boundary effects and double counting. In a postprocessing step, all individual AuNP concentrations were identified via connected-component analysis, allowing to assess their individual sizes.

The deep neural network follows a U-net like architecture and consists of 4 levels of en- and decoding units. Each layer of encoding units doubles the number of feature channels, starting from 16 and ending at 265 at the deepest [16] level. The network was trained for 10 epochs on a training set of ca. 5000 patches. Details of architecture, implementation, and training procedure follow a previously described protocol [34].

5. Conclusions

Herein, we show that the visualization of tumor cells with AuNPs by addressing membrane Hsp70 is feasible. We present data showing a superior uptake of cmHsp70.1-AuNPs inside Hsp70 membrane-positive tumor cells. Inside the tumor cells, these particles accumulated in the perinuclear region within 24 h. The Hsp70 specificity was shown since unconjugated nanoparticles and nanoparticles conjugated with an irrelevant control antibody were not taken up into Hsp70 membrane-positive tumor cells. Furthermore, Hsp70 knockout tumor cells that do not express Hsp70 in the cytosol and on the plasma membrane showed no uptake of the cmHsp70.1-conjugated nanoparticles [16]. Quantification of the internalized cmHsp70.1-conjugated AuNPs reveals a high sensitivity for the detection of single cells. Experiments are ongoing to study the capability of cmHsp70.1-AuNPs for spectral CT imaging of further Hsp70 membrane-positive and negative tumor models and whether these NPs can be exploited for therapeutic approaches. In the future, these antibody-conjugated AuNPs might be useful for the diagnosis of tumors and for radiotherapeutic interventions.

Author Contributions: Conceptualization, M.A.K. and S.S.; Data curation, M.A.K., M.S., C.W. and S.S.; Formal analysis, M.A.K., C.W., B.H.M., G.M. and S.S.; Funding acquisition, M.A.K., G.M. and S.S.; Investigation, M.S. and S.S.; Methodology, M.A.K., C.W., W.S., W.Z., O.S., R.P., O.B., M.M. and S.S.; Project administration, G.M. and S.S.; Resources, G.M. and S.S.; Supervision, B.H.M., E.J.R., G.M. and S.S.; Validation, M.A.K., C.W., O.S. and S.S.; Visualization, M.A.K., R.P. and S.S.; Writing—original draft, M.A.K. and S.S.; Writing—review and editing, M.A.K., M.S., C.W., W.S., W.Z., O.S., B.H.M., E.J.R., R.P., M.M., G.M. and S.S. All authors were involved in drafting the article or in revising it critically for important intellectual content. All authors have read and agreed to the published version of the manuscript.

Appendix A

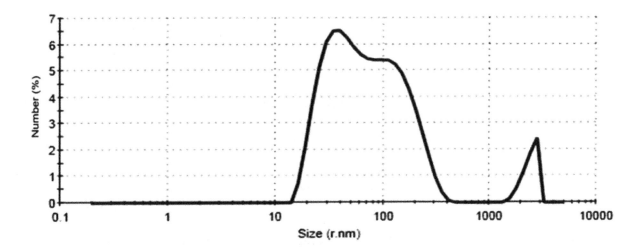

Figure A1. Size distribution of cmHsp70.1-AuNPs after 2 weeks at 4 °C: Size distribution is given in size by number histogram.

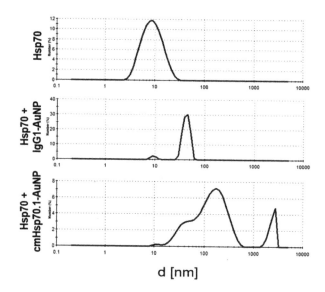

d [nm]

Figure A2. Size distribution of recombinant Hsp70 (upper panel) as well as IgG1-AuNPs (middle panel) and cmHsp70.1-AuNPs (lower panel) following incubation with recombinant Hsp70 for 4 h: Size distribution is given in size by number histograms.

References

1. Vanderstraeten, B.; Duthoy, W.; De Gersem, W.; De Neve, W.; Thierens, H. [18F]fluoro-deoxy-glucose positron emission tomography ([18F]FDG-PET) voxel intensity-based intensity-modulated radiation therapy (IMRT) for head and neck cancer. *Radiother. Oncol.* **2006**, *79*, 249–258. [CrossRef] [PubMed]

2. Bal, H.; Guerin, L.; Casey, M.E.; Conti, M.; Eriksson, L.; Michel, C.; Fanti, S.; Pettinato, C.; Adler, S.; Choyke, P. Improving PET spatial resolution and detectability for prostate cancer imaging. *Phys. Med. Biol.* **2014**, *59*, 4411–4426. [CrossRef]

3. Cormode, D.P.; Naha, P.C.; Fayad, Z.A. Nanoparticle contrast agents for computed tomography: A focus on micelles. *Contrast Media Mol. Imaging* **2014**, *9*, 37–52. [CrossRef]

4. Anjomrouz, M.; Shamshad, M.; Panta, R.K.; Broeke, L.V.; Schleich, N.; Atharifard, A.; Aamir, R.; Bheesette, S.; Walsh, M.F.; Goulter, B.P.; et al. Beam profile assessment in spectral CT scanners. *J. Appl. Clin. Med. Phys.* **2018**, *19*, 287–297. [CrossRef]

5. Chen, W.H.; Chen, J.X.; Cheng, H.; Chen, C.S.; Yang, J.; Xu, X.D.; Wang, Y.; Zhuo, R.X.; Zhang, X.Z. A new anti-cancer strategy of damaging mitochondria by pro-apoptotic peptide functionalized gold nanoparticles. *Chem. Commun.* **2013**, *49*, 6403–6405. [CrossRef]

6. Cormode, D.P.; Roessl, E.; Thran, A.; Skajaa, T.; Gordon, R.E.; Schlomka, J.P.; Fuster, V.; Fisher, E.A.; Mulder, W.J.; Proksa, R.; et al. Atherosclerotic plaque composition: Analysis with multicolor CT and targeted gold nanoparticles. *Radiology* **2010**, *256*, 774–782. [CrossRef] [PubMed]

7. Shevtsov, M.; Zhou, Y.; Khachatryan, W.; Multhoff, G.; Gao, H. Recent Advances in Gold Nanoformulations for Cancer Therapy. *Curr. Drug Metab.* **2018**, *19*, 768–780. [CrossRef] [PubMed]

8. Sherman, M.; Multhoff, G. Heat shock proteins in cancer. *Ann. N. Y. Acad. Sci.* **2007**, *1113*, 192–201. [CrossRef]

9. Stangl, S.; Gehrmann, M.; Riegger, J.; Kuhs, K.; Riederer, I.; Sievert, W.; Hube, K.; Mocikat, R.; Dressel, R.; Kremmer, E.; et al. Targeting membrane heat-shock protein 70 (Hsp70) on tumors by cmHsp70.1 antibody. *Proc. Natl. Acad. Sci. USA* **2011**, *108*, 733–738. [CrossRef]

10. Hantschel, M.; Pfister, K.; Jordan, A.; Scholz, R.; Andreesen, R.; Schmitz, G.; Schmetzer, H.; Hiddemann, W.; Multhoff, G. Hsp70 plasma membrane expression on primary tumor biopsy material and bone marrow of leukemic patients. *Cell Stress Chaperones* **2000**, *5*, 438–442. [CrossRef]

11. Stangl, S.; Tontcheva, N.; Sievert, W.; Shevtsov, M.; Niu, M.; Schmid, T.E.; Pigorsch, S.; Combs, S.E.; Haller, B.; Balermpas, P.; et al. Heat shock protein 70 and tumor-infiltrating NK cells as prognostic indicators for patients with squamous cell carcinoma of the head and neck after radiochemotherapy: A multicentre retrospective study of the German Cancer Consortium Radiation Oncology Group (DKTK-ROG). *Int. J. Cancer* **2018**, *142*, 1911–1925. [CrossRef] [PubMed]

12. Farkas, B.; Hantschel, M.; Magyarlaki, M.; Becker, B.; Scherer, K.; Landthaler, M.; Pfister, K.; Gehrmann, M.; Gross, C.; Mackensen, A.; et al. Heat shock protein 70 membrane expression and melanoma-associated marker phenotype in primary and metastatic melanoma. *Melanoma Res.* **2003**, *13*, 147–152. [CrossRef] [PubMed]

13. Steiner, K.; Graf, M.; Hecht, K.; Reif, S.; Rossbacher, L.; Pfister, K.; Kolb, H.J.; Schmetzer, H.M.; Multhoff, G. High HSP70-membrane expression on leukemic cells from patients with acute myeloid leukemia is associated with a worse prognosis. *Leukemia* **2006**, *20*, 2076–2079. [CrossRef] [PubMed]

14. Gehrmann, M.; Radons, J.; Molls, M.; Multhoff, G. The therapeutic implications of clinically applied modifiers of heat shock protein 70 (Hsp70) expression by tumor cells. *Cell Stress Chaperones* **2008**, *13*, 1–10. [CrossRef] [PubMed]

15. Stangl, S.; Gehrmann, M.; Dressel, R.; Alves, F.; Dullin, C.; Themelis, G.; Ntziachristos, V.; Staeblein, E.; Walch, A.; Winkelmann, I.; et al. In vivo imaging of CT26 mouse tumours by using cmHsp70.1 monoclonal antibody. *J. Cell. Mol. Med.* **2011**, *15*, 874–887. [CrossRef] [PubMed]

16. Gehrmann, M.K.; Kimm, M.A.; Stangl, S.; Schmid, T.E.; Noel, P.B.; Rummeny, E.J.; Multhoff, G. Imaging of Hsp70-positive tumors with cmHsp70.1 antibody-conjugated gold nanoparticles. *Int. J. Nanomed.* **2015**, *10*, 5687–5700. [CrossRef]

17. Shevtsov, M.; Stangl, S.; Nikolaev, B.; Yakovleva, L.; Marchenko, Y.; Tagaeva, R.; Sievert, W.; Pitkin, E.; Mazur, A.; Tolstoy, P.; et al. Granzyme B Functionalized Nanoparticles Targeting Membrane Hsp70-Positive Tumors for Multimodal Cancer Theranostics. *Small* **2019**, *15*, e1900205. [CrossRef]

18. Schlomka, J.P.; Roessl, E.; Dorscheid, R.; Dill, S.; Martens, G.; Istel, T.; Baumer, C.; Herrmann, C.; Steadman, R.; Zeitler, G.; et al. Experimental feasibility of multi-energy photon-counting K-edge imaging in pre-clinical computed tomography. *Phys. Med. Biol.* **2008**, *53*, 4031–4047. [CrossRef]

19. Ashton, J.R.; Clark, D.P.; Moding, E.J.; Ghaghada, K.; Kirsch, D.G.; West, J.L.; Badea, C.T. Dual-energy micro-CT functional imaging of primary lung cancer in mice using gold and iodine nanoparticle contrast agents: A validation study. *PLoS ONE* **2014**, *9*, e88129. [CrossRef]

20. Hirsh, M.I.; Hashiguchi, N.; Chen, Y.; Yip, L.; Junger, W.G. Surface expression of HSP72 by LPS-stimulated neutrophils facilitates gammadeltaT cell-mediated killing. *Eur. J. Immunol.* **2006**, *36*, 712–721. [CrossRef]

21. Stangl, S.; Tei, L.; De Rose, F.; Reder, S.; Martinelli, J.; Sievert, W.; Shevtsov, M.; Ollinger, R.; Rad, R.; Schwaiger, M.; et al. Preclinical Evaluation of the Hsp70 Peptide Tracer TPP-PEG24-DFO[(89)Zr] for Tumor-Specific PET/CT Imaging. *Cancer Res.* **2018**, *78*, 6268–6281. [CrossRef]

22. Stangl, S.; Varga, J.; Freysoldt, B.; Trajkovic-Arsic, M.; Siveke, J.T.; Greten, F.R.; Ntziachristos, V.; Multhoff, G. Selective in vivo imaging of syngeneic, spontaneous, and xenograft tumors using a novel tumor cell-specific hsp70 peptide-based probe. *Cancer Res.* **2014**, *74*, 6903–6912. [CrossRef] [PubMed]

23. Cormode, D.P.; Si-Mohamed, S.; Bar-Ness, D.; Sigovan, M.; Naha, P.C.; Balegamire, J.; Lavenne, F.; Coulon, P.; Roessl, E.; Bartels, M.; et al. Multicolor spectral photon-counting computed tomography: In vivo dual contrast imaging with a high count rate scanner. *Sci. Rep.* **2017**, *7*, 4784. [CrossRef] [PubMed]

24. Si-Mohamed, S.; Cormode, D.P.; Bar-Ness, D.; Sigovan, M.; Naha, P.C.; Langlois, J.B.; Chalabreysse, L.; Coulon, P.; Blevis, I.; Roessl, E.; et al. Evaluation of spectral photon counting computed tomography K-edge imaging for determination of gold nanoparticle biodistribution in vivo. *Nanoscale* **2017**, *9*, 18246–18257. [CrossRef] [PubMed]

25. Schubertova, V.; Martinez-Veracoechea, F.J.; Vacha, R. Influence of ligand distribution on uptake efficiency. *Soft Matter* **2015**, *11*, 2726–2730. [CrossRef] [PubMed]

26. Lammers, T.; Kiessling, F.; Hennink, W.E.; Storm, G. Drug targeting to tumors: Principles, pitfalls and (pre-)clinical progress. *J. Control. Release* **2012**, *161*, 175–187. [CrossRef] [PubMed]

27. Zhang, X.D.; Wu, D.; Shen, X.; Liu, P.X.; Yang, N.; Zhao, B.; Zhang, H.; Sun, Y.M.; Zhang, L.A.; Fan, F.Y. Size-dependent in vivo toxicity of PEG-coated gold nanoparticles. *Int. J. Nanomed.* **2011**, *6*, 2071–2081. [CrossRef]

28. Alkilany, A.M.; Murphy, C.J. Toxicity and cellular uptake of gold nanoparticles: What we have learned so far? *J. Nanopart. Res.* **2010**, *12*, 2313–2333. [CrossRef]

29. Zhang, X.D.; Wu, H.Y.; Wu, D.; Wang, Y.Y.; Chang, J.H.; Zhai, Z.B.; Meng, A.M.; Liu, P.X.; Zhang, L.A.; Fan, F.Y. Toxicologic effects of gold nanoparticles in vivo by different administration routes. *Int. J. Nanomed.* **2010**, *5*, 771–781. [CrossRef]

30. Dorsey, J.F.; Sun, L.; Joh, D.Y.; Witztum, A.; Kao, G.D.; Alonso-Basanta, M.; Avery, S.; Hahn, S.M.; Al Zaki, A.; Tsourkas, A. Gold nanoparticles in radiation research: Potential applications for imaging and radiosensitization. *Transl. Cancer Res.* **2013**, *2*, 280–291. [CrossRef]

31. Muddineti, O.S.; Ghosh, B.; Biswas, S. Current trends in using polymer coated gold nanoparticles for cancer therapy. *Int. J. Pharm.* **2015**, *484*, 252–267. [CrossRef]

32. Hainfeld, J.F.; Dilmanian, F.A.; Zhong, Z.; Slatkin, D.N.; Kalef-Ezra, J.A.; Smilowitz, H.M. Gold nanoparticles enhance the radiation therapy of a murine squamous cell carcinoma. *Phys. Med. Biol.* **2010**, *55*, 3045–3059. [CrossRef]

33. Rothammer, A.; Sage, E.K.; Werner, C.; Combs, S.E.; Multhoff, G. Increased heat shock protein 70 (Hsp70) serum levels and low NK cell counts after radiotherapy—Potential markers for predicting breast cancer recurrence? *Radiat. Oncol.* **2019**, *14*, 78. [CrossRef]

34. Pan, C.; Schoppe, O.; Parra-Damas, A.; Cai, R.; Todorov, M.I.; Gondi, G.; von Neubeck, B.; Bogurcu-Seidel, N.; Seidel, S.; Sleiman, K.; et al. Deep Learning Reveals Cancer Metastasis and Therapeutic Antibody Targeting in the Entire Body. *Cell* **2019**, *179*, 1661–1676. [CrossRef]

Permissions

The contributors of this book come from diverse backgrounds, making this book a truly international effort. This book will bring forth new frontiers with its revolutionizing research information and detailed analysis of the nascent developments around the world.

We would like to thank all the contributing authors for lending their expertise to make the book truly unique. They have played a crucial role in the development of this book. Without their invaluable contributions this book wouldn't have been possible. They have made vital efforts to compile up to date information on the varied aspects of this subject to make this book a valuable addition to the collection of many professionals and students.

This book was conceptualized with the vision of imparting up-to-date information and advanced data in this field. To ensure the same, a matchless editorial board was set up. Every individual on the board went through rigorous rounds of assessment to prove their worth. After which they invested a large part of their time researching and compiling the most relevant data for our readers.

The editorial board has been involved in producing this book since its inception. They have spent rigorous hours researching and exploring the diverse topics which have resulted in the successful publishing of this book. They have passed on their knowledge of decades through this book. To expedite this challenging task, the publisher supported the team at every step. A small team of assistant editors was also appointed to further simplify the editing procedure and attain best results for the readers.

Apart from the editorial board, the designing team has also invested a significant amount of their time in understanding the subject and creating the most relevant covers. They scrutinized every image to scout for the most suitable representation of the subject and create an appropriate cover for the book.

The publishing team has been an ardent support to the editorial, designing and production team. Their endless efforts to recruit the best for this project, has resulted in the accomplishment of this book. They are a veteran in the field of academics and their pool of knowledge is as vast as their experience in printing. Their expertise and guidance has proved useful at every step. Their uncompromising quality standards have made this book an exceptional effort. Their encouragement from time to time has been an inspiration for everyone.

The publisher and the editorial board hope that this book will prove to be a valuable piece of knowledge for researchers, students, practitioners and scholars across the globe.

List of Contributors

Kehinde Aruleba, George Obaido and Blessing Ogbuokiri
School of Computer Science and Applied Mathematics, University of the Witwatersrand, Johannesburg 2001, South Africa

Adewale Oluwaseun Fadaka and Ashwil Klein
Department of Biotechnology, Faculty of Natural Sciences, University of the Western Cape, Private Bag X17, Bellville, Cape Town 7535, South Africa

Tayo Alex Adekiya
Department of Pharmacy and Pharmacology, School of Therapeutic Science, Faculty of Health Sciences, University of the Witwatersrand, Johannesburg, 7 York Road, Parktown 2193, South Africa

Raphael Taiwo Aruleba
Department of Molecular and Cell Biology, Faculty of Science, University of Cape Town, Cape Town 7701, South Africa

Emanuele Torti, Marco La Salvia, Giordana Florimbi and Francesco Leporati
Department of Electrical, Computer and Biomedical Engineering, University of Pavia, 27100 Pavia, Italy

Raquel Leon, Beatriz Martinez-Vega, Himar Fabelo, Samuel Ortega and Gustavo M. Callicó
Institute for Applied Microelectronics (IUMA), University of Las Palmas de Gran Canaria (ULPGC), 35017 Las Palmas de Gran Canaria, Spain

Frederick R. Ueland
Department of Obstetrics and Gynecology, Division of Gynecologic Oncology and the Markey Cancer Center, University of Kentucky College of Medicine, Lexington, KY 40515, USA
Division of Gynecologic Oncology, Department of Obstetrics and Gynecology, University of Kentucky Chandler Medical Center-Markey Cancer Center, Lexington, KY 40536-0293, USA

Angelo Castello and Egesta Lopci
Nuclear Medicine, Humanitas Clinical and Research Center-IRCCS, 20089 Rozzano, Italy

Francesco Giuseppe Carbone
Anatomy and Histopathology, Santa Chiara Hospital, 38122 Trento, Italy

Sabrina Rossi and Luca Toschi
Oncology and Hematology, Humanitas Clinical and Research Center-IRCCS, 20089 Rozzano, Italy

Simona Monterisi
Immunology and Inflammation, Humanitas Clinical and Research Center-IRCCS, 20089 Rozzano, Italy

Davide Federico
Pathology, Humanitas Clinical and Research Center-IRCCS, 20089 Rozzano, Italy

Serena Monti, Valentina Brancato, Luca Basso, Concetta Schiano, Nunzia Garbino and Carlo Cavaliere
IRCCS SDN, 80143 Naples, Italy

Rossana Castaldo, Katia Pane, Emanuele Nicolai, Marco Salvatore and Monica Franzese
IRCCS SDN, Via E. Gianturco, 113, 80143 Naples, Italy

Giuseppe Di Costanzo, Marta Puglia and Alfonso Ragozzino
Ospedale S. Maria delle Grazie, 80078 Pozzuoli, Italy

Masafumi Koshiyama
Department of Gynecology and Obstetrics, Kyoto University, Graduate School of Medicine, Sakyo-ku, Kyoto 606-8507, Japan
Department of Women's Health, Graduate School of Human Nursing, The University of Shiga Prefecture, 2500 Hassakacho, Hikone, Shiga 522-8533, Japan

Noriomi Matsumura
Department of Gynecology and Obstetrics, Kyoto University, Graduate School of Medicine, Sakyo-ku, Kyoto 606-8507, Japan

Ikuo Konishi
Department of Gynecology and Obstetrics, Kyoto University, Graduate School of Medicine, Sakyo-ku, Kyoto 606-8507, Japan
Department of Obstetrics and Gynecology, National Hospital Organization Kyoto Medical Center, Fushimi-ku, Kyoto 612-8555, Japan

Domenico Albano and Rexhep Durmo
Nuclear Medicine, University of Brescia, Spedali Civili Brescia, 25123 Brescia, Italy

Riccardo Laudicella
Nuclear Medicine Unit, Department of Biomedical and Dental Sciences and Morpho-Functional Imaging, University of Messina, 98125 Messina, Italy

Paola Ferro
Nuclear Medicine Department, IRCCS San Raffaele Hospital, 20132 Milan, Italy

Michela Allocca, Elisabetta Abenavoli and Flavia Linguanti
Nuclear Medicine Unit, Department of Experimental and Clinical Biomedical Sciences, University of Florence, 50134 Florence, Italy

Ambra Buschiazzo
Nuclear Medicine Department, S. Croce e Carle Hospital Cuneo, 12100 Cuneo, Italy

Alessia Castellino
Hematology Division, S. Croce e Carle Hospital Cuneo, 12100 Cuneo, Italy

Agostino Chiaravalloti
Department of Biomedicine and Prevention, University Tor Vergata, 00133 Rome, Italy
IRCCS Neuromed, 86077 Pozzilli, Italy

Annarosa Cuccaro
Istituto di Ematologia, Fondazione Policlinico Universitario A. Gemelli IRCCS, Università Cattolica del Sacro Cuore, 00168 Rome, Italy

Lea Cuppari
Nuclear Medicine and Molecular Imaging Unit, Veneto Institute of Oncology IOV-IRCCS, 35128 Padua, Italy

Laura Evangelista
Nuclear Medicine Unit, Department of Medicine – DIMED, University of Padua, 35121 Padua, Italy

Viviana Frantellizzi
Department of Molecular Medicine, Sapienza University of Rome, 00185 Rome, Italy

Sofya Kovalchuk
Hematology Unit, Department of Experimental and Clinical Biomedical Sciences, University of Florence, 50134 Florence, Italy

Giulia Santo
Nuclear Medicine Unit, Department of Interdisciplinary Medicine, University of Bari Aldo Moro, 70124 Bari, Italy

Matteo Bauckneht
Nuclear Medicine, IRCCS Policlinico San Martino, 16132 Genova, Italy

Salvatore Annunziata
Institute of Nuclear Medicine, Fondazione Policlinico Universitario A. Gemelli IRCCS, Università Cattolica del Sacro Cuore, 00168 Rome, Italy

Robert M. Ore, Lauren Baldwin, Dylan Woolum, Erika Elliott, Christiaan Wijers, Chieh-Yu Chen, Rachel W. Miller, Christopher P. DeSimone, John R. van Nagell and Edward J. Pavlik
Division of Gynecologic Oncology, Department of Obstetrics and Gynecology, University of Kentucky Chandler Medical Center-Markey Cancer Center, Lexington, KY 40536-0293, USA

Richard J. Kryscio
Department of Statistics, University of Kentucky Chandler Medical Center-Markey Cancer Center, Lexington, KY 40536-0293, USA

Andrea Soricelli
IRCCS SDN, 80134 Naples, Italy
Department of Motor Sciences and Healthiness, University of Naples Parthenope, 80134 Naples, Italy

Filomena de Nigris
Department of Precision Medicine, University of Campania "Luigi Vanvitelli", 80138 Naples, Italy

Claudio Napoli
IRCCS SDN, 80134 Naples, Italy
Department of Advanced Medical and Surgical Sciences, University of Campania "Luigi Vanvitelli", 80138 Naples, Italy

Christopher Montemagno, Mitra Ahmadi, Sandrine Bacot, Marlène Debiossat, Audrey Soubies, Loic Djaïleb, Julien Leenhardt, Nicolas De Leiris, Pascale Perret, Laurent Riou, Daniel Fagret, Catherine Ghezzi and Alexis Broisat
Laboratory of Bioclinical Radiopharmaceutics, Universite Grenoble Alpes, Inserm, CHU Grenoble Alpes, LRB, 38000 Grenoble, France

Laurent Dumas
Laboratory of Bioclinical Radiopharmaceutics, Universite Grenoble Alpes, Inserm, CHU Grenoble Alpes, LRB, 38000 Grenoble, France
Advanced Accelator Applications, 01630 Saint-Genis-Pouilly, France

Pierre Cavaillès
Natural Barriers and Infectiosity, Universite Grenoble Alpes, CNRS, CHU Grenoble Alpes, TIMC-IMAG, 38000 Grenoble, France

Maeva Dufies
Biomedical Department, Centre Scientifique de Monaco, 980000 Monaco, Monaco

Gilles Pagès
Biomedical Department, Centre Scientifique de Monaco, 980000 Monaco, Monaco
Institute for Research on Cancer and Aging of Nice, Universite Cote d'Azur, CNRS UMR 7284, INSERM U1081, Centre Antoine Lacassagne, 061489 Nice, France

Sophie Hernot and Nick Devoogdt
Laboratory of In Vivo Cellular and Molecular Imaging, ICMI-BEFY, Vrije Universiteit Brussel, Laarbeeklan 103, B-1090 Brussels, Belgium

Anna Myriam Perrone, Giulia Dondi, Marco Tesei and Pierandrea De Iaco
Gynecologic Oncology Unit, Sant'Orsola-Malpighi Hospital, 40138 Bologna, Italy
Centro di Studio e Ricerca delle Neoplasie Ginecologiche (CSR) University of Bologna, 40138 Bologna, Italy

Manuela Coe
Department of Specialized, Diagnostic, and Experimental Medicine, Sant'Orsola-Malpighi Hospital, 40138 Bologna, Italy

Martina Ferioli
Radiotherapy Unit, Sant'Orsola-Malpighi Hospital, 40138 Bologna, Italy

Silvi Telo
Nuclear Medicine Unit, Sant'Orsola-Malpighi Hospital, 40138 Bologna, Italy

Andrea Galuppi and Alessio G. Morganti
Centro di Studio e Ricerca delle Neoplasie Ginecologiche (CSR) University of Bologna, 40138 Bologna, Italy
Radiotherapy Unit, Sant'Orsola-Malpighi Hospital, 40138 Bologna, Italy

Eugenia De Crescenzo
Gynecologic Oncology Unit, Sant'Orsola-Malpighi Hospital, 40138 Bologna, Italy

Paolo Castellucci and Cristina Nanni
Nuclear Medicine Unit, Sant'Orsola-Malpighi Hospital, 40138 Bologna, Italy

Stefano Fanti
Centro di Studio e Ricerca delle Neoplasie Ginecologiche (CSR) University of Bologna, 40138 Bologna, Italy
Nuclear Medicine Unit, Sant'Orsola-Malpighi Hospital, 40138 Bologna, Italy

Francesco Fiz, Helmut Dittmann, Matthias Weissinger and Matthias Reimold
Department of Nuclear Medicine and Clinical Molecular Imaging, University Hospital Tübingen, 72076 Tübingen, Germany

Cristina Campi
Department of Medicine-DIMED, Nuclear Medicine Unit, University Hospital of Padua, 35128 Padua, Italy

Samine Sahbai
Nuclear Medicine Unit, Hospital Universitaire Henri Mondor, 94010 Créteil, France

Arnulf Stenzl
Department of Urology, University Hospital Tübingen, 72076 Tübingen, Germany

Michele Piana
Department of Mathematics, University of Genoa, 16146 Genoa, Italy

Gianmario Sambuceti
Department of Health Sciences, Nuclear Medicine Unit, University of Genoa, 16146 Genoa, Italy

Christian la Fougère
Department of Nuclear Medicine and Clinical Molecular Imaging, University Hospital Tübingen, 72076 Tübingen, Germany
iFIT Cluster of Excellence, University of Tübingen, 72076 Tübingen, Germany

Eleanor L. Ormsby
Department of Radiology, University of California Davis Medical Center, 4860 Y Street, Suite 3100, Sacramento, CA 95817, USA
Department of Radiology, Kaiser Permanente Sacramento, 2025 Morse Ave, CA 95825, USA

John P. McGahan
Department of Radiology, University of California Davis Medical Center, 4860 Y Street, Suite 3100, Sacramento, CA 95817, USA

Melanie A. Kimm and Ernst J. Rummeny
Department of Diagnostic and Interventional Radiology, Klinikum rechts der Isar der Technischen Universität München, 81675 Munich, Germany

Caroline Werner, Wolfgang Sievert, Wu Zhiyuan, Gabriele Multhoff and Stefan Stangl
Central Institute for Translational Cancer Research (TranslaTUM), Klinikum rechts der Isar der Technischen Universität München, 81675 Munich, Germany

Maxim Shevtsov
Central Institute for Translational Cancer Research
(TranslaTUM), Klinikum rechts der Isar der Technischen
Universität München, 81675 Munich, Germany
Pavlov First Saint Petersburg State Medical University,
197022 St. Petersburg, Russia
Institute of Cytology of the Russian Academy of
Sciences (RAS), 194064 St. Petersburg, Russia

Oliver Schoppe and Bjoern H. Menze
Central Institute for Translational Cancer Research
(TranslaTUM), Klinikum rechts der Isar der Technischen
Universität München, 81675 Munich, Germany
Institute for Advanced Studies, Department of
Informatics, Technical University of Munich, 85748
Garching, Germany

Roland Proksa
Philips GmbH Innovative Technologies, Research
Laboratories, 22335 Hamburg, Germany

Olga Bystrova and Marina Martynova
Institute of Cytology of the Russian Academy of
Sciences (RAS), 194064 St. Petersburg, Russia

**Noriyuki Fujima, Yukie Shimizu, Daisuke Yoshida
and Kohsuke Kudo**
Department of Diagnostic and Interventional
Radiology, Hokkaido University Hospital, Sapporo
060-8638, Hokkaido, Japan

**Satoshi Kano, Takatsugu Mizumachi and Akihiro
Homma**
Department of Otolaryngology-Head and Neck
Surgery, Hokkaido University Graduate School of
Medicine, Sapporo 060-8638, Hokkaido, Japan

Koichi Yasuda and Rikiya Onimaru
Department of Radiation Medicine, Hokkaido
University Graduate School of Medicine, Sapporo 060-
8638, Hokkaido, Japan

Osamu Sakai
Departments of Radiology, Otolaryngology-Head
and Neck Surgery, and Radiation Oncology, Boston
Medical Center, Boston University School of Medicine,
Boston, MA 02118, USA

Hiroki Shirato
Department of Radiation Medicine, Hokkaido
University Graduate School of Medicine, Sapporo 060-
8638, Hokkaido, Japan
The Global Station for Quantum Medical Science
and Engineering, Global Institution for Collaborative
Research and Education, Sapporo 060-0808, Hokkaido,
Japan

Index

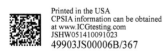

Printed in the USA
CPSIA information can be obtained
at www.ICGtesting.com
JSHW051410091023
49903JS00006B/367